EDITOR-IN-CHIEF

SALLY MILLAR, R.N., CCRN

Head Nurse, Respiratory/Surgical Intensive Care Unit
Massachusetts General Hospital
Boston, Massachusetts

EDITORS

LESLIE K. SAMPSON, R.N., CCRN

Patient Care Coordinator
Intensive Care Unit, Emergency Unit and Recovery Room
Albert Einstein Medical Center, Northern Division
Philadelphia, Pennsylvania

SISTER MAURITA SOUKUP, R.S.M., R.N., M.S.N.

Critical-Care Clinical Nursing Specialist
St. Luke's Hospital
Cedar Rapids, Iowa

Formerly, Critical Care Clinical Nursing Specialist
St. Joseph's Hospital;
and Assistant Clinical Professor
Marquette University
Milwaukee, Wisconsin

SYLVAN LEE WEINBERG, M.D.

Clinical Professor of Medicine and Co-Director, Group in Cardiology
Wright State University School of Medicine

Director, Coronary Care Unit
Chairman, Cardiology Section
Good Samaritan Hospital
Dayton, Ohio

METHODS IN CRITICAL CARE

THE AACN MANUAL

by

The American Association of Critical-Care Nurses

W. B. SAUNDERS COMPANY   Philadelphia London Toronto   1980

W. B. Saunders Company: West Washington Square
Philadelphia, PA   19105

1 St. Anne's Road
Eastbourne, East Sussex BN21, 3UN, England

1 Goldthorne Avenue
Toronto, Ontario M8Z 5T9, Canada

Front and back cover illustrations are modified from illustrations appearing in
Victorian Stained Glass Pattern Book, by Ed Sibbett, Jr.,
published by Dover Publications, Inc., New York, 1979.

Methods in Critical Care   ISBN   0-7216-1006-4

Last digit is the print number: 9   8   7   6   5   4   3   2   1

DEDICATION

As critical care nurses we will be faced with ever-increasing automation and computerization. An important challenge will be to prevent dehumanization in patient care.

Dorothy Voorman, R.N., B.S.N., CCRN
President, AACN, 1975–1976
Heart and Lung, 5:364, 1976

CONTRIBUTORS

ELAINE BROGDEN, R.N., B.S.N.
Staff Nurse, Critical Care Unit
Swedish Hospital Medical Center
Seattle, Washington

JANICE M. CASPER, R.N., B.S.N.
Head Nurse
Intensive Care Unit
St. Joseph's Hospital
Milwaukee, Wisconsin

CAROLYN B. CHALKLEY, R.N., M.S.N.
Clinical Director
Cardiovascular Nursing Programs
and Services
Brookwood Medical Center
Birmingham, Alabama

Clinical Instructor, School of
Nursing, University of Alabama
in Birmingham
Birmingham, Alabama

RITA COLLEY, R.N.
Clinical Nurse Specialist
Hyperalimentation Unit
Cincinnati General Hospital
Cincinnati, Ohio

RUTH M. DELOOR, R.N., M.S.N.
Instructor, Nursing Education
Atlanta Veterans Administration
Hospital
Atlanta, Georgia

BARBARA FELLOWS, R.N., M.A.
Clinical Assistant Professor
University of Washington
School of Nursing
Renal Nurse Clinician
University of Washington Hospital
Seattle, Washington

PENNY J. FORD, R.N., M.S.
Cardiac Clinician, Intensive Care
Nursing Service
Massachusetts General Hospital
Boston, Massachusetts

DOREEN GARDNER, R.N.
Clinical Leader, Neuromedical/
Neurosurgical Nursing Service
Massachusetts General Hospital
Boston, Massachusetts

JUDITH J. HENDERSON, R.N.,
M.S.N.
Cardiovascular Clinical Nursing
Specialist
Mary Hitchcock Hospital
Hanover, New Hampshire

KAREN C. JOHNSON, R.N., M.S.,
CCRN
Lecturer, San Francisco State
University School of Nursing
San Francisco, California

ELAINE LARSON, R.N., M.A.
Clinical Assistant Professor
University of Washington
School of Nursing
Nurse Coordinator, Staff
Development
University of Washington
Hospital
Seattle, Washington

ANNA J. LAVELLE, R.N., B.S.N.
Former Assistant Head Nurse,
Renal Transplant and Dialysis
Unit
University Hospital
University of Washington
Currently enrolled in Master of
Nursing Program
Seattle, Washington

JEANNETTE McCANN McHUGH,
R.N., M.S.N.
Pulmonary Clinical Nurse
Specialist
Eden, New York

KAREN M. MILLER, R.N., M.S.N.
Cardiovascular Clinical Nurse
Specialist
St. Luke's Hospital
Milwaukee, Wisconsin

NEIL MILLER, Ph.D.
Director, Hospital Services
Emergency Care Research
Institute Shared Services
Plymouth Meeting, Pennsylvania

NORMA L. MOCK, R.N., B.S.N.
Chief Cardiovascular Clinical
Technologist and Coordinator
of Cardiac Hemodynamic
Monitoring, Cardiac Pace-
makers, and Intra-Aortic
Balloon Pump Services
Cardiovascular Laboratory
Broward General Medical Center
Fort Lauderdale, Florida

KATHY MOSSING, R.N., M.A.
Critical Care Clinical Specialist
Swedish Hospital Medical Center
Seattle, Washington

BETTY NORRIS, R.N., M.S.N.
Adjunct Associate Professor
Sanford University School of
Nursing
Cardiovascular Nurse Specialist
Baptist Medical Center-Montclair
Birmingham, Alabama

SANDRA J. PFAFF, R.N., B.S.N.
Nurse Consultant
South Florida Hospital Consor-
tium for Infection Control, Inc.
Miami, Florida

REBECCA A. PRESTON, R.N.,
B.S.N.
Unit Teacher, Cardiac Surgical
Intensive Care Unit
Massachusetts General Hospital
Boston, Massachusetts

PEGGY J. REILEY, R.N., M.S.
Formerly Transplantation
Coordinator
Interhospital Organ Bank of
New England
Boston, Massachusetts
Presently Orientation/Special
Program Coordinator
Beth Israel Hospital
Boston, Massachusetts

MARILYN M. RICCI, R.N., M.S.,
C.N.R.N.
Clinical Nurse Specialist,
Neurology/Neurosurgery
Barrow Neurological Institute
St. Joseph's Hospital and Medical
Center
Phoenix, Arizona
Assistant Professor
Arizona State University

BRENDA SANZOBRINO, R.N.,
B.S.N.
  Cardiovascular Nurse Clinician
  Broward General Medical Center
  Fort Lauderdale, Florida

MARY JO SCHREIBER, R.N.,
M.S.N.
  Cardiovascular Clinical Specialist
  Winter Haven Hospital
  Winter Haven, Florida

MARTHA SPENCE, R.N., M.N.
  Lecturer, University of Miami
  Graduate School of Nursing
  Staff Nurse, Critical Care Unit
  Inservice Instructor
  Department of Clinical Nursing
  Education
  Baptist Hospital
  Miami, Florida

KIT STAHLER, R.N., M.S.N.
  Research Nurse, Division of
  Neonatology
  Children's Hospital of
  Philadelphia
  Philadelphia, Pennsylvania

LANI MOSKOWITZ STROM, R.N.,
M.S., C.E.T.
  Cardiopulmonary Clinical
  Specialist
  Sequoia Hospital
  Redwood City, California

BARBARA TABOR, R.N., B.S.N.
  Head Nurse, Emergency Room
  Harborview Medical Center
  Seattle, Washington

CAROLYN A. TAMER, R.N., E.T.
  Enterostomal Therapist
  Ostomy Clinician
  Massachusetts General Hospital
  Boston, Massachusetts

KAREN WHEELOCK, R.N., M.A.
  Director of In-Service Education
  St. Olaf Hospital
  Austin, Minnesota
  Former Assistant Professor
  Department of Nursing
  Mt. Mercy College
  Cedar Rapids, Iowa

CHERYL TOMICH WYMAN, R.N.,
B.S.N.
  Renal Dialysis Educational
  Coordinator
  Renal Transplant and Dialysis
  Unit
  University of Washington Hospital
  Seattle, Washington

PATRICIA A. YANUL, R.N.
  Assistant Nurse Leader,
  Coronary Care Unit
  Tufts-New England Medical
  Center
  Boston, Massachusetts

PREFACE

The American Association of Critical-Care Nurses endorses the philosophy that each critically ill person has the right to expect nursing care provided by a critical care nurse. Critical care nursing practice requires the utilization of various methodologies in the prevention of and intervention in life-threatening situations.

Methods in Critical Care—The AACN Manual has been written to provide the critical care nurse with specific procedural guidelines that can be used rapidly in adult critical care areas. This text can also be utilized by floor nurses who are often caring for critically ill patients. In addition, it will be valuable in teaching entry-level and continuing education courses in critical care. *Methods in Critical Care* may also be used by institutions in the preparation of their own procedural manuals or be adopted in its entirety for use in courses to fulfill licensure or accreditation requirements.

Much has been written since the advent of critical care as a specialty. This manual presents a specific part of the most pertinent information. The methods follow a consistent format: Overview and Instrumentation (as appropriate), Objectives, Special Equipment, Method, Precautions, Related Care, and Complications. Illustrations are used throughout. If the user requires additional theoretical background information, a sampling of references from the literature is included. Finally, a list of suppliers follows each method. Because equipment utilized within the critical care setting is constantly changing, it is a formidable, if not impossible, task to include all the manufacturers of equipment that can be utilized in critical care areas.

In addition, there are certain expectations common to the performance of the majority of the methods. These expectations are that the critical care nurse will:

- Read the equipment operator manuals so as to become familiar with specific controls, functions, safety devices, trouble-shooting techniques, and precautions.
- Provide patients or family or both with appropriate explanations of the methods and make sure they understand them. Emotional and intellec-

tual preparation may lessen anxiety and increase cooperation. In some instances, the patient or family will require more detail and an educational process will have to be completed.

- Obtain a physician's order when required by the institution.
- Obtain permits signed by the patient or person legally permitted to sign when indicated. This process must be carried out carefully in light of legal requirements for informed consent.
- Ascertain the patient's allergy history to prevent unfavorable reactions to prep solutions, anesthetic agents, or drugs.
- Collect, organize, and set up equipment and supplies necessary for the efficient completion of the method.
- Wash hands prior to beginning of each method. This is one of the most significant and effective means of preventing nosocomial infections.
- Strictly adhere to sterile technique and assume an active assertive role in implementing it.
- Integrate emotional support into each method. Many of the methods cause discomfort or anxiety and will require use of touch or contact with the patient, frequent explanations, and an understanding of responses. Premedicating patients prior to initiating some of the methods may also lessen the discomfort or anxiety.

It is important to note that these methods are most appropriately carried out in the critical care environment. Support personnel, supplies, and emergency equipment must be immediately available.

There are some constraints imposed on *Methods in Critical Care* by the diverse nature of critical care practice. Identification of personnel who are permitted to perform the methods is not included here because of varying institutional and state policies and regulations. There may also be differing requirements for certification or authorization by professional organizations. In addition, specific subspecialty methods (e.g., pediatrics, neonatology, and others) have not been included.

These methods have been written in light of what is accepted methodology supported by current literature. However, the only constant is change, and the fields of nursing and medicine are so broad that all acceptable modalities cannot be anticipated or be presented. The user must evaluate regional or institutional variability against established, acceptable principles.

Finally, there is a risk involved in writing a book like *Methods in Critical Care*. This is a manual oriented to technical tasks. It *cannot* be considered as a sole resource that, if followed, will result in competent critical care practice. These methods are not meant to be used in a vacuum. They are only one part of the holistic approach to critical care nursing, an approach based on a specific and thorough knowledge of the interrelatedness of body systems, the dynamic nature of the life process, and a recognition and appreciation of the individual's wholeness, uniqueness, and significant social and environmental relationships.

SALLY MILLAR
LESLIE K. SAMPSON
SISTER MAURITA SOUKUP
SYLVAN WEINBERG

ACKNOWLEDGMENTS

We would like to acknowledge the work done by our illustrator, Steve Reed, of Newton, Massachusetts; our photographers, Scott Savage of Milwaukee, Wisconsin, Robert Sheen of Seattle, Washington, and Stephen Smith of Boston, Massachusetts; and our typists, Gail Bor, of Needham, Massachusetts, and Patricia Marciniak of Milwaukee, Wisconsin.

CONTENTS

THE CARDIOVASCULAR SYSTEM _____ 1a

ELECTROCARDIOGRAM (ECG)   1

Norma Mock, R.N., and Brenda Sanzobrino, R.N., B.S.N.

    12-Lead ECG   8
    Lead Systems   16
    Telemetry   26

CARDIOVERSION   30

Martha Spence, R.N., M.N.

DEFIBRILLATION   37

Martha Spence, R.N., M.N.

VASCULAR INVASIVE TECHNIQUES   43

Karen M. Miller, R.N., M.S.N.

    Venipuncture   43
    Arterial Puncture   49

HEMODYNAMIC MONITORING   57

_Karen C. Johnson, R.N., M.S., CCRN, and Lani Moskowitz Strom,
R.N., M.S., C.E.T._

    Single Pressure Transducer System   61
    Multiple Pressure Transducer System   68
    Central Venous Pressure   75
    Pulmonary Artery Pressure   82
    Arterial Pressure   91
    Left Atrial Pressure   96
    Cardiac Output   100
    Automatic Blood Pressure Monitoring   105

CIRCULATORY ASSIST DEVICES 108

Penny Ford, R.N., M.S., and Rebecca Preston, R.N., B.S.N.

Intra-Aortic Balloon Pump Management 108
External Pressure Circulatory Assist 116
Penny Ford, R.N., M.S., Rebecca Preston, R.N., B.S.N., and
Patricia A. Yanul, R.N.

External Counterpressure with G-Suit 123
Penny Ford, R.N., M.S., and Rebecca Preston, R.N., B.S.N.

TEMPORARY PACEMAKER MANAGEMENT 127

Betty Norris, R.N., M.S.N.

Emergency Insertion of a Temporary Pacing Electrode (Assisting with) 129
Initiating Temporary Epicardial Pacing 134
Conversion from Bipolar to Unipolar System with Temporary Pacing 138
Atrial ECG with Temporary Atrial Pacing Electrode 140
Overdrive Atrial Pacing 142
Assessing Temporary Pacemaker Function 144

PERMANENT PACEMAKER MANAGEMENT 149

Carolyn Chalkley, R.N., M.S.N.

Assessing Select Parameters of a Permanent Pacing System 149
Inhibition of a Permanent Pacemaker 161
Reprogramming a Permanent Pacemaker 163
Use of a Magnet 165

NONINVASIVE PERIPHERAL VASCULAR BLOOD FLOW
MEASUREMENT 169

Karen Wheelock, R.N., M.A.

Ultrasound Blood Flow Detector 169
Pulse Volume Recorder 172
Strain Gauge Plethysmography 175

ROTATING TOURNIQUETS 178

Karen Wheelock, R.N., M.A.

THERAPEUTIC PHLEBOTOMY 183

Janice Casper, R.N., B.S.N.

CARDIOCENTESIS (ASSISTING WITH) 186

Karen Wheelock, R.N., M.A.

THE PULMONARY SYSTEM 189

AIRWAY MANAGEMENT 191

Jeannette McCann McHugh, R.N., M.S.N.

Esophageal Obturator Airway Insertion 194
Endotracheal Intubation 196
Endotracheal Suctioning 200
Blind Endotracheal Suctioning 204
Tracheostomy Care 208
Prevention of Tracheal Injuries 211
Securing Airways 214
Extubation 216

VENTILATORY MANAGEMENT 220

Jeanette McCann McHugh, R.N., M.S.N.

Instituting Mechanical Ventilation 220
Weaning from Mechanically Assisted Ventilation 226
Ambuing with Positive End Airway Pressure (PEEP) 229
Continuous Positive Airway Pressure (CPAP) 231

CHEST TUBE MANAGEMENT 236

Jeanette McCann McHugh, R.N., M.S.N.

Chest Tube Placement (Assisting with) 236
Three-Bottle Closed Chest Drainage System 239
Disposable Chest Drainage Unit 244

CHEST PHYSIOTHERAPY 246

Janice Casper, R.N., B.S.N.

THORACENTESIS (ASSISTING WITH) 252

Janice Casper, R.N., B.S.N.

THE RENAL SYSTEM **257**

ACUTE HEMODIALYSIS 259

Anna J. Lavelle, R.N., B.S.N., and Cheryl Tomich Wyman, R.N., B.S.N.

Initiating Hemodialysis 264
Monitoring Hemodialysis 268
Terminating Hemodialysis 271
Hemodialysis Cannula and Site Care 273

PERITONEAL DIALYSIS 277

Elaine Larson, R.N., M.A., and Barbara Fellows, R.N., M.A.

Insertion of Peritoneal Dialysis Catheter (Assisting with) 278
Peritoneal Dialysis Catheter Site Care 282
Monitoring Peritoneal Dialysis 283

THE NEUROLOGIC SYSTEM **289**

INTRACRANIAL PRESSURE MONITORING 291

Doreen Gardner, R.N.

LUMBAR AND CISTERNAL PUNCTURES (ASSISTING WITH)   296

Marilyn Ricci, R.N., M.S., C.N.R.N.

HYPOTHERMIA AND HYPERTHERMIA   301

Marilyn Ricci, R.N., M.S., C.N.R.N.

THE GASTROINTESTINAL SYSTEM   307

MANAGEMENT OF UPPER GASTROINTESTINAL HEMORRHAGE   309

*Elaine Brogdon, R.N., B.S.N., Kathy Mossing, R.N., M.A., and
Barbara Tabor, R.N., B.S.N.*

    Nasogastric Tube Insertion   309
    Gastric Lavage   312
    Sengstaken/Blakemore Tube   315
    Linton Tube   321
    Mesenteric Artery Line and Pitressin Infusion   325

GASTRIC LAVAGE IN OVERDOSE   328

*Elaine Brogdon, R.N., B.S.N., Kathy Mossing, R.N., M.A., and
Barbara Tabor, R.N., B.S.N.*

PARACENTESIS (ASSISTING WITH)   331

*Elaine Brogdon, R.N., B.S.N., Kathy Mossing, R.N., M.A., and
Barbara Tabor, R.N., B.S.N.*

STOMA/FISTULA MANAGEMENT   334

Carolyn A. Tamer, R.N., E.T.

    Ostomy/Fistula Containment   335
    Fistula/Drain Site Care   342
    Colostomy Irrigation   344
    Ostomy/Fistula Skin Care   346
    Ostomy/Fistula Odor Control   349
    Obtaining Urine Specimen for Culture and Sensitivity from
      Ileal Loop Stoma   350

THE HEMATOLOGIC SYSTEM   353

BLOOD AND BLOOD COMPONENT ADMINISTRATION   355

Ruth DeLoor, R.N., M.S.N., and Mary Jo Schreiber, R.N., M.S.N.

TRANSFUSION REACTION   367

Ruth DeLoor, R.N., M.S.N., and Mary Jo Schreiber, R.N., M.S.N.

AUTOTRANSFUSION   370

Ruth DeLoor, R.N., M.S.N., and Mary Jo Schreiber, R.N., M.S.N.

BLOOD WARMING   373

Ruth DeLoor, R.N., M.S.N., and Mary Jo Schreiber, R.N., M.S.N.

USE OF A BLOOD PUMP   376

Ruth DeLoor, R.N., M.S.N., and Mary Jo Schreiber, R.N., M.S.N.

THE INTEGUMENTARY SYSTEM   379

WOUND MANAGEMENT: CLEAN WOUNDS   381

Sandra J. Pfaff, R.N., B.S.N.

WOUND MANAGEMENT: CONTAMINATED WOUNDS   385

Sandra J. Pfaff, R.N., B.S.N.

  Dressing Wounds with Drains   385
  Dressing Open Wounds   387
  Wound Irrigation   388
  Wound Cultures   389

WOUND MANAGEMENT: DECUBITI   393

Sandra J. Pfaff, R.N., B.S.N.

  Prevention of Decubiti   393
  Management of Decubiti   394

WOUND MANAGEMENT: BURNS   397

Sandra J. Pfaff, R.N., B.S.N.

  Care of First-Degree Burns   397
  Care of Open Burns   398
  Care of Intact Second-Degree Burns (Unbroken Blisters)   398
  Care of Nonintact Second-Degree Burns (Broken Blisters)   399
  Care of Third-Degree Burns (Full-Thickness Burns)   400

INVASIVE SITE CARE (VENOUS AND ARTERIAL)   403

Judith Henderson, R.N., M.S.N.

  Short Venous Indwelling Catheter Site Care   403
  Long Venous and Arterial Indwelling Catheter Site Care   406

NUTRITIONAL SUPPORT   415

TOTAL PARENTERAL NUTRITION   417

Rita Colley, R.N.

  Insertion of a Total Parenteral Nutrition Catheter (Assisting with)   418
  Monitoring Daily Infusion of Total Parenteral Nutrition Therapy   423
  Total Parenteral Nutrition Catheter Site Care   425

Total Parenteral Nutrition Intravenous Tubing and Filter Change 430
Removal of Subclavian Total Parenteral Nutrition Catheter 433
Culturing a Total Parenteral Nutrition Subclavian Venous Catheter 435

LIPID THERAPY 438

Rita Colley, R.N.

Administration of Intravenous Lipids 438

SAFETY 441

INFECTION SURVEILLANCE IN THE CRITICAL CARE UNIT 443

Elaine Larson, R.N., M.A.

INFECTION CONTROL IN THE CRITICAL CARE UNIT 447

Elaine Larson, R.N., M.A.

Infection Control Measures: Personnel 447
Infection Control Measures: Environment 451
Infection Control Measures: Equipment 452

ELECTRICAL SAFETY 454

Kit Stahler, R.N., M.S.N., and Neil Miller, Ph.D.

Electrical Safety for Patients and Medical Device Operators 454
Electrical Safety Precautions for Patients with Direct
  Conduction Pathways to Myocardium 458

ORGAN DONATION 461

ORGAN DONATION 463

Peggy J. Reiley, R.N., B.S.N.

Recognizing Potential Organ Donors 464
Facilitating Organ Donation 466
Organ Preparation 468

APPENDIX: SAMPLE FLOW SHEETS AND LOGS 471

APPENDIX 1-A.   INTRA-AORTIC BALLOON PUMP
                FLOW SHEET 473

APPENDIX 1-B.   HEMODIALYSIS ORDERS 474

APPENDIX 1-C.   HEMODIALYSIS — COMPOSITE 475

APPENDIX 1-D.   HEMODIALYSIS LOG 476

APPENDIX 1-E.   PERITONEAL DIALYSIS   477

APPENDIX 1-F.   PERITONEAL DIALYSIS LOG   478

APPENDIX 1-G.   HYPERALIMENTATION MONITORING
               FLOWSHEET   479

INDEX _____ **481**

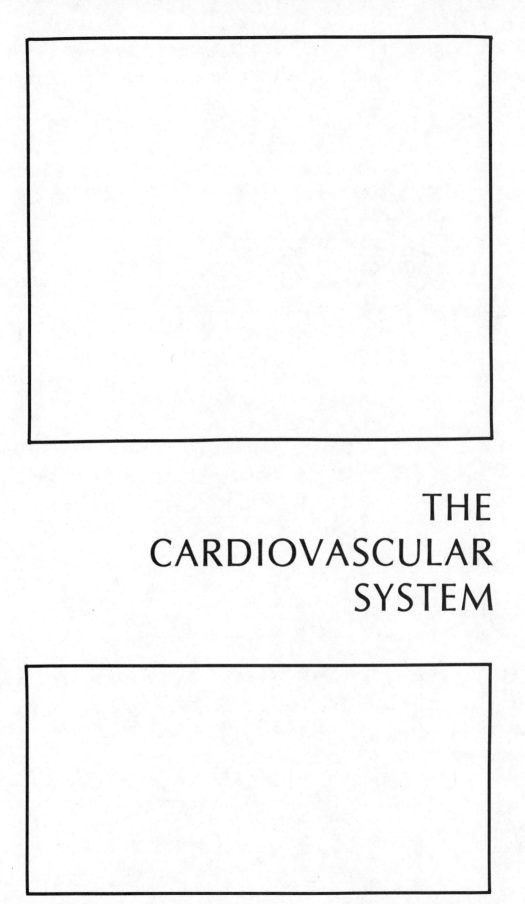

THE
CARDIOVASCULAR
SYSTEM

ELECTROCARDIOGRAM (ECG)

Norma Mock, R.N., and
Brenda Sanzobrino, R.N.

OVERVIEW

Within the field of critical care, electrocardiogram (ECG) monitoring is a required competency of the multidisciplinary health team. It may be done by using serial 12-lead ECG's, an isolated but continuous ECG lead system, and/or a computerized system that correlates multiple physiologic parameters. Select ECG monitoring is also available for the ambulatory patient.

12-Lead Electrocardiogram. The 12-lead electrocardiogram is a graphic recording of the electrical potential generated by the electrical activity of the heart. The electrical impulses generated by the heart's conduction system produce electrical currents which diffuse throughout the body. Electrodes, placed up on the surface of the body and connected to an electrocardiographic apparatus, record the mean electrical currents of the heart and produce the electrocardiogram. The primary purpose of the 12-lead ECG is to provide data related to the patient's cardiac electrical activity to help diagnose select pathologic conditions.

The 12-lead ECG may be useful in many ways to the critical care nurse. The areas in which the 12-lead ECG is most significant are summarized below.

MAJOR AREAS	IMPORTANCE
Dysrhythmia detection	Supraventricular, ventricular, and AV block of dysrhythmias
Cardiac electrical axis	Establishing presence of left anterior hemiblock and left posterior hemiblock; pacemaker tip location
Electrical changes associated with acute myocardial infarction	Current of injury, ischemia, necrosis
Electrical changes associated with bundle branch block	Identifying left bundle branch block and right bundle branch block
Electrical changes associated with hypertrophy	Identifying left ventricular hypertrophy and right ventricular hypertrophy

Two basic 12-lead ECG recorders are commonly used, the single-channel and three-channel ECG recorders. The single-channel ECG recorder

(Fig. 1) is directly controlled by the operator, thus allowing individual lead selection and variable lengths of lead recordings. The three-channel ECG recorder (Fig. 2) documents three consecutive leads simultaneously. Once the three-channel ECG recorder begins to operate, the 12-lead ECG is recorded without further input from the operator.

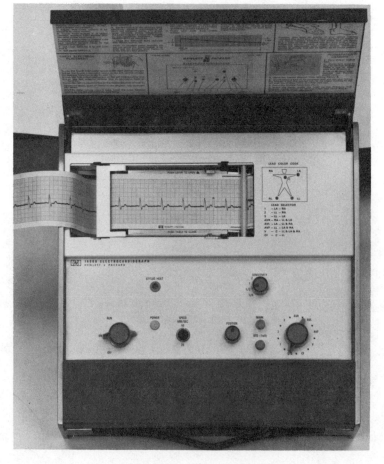

Figure 1. Single-channel ECG recorder. Reprinted with permission of Hewlett-Packard Company.

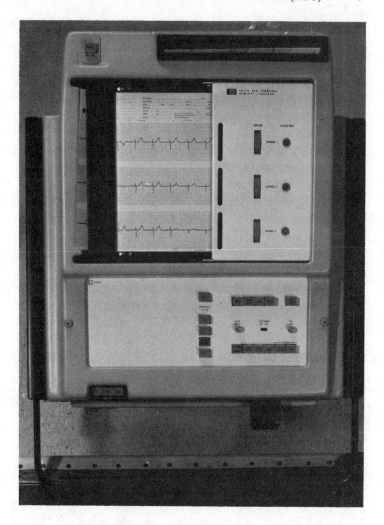

Figure 2. Three-channel ECG recorder. Reprinted with permission of Hewlett-Packard Company.

Both the single channel and three-channel ECG recorders record 12-lead ECG's accurately; however, there are some situations in which selection of a specific recorder is advantageous. The single-channel ECG recorder is preferred when recording ECG's for uncooperative patients and in arrest situations. For patients who are unable to cooperate, frequent stops and restarts may be necessary. The single-channel ECG recorder offers the operator more control over the resultant ECG. In arrest situations, paper use is voluminous. The single-lead ECG recorder minimizes this volume in comparison to that which the three-channel ECG recorder would use, since the operator has control over the ECG machine. Use of the three-channel ECG recorder is advantageous when recording ECG's for routine 12-lead ECG's and/or evaluating ectopy or dysrhythmia, since the recording is obtained rapidly and one copy may be left for the patient's chart, thus omitting any delay due to mounting and interpreting. Also, simultaneous leads are advantageous in the diagnosis of difficult dysrhythmias and the determination of the origin of ventricular ectopy with more accuracy.

Bedside ECG Monitoring System. The bedside ECG monitoring system (Fig. 3) permits observation of the ECG and relays information to the central monitoring station. An ECG lead system transmits the ECG signal from the patient's electrodes to the monitor. The location of the electrodes on the chest wall and the connecting lead system determines the QRS morphology, which is displayed on the bedside oscilloscope. While detailed instructions for specific bedside monitoring ECG systems can be found in the information manuals accompanying the system, standard components should be recognized:

Power—off/on switch.

Oscilloscope—permits direct visual observation of the ECG signal.

Gain control—allows adjustment of amplitude for the QRS signal, usually set at 1 mV.

Position control—permits the ECG tracing to be adjusted to the top, bottom, or central area of the screen.

Sweep control—regulates the rate at which the ECG signal travels across the oscilloscope. The usual setting is 25 mm./sec. A setting of 50 mm./sec. may be used to visualize the QRS morphology more adequately.

Rate indicator—averages and shows heart rate per minute, using a digital number or a rate meter.

Alarm system—integrated with the rate indicator, operates according to preset levels.

Additional components may include:

Lead selector—allows lead selection for monitoring; usually accompanies a five-lead cable system.

Synchronizer jack—used to connect to the defibrillator for cardio-

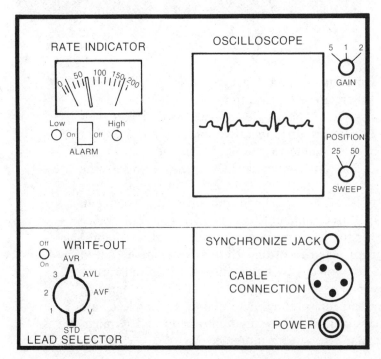

Figure 3. Bedside ECG monitoring.

version; located in the front or rear of the monitor.

Write-out—facilitates manual operation of the ECG recorder at a central nurses' station.

Central Monitoring Station. The central monitoring station (Fig. 4) receives data from the bedside monitors, allows observation of several patients' ECG at one time in a central area, provides the ability to document the ECG tracing away from the bedside automatically or manually, and reduces the number of staff members required to monitor a large number of patients' ECG recordings individually.

Components of the central console may include:

"Slave" oscilloscope—for continuous display of each patient's ECG rhythm, showing several patients at one time.

Direct recorder—for manual or automatic response in providing ECG recordings.

Memory tape loop—to record and later play back events immediately prior to and following an alarm situation.

Dysrhythmia detector—to "sense" QRS alterations in R-to-R intervals and institute an alarm.

Lead failure signal—to indicate *mechanical* failure in the monitoring cable system, differentiating from a patient alarm situation.

Timer-date marker—to mark the ECG tracing automatically; may also include a bed identification number.

Alarm system—to alert the staff of a patient emergency; this system is dependent upon information from the bedside monitor.

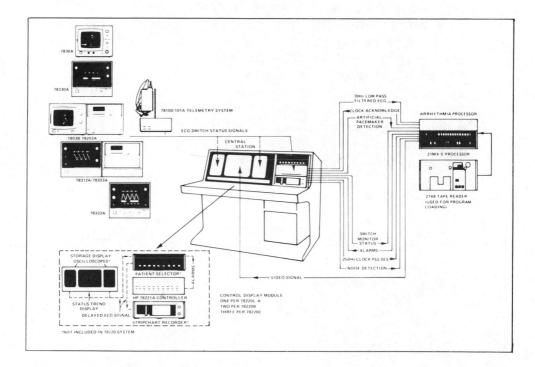

Figure 4. Central monitoring station. Reprinted with permission of Hewlett-Packard Company.

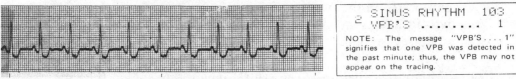

Figure 5. Status displays from computerized dysrhythmia system. Reprinted with permission of Hewlett-Packard Company.

Computerized ECG Monitoring. The application of computer microprocessor techniques in the management of cardiac patients may be used for ECG monitoring in many ways. Computerized dysrhythmia systems provide periodic and demand ECG monitoring, a continuous scanning of ECG rhythms and patterns, an accumulation of data for review, and a system of audible and visual alarms in life-threatening situations. It must be borne in mind, however, that even though computers are valuable adjuncts to the nursing staff, they do not replace a staff member's ability to discern between a false alarm and a real emergency. Yet, computers do direct attention to cardiac rhythm variations which might otherwise go unnoticed. Computerized monitoring is advantageous for its processing power, which illustrates trends of the heart rate, PVC's, and other dysrhythmias.

Features of computerized ECG monitoring may include:

Continuous monitoring—performs a round-the-clock observation of rhythm and QRS patterns, providing a diagnosis as often as every minute.

Automatic detection of dysrhythmias—examines the morphology of the QRS as well as the rate and rhythm; detects ventricular dysrhythmias, supraventricular premature beats, and irregular rhythms.

Priority alarm system—alerts the nurse according to the severity of the condition, since alarms are coded for specific events. This also initiates operation of the strip chart recorder.

Detection of paced rhythms—displays a total number of paced and nonpaced beats/minute; signals pacemaker nonfunction.

Status displays—provide continuous displays of heart rate, ectopic activity, rhythm and monitoring status (Fig. 5).

Trend charts—provide instant display of significant events in a trend plot form, provided on demand (Fig. 6).

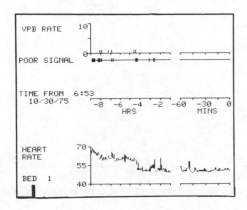

Figure 6. Trend recording. Reprinted with permission of Hewlett-Packard Company.

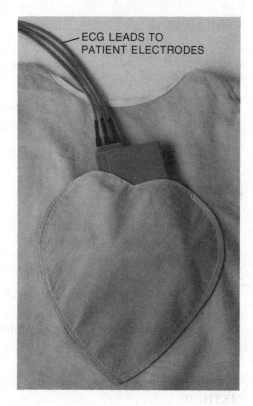

ECG LEADS TO
PATIENT ELECTRODES

Figure 7. Telemetry unit secured in patient's gown pocket. (Courtesy of St. Joseph's Hospital, Milwaukee, Wisconsin.)

Telemetry.   ECG telemetry allows transmission of the ECG without requiring that the patient be attached to a monitor by lead wires. It is especially practical for an ambulatory cardiac patient or a patient resuming progressive activity. Telemetry monitoring involves attaching a two-lead system to the patient, connecting it to a small transmitter about the size of a small transistor radio, and securing the transmitter in a pocket (Fig. 7).

Components of a telemetry system include:

Transmitter—emits a signal to a receiver with which it is paired. (This signal may be lost or interfered with for various reasons. Check the manual or contact a service representative if this occurs.)

Antenna—usually incorporated into the lead wires. Transmission may be further enhanced by the installation of an antenna at the acute health care facility.

Receiver—usually located at a central station, along with an oscilloscope, for monitoring several patients at one time. It can pick up several transmitting signals simultaneously.

Special features offered by a telemetry system include the ability to switch from a monitor to a diagnostic trace, the ability to be converted to a regular cable or "hard wire" system, a signal indicating battery depletion, a special jack to transmit the signal over the telephone, and a delay switch to minimize false alarms.

The critical care nurse assumes multidimensional responsibility for ECG monitoring. This section describes methods for a 12-lead ECG, lead systems, and telemetry.

12-LEAD ECG

OBJECTIVE

To provide data regarding the patient's electrical cardiac activity for diagnostic purposes, utilizing a single-channel or three-channel ECG recorder.

SPECIAL EQUIPMENT

ECG recorder:single-channel or three-channel ECG recorder
ECG recording paper
Electrode cable
Four limb electrode plates with electrode straps
Chest suction cup for single-channel ECG recorder

Six chest suction cups for three-channel ECG recorder
ECG electrode gel
Alcohol prep pads
Gauze pads

METHOD

ACTION	RATIONALE
1. Prepare ECG recorder.	
A. Select single-channel or three-channel ECG recorder.	A. See "Overview" for advantages.
B. Plug in grounded ECG recorder.	
C. Activate power on ECG recorder.	
2. Prepare patient.	
A. Place patient in supine position in the center of the bed for adequate support to all limbs.	
B. Expose the forearms, forelegs, and chest.	
C. Check that feet do not touch foot board of bed.	
3. Apply limb leads (Fig. 8).	
A. Use one ECG electrode plate for inner aspect of each forearm and for medial aspect of each lower leg.	A. The skin sites selected should ensure good contact and stabilization of the ECG electrode plate.

ACTION	RATIONALE

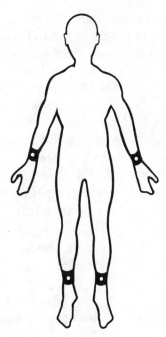

Figure 8. Limb lead location for 12-lead ECG.

B. Cleanse skin site with alcohol prep pad.

B. Removing oil from the skin surfaces enhances ECG electrode contact and controls for artifact.

C. Apply electrode gel to skin site and rub onto the ECG electrode plate to ensure good contact.

D. Secure ECG electrode plates with electrode straps; check tension.

D. Straps that are too tight may induce artifacts on tracing; electrodes should be placed so that the patient cable may be attached without bending or pulling the individual lead wires.

E. Attach limb lead cable wires to appropriate ECG electrodes.
   (1) Use white for right arm.
   (2) Use black for left arm.
   (3) Use red for left leg.
   (4) Use green for right leg.
   (5) Use brown for chest lead.

E. The tip of each lead cable wire is lettered and color-coded for easy identification.

F. Verify that each limb lead ECG electrode is positioned properly and secured on the correct extremities.

F. Avoid draping the cable over the abdomen, as this will cause respiratory artifact.

ACTION   **RATIONALE**

4. Apply chest leads (Fig. 9).
    A. Single-channel ECG recorder:
        (1) Place chest suction cup
            electrode on brown tip of
            patient cable marked "C."
        (2) Cleanse sites with alcohol
            prep pads.
        (3) Apply electrode gel to
            chest lead sites.
            (a) Use fourth inter-
                costal space, right
                sternal border, for V_1.
            (b) Use fourth inter-
                costal space, left
                sternal border, for
                V_2.
            (c) Use location midway
                between V_2 and V_4 for
                V_3.

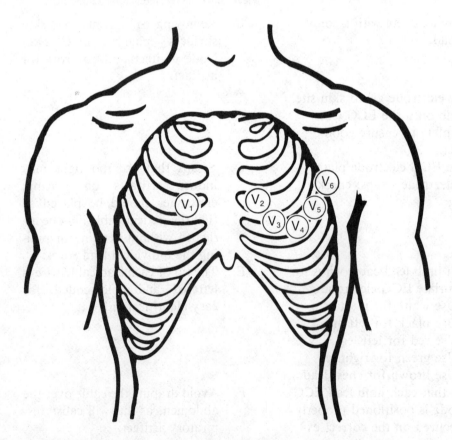

Figure 9. Standard chest lead positions for 12-lead ECG.

ACTION

RATIONALE

 (d) Use fifth intercost-
  al space, left of sternum, midclavicular
  line, for V₄.

 (e) Use fifth intercostal
  space, left of sternum,
  anterior axillary line,
  for V₅.

 (f) Use fifth intercostal
  space, left of sternum,
  midaxillary line, for
  V₆.

 (4) Secure suction cup to predetermined site to record
  individual chest leads.

B. Three-channel ECG recorder:

 (1) Place all six suction cups
  on appropriate six chest
  lead tips of the patient
  cable as described for
  single-channel recorder.

 (2) Apply electrode gel to
  chest lead sites.

 (3) Secure all six suction cups
  to predetermined and
  gelled sites.

5. Record the ECG.

A. Single-channel ECG recorder
 (Fig. 10).

 (1) Turn power switch to
  "run." ECG recording
  paper should feed
  correctly.

 (2) Turn lead selector switch
  to "standard" (STD
  position).

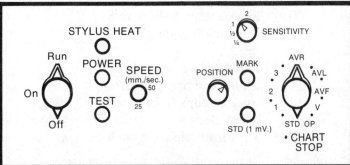

Figure 10. Single-channel ECG recorder.

ACTION	RATIONALE

(3) Center the stylus on the ECG paper using position control; adjust heat control.

(4) Press the STD 1mV. button.
  (a) Observe for deflection.
  (b) Adjust to 1 millivolt (mV.) if standardization is not correct.

(4) The ECG is standardized to assure that at 1 mV. the deflection will be 10 mm.; at ½ mV. the deflection will be 5 mm. (Each small square on the recording paper equals 1 mm.)

(5) Press marker button; note code on lower or upper edge of ECG paper.

(6) Return power switch to "on" to stop paper flow.

(7) Place lead selector to Lead I.

(8) Turn power switch to "run" and record approximately 10 beats.

(9) Mark Lead I with appropriate code. Suggested code:

Lead I —
Lead II — —
Lead III — — —
AVR ——
AVL —— ——
AVF —— —— ——
V₁ —— —
V₂ —— — —
V₃ —— — — —
V₄ —— — — —
V₅ —— — — — —
V₆ —— — — — — —

(10) Repeat steps 5 through 8 for each frontal plane lead.

(11) Return power switch to "on" and apply chest suction cups to brown chest electrode.

(12) Turn lead selector switch

ACTION	RATIONALE

to "V" and record all chest leads.

(13) Apply electrode gel to the six chest lead sites.

(14) Place the suction cup on V_1 site.

(15) Turn power switch to "run" and record.

(16) Repeat process for each chest lead, moving the suction cup appropriately.

B. Three-channel ECG recorder (Fig. 11):

(1) Position all leads, including the six chest leads, before the recording process is started.

(2) Standardize to 1 mV.

(3) Turn paper speed to 25 mm. per second.

(4) Turn on automatic marking.

(5) Depress AUTO-RUN button to record 12 leads in approximately 12 to 30 seconds.

(a) To interrupt an ECG recording, press the reset button and AUTO-RUN for a new ECG recording.

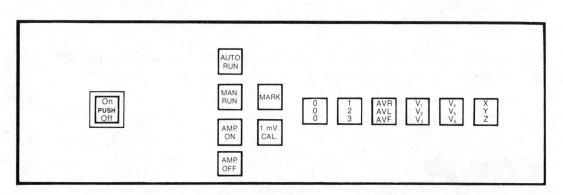

Figure 11. Three-channel ECG recorder.

ACTION	RATIONALE

     (b) Use manual mode as an option for further studies of select leads or for dysrhythmia recordings.

6. Turn off ECG recorder.

7. Remove ECG electrodes from patient; cleanse site and equipment.

8. Label ECG recording with patient's name, medical record number, date, and time; mount ECG recording appropriately.

PRECAUTIONS

1. Follow electrical safety guidelines. Ground ECG recorder and any electrical equipment in direct contact with patient for safety and to enhance the quality of the ECG recording.
2. Check accuracy of lead placement. Inaccurate chest lead placement may misrepresent the anterior surface of the heart. If the leads are mistakenly placed below the fifth intercostal space, a horizontal plane lead may be inadvertently transposed into a frontal plane lead.

RELATED CARE

1. Assess 12-lead ECG recording for warning of lethal dysrhythmias; provide prompt intervention.
2. Assess ECG recording for electrical or mechanical interference, or improper electrode placement:
   A. Electrical, AC or 60-cycle interference (as seen in Fig. 12); AC interference may be caused by improperly grounded equipment in the patient's room, such as a ventilator or an intravenous infusion pump. The interference may be eliminated by grounding each electrical apparatus properly.
   B. Mechanical interference, muscle tremor, singultus, or seizure activity may cause mechanical interference (as shown in Fig. 13).

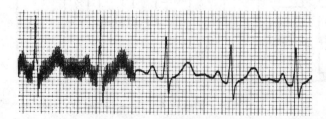

Figure 12. AC interference.

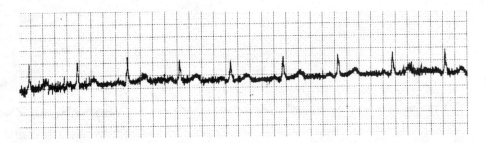

Figure 13. Mechanical interference.

Mechanical interference may be eliminated by treating the cause; e.g., if muscle tremor is due to shivering or chilling, provide a warm environment.

C. Improper electrode placement in the limb leads is usually seen on Lead I, where the left arm and the right arm may have been accidentally reversed. Lead reversal is demonstrated in Figure 14; correct lead placement is shown in Figure 15.

3. Note adjustments in recordings of ½ or 2 mV. by providing calibration marking on 12-lead ECG.

4. Adjust paper speed to enable better examination of complexes during periods of rapid heart rate.

5. In the case of an amputee, apply electrode to stump of affected extremity.

6. Apply electrodes high on extremities for patient with involuntary trembling.

7. Use minimal suction with suction cups when patient is being anticoagulated.

COMPLICATIONS

Dysrhythmias	Altered skin integrity
Electromicroshock	Equipment malfunction

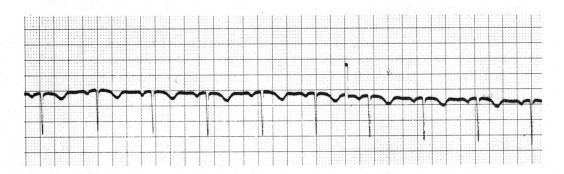

Figure 14. Lead reversal.

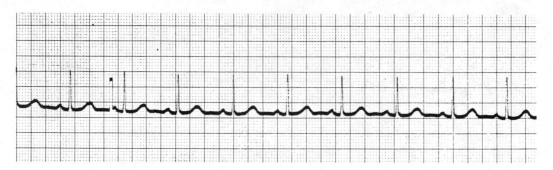

Figure 15.   Correct lead placement.

REFERENCES

Andreoli, K.G., et al.: *Comprehensive Cardiac Care* 4th ed. St. Louis, C. V. Mosby, 1979, pp. 87–127.

Brunner, L.S., et. al.: *The Lippincott Manual of Nursing Practice*, 2nd. edition, Philadelphia, J.B. Lippincott Co., 1978, pp. 383–385, p. 458.

Burdick Instruction Manual on EK-6, 3-Channel Cardiograph. Milton, Wisconsin, The Burdick Corporation, 1974, pp. 1-37.

Hewlett-Packard Company 3-Channel Automatic Cardiograph. Waltham, Massachusetts. The Hewlett Packard Company, 1975, pp. 1-37.

LEAD SYSTEMS

OBJECTIVES

1. To determine the appropriate ECG lead system for therapeutic ECG monitoring of select patients.
2. To provide an adequate and stable QRS complex and signal voltage, ensuring both visual observation and optimal monitoring operation.
3. To enhance individualization and flexibility among lead selections in order to recognize and diagnose electrical cardiac abnormalities.

SPECIAL EQUIPMENT

ECG monitor
Electrodes (pregelled disposable or nondisposable and electrode gel)
Razor

Sterile gauze pads
Alcohol prep pads
Computerized monitoring equipment (optional)

METHOD

ACTION

1. Prepare bedside ECG monitor and central monitoring station as directed by manufacturer.
2. Apply ECG electrodes to preselected and prepared skin sites.

   A. Choose sites for electrode placement (see 3, below, for options).

   B. Shave a 4-×4-inch square site for each electrode.

   C. Clean areas with alcohol prep pad, rubbing dry with sterile gauze pads and abrading the skin lightly.
   D. Connect electrode to lead wire.
   E. Apply gel-coated electrode to predetermined sites, pressing firmly in a circular pattern.

3. Select lead system (options).
   A. Three-lead system:

RATIONALE

2. Proper application of electrodes will enhance quality of ECG recording, with a distinct R wave.
   A. Care should be taken to avoid skeletal muscle by using the hollow of the clavicles and the lower sides of the thoracic cage.
   B. Removal of hair will minimize patient discomfort and facilitate conduction.
   C. Removal of skin oils and debris reduces the barrier to electrical flow.

   E. Pressure applied on electrode center may cause disbursement of gel with poor adhesive contact.

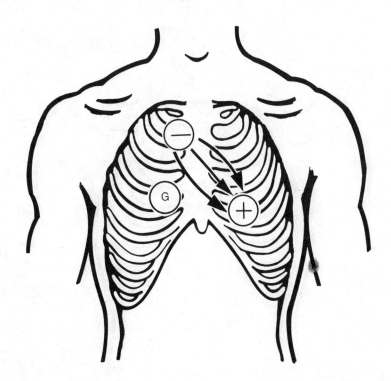

Figure 16. Lead II.

ACTION	RATIONALE
(1) Lead II (Fig. 16):	(1) This is best utilized for a positive and tall QRS complex, and normally has a good positive P wave. Also, this may be used for observation of QRS axis change denoting left anterior hemiblock.
(a) Apply negative electrode to first intercostal space, right sternal border.	
(b) Apply positive electrode to fourth intercostal space, left midclavicular line.	
(c) Apply ground electrode at fourth intercostal space, right sternal border.	
(2) MCL$_1$(modified chest lead V$_1$) (Fig. 17):	(2) This is an excellent lead for interpreting QRS axis, the differential diagnosis of ventricular ectopy, conduction disturbances, and a shift in pacing catheter electrode sites. It produces variable P-wave polarity and a negative QRS complex.
(a) Apply negative electrode just inferior to left clavicle, midclavicular line.	
(b) Apply positive electrode at fourth intercostal space, right sternal border.	
(c) Apply ground electrode just inferior to	

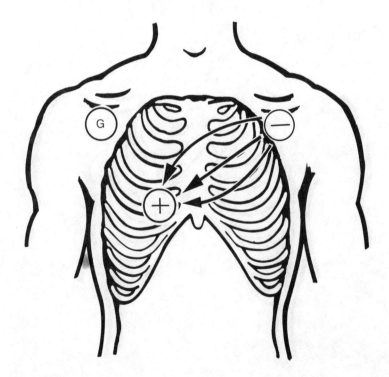

Figure 17. Modified chest Lead I .

ACTION　　　　　　　　　　　　　　　RATIONALE

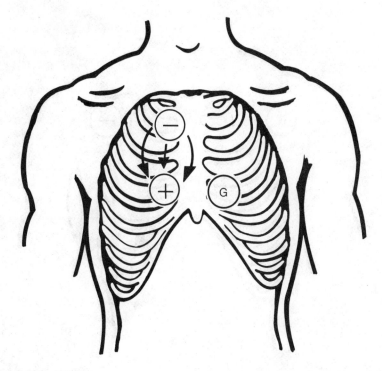

Figure 18. Lewis Lead.

right clavicle, midcla-
vicular line.

(3)　Lewis lead (Fig. 18):　　　(3)　This produces good P
　　(a)　Apply negative elec-　　　　waves and is used in atrial
　　　　trode at first inter-　　　　dysrhythmia identification.
　　　　costal space, right
　　　　sternal border.
　　(b)　Apply positive elec-
　　　　trode at fourth inter-
　　　　costal space, right
　　　　sternal border.
　　(c)　Apply ground elec-
　　　　trode at fourth inter-
　　　　costal space, left
　　　　sternal border.

(4)　MCL₃ (modified chest　　　(4)　This offers another lead
　　Lead 3) (Fig. 19):　　　　　　position for a positive QRS
　　(a)　Apply negative elec-　　　complex.
　　　　trode just inferior to
　　　　left clavicle, midcla-
　　　　vicular line.
　　(b)　Apply positive elec-
　　　　trode on last left in-
　　　　tercostal space, mid-
　　　　clavicular line.

ACTION   **RATIONALE**

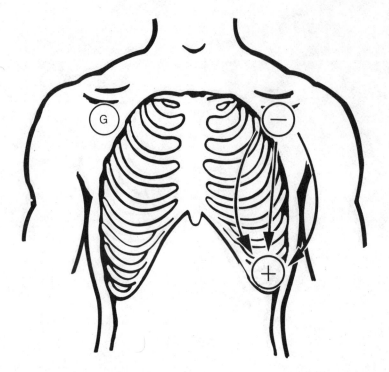

Figure 19.   Modified Lead III.

    (c) Apply ground electrode inferior to right clavicle, midclavicular line.

(5) MCL$_6$ (modified chest lead 6) (Fig. 20):

    (a) Apply negative electrode inferior to left clavicle, midclavicular line.

    (b) Apply positive electrode to fifth intercostal space, midclavicular line.

    (c) Apply ground electrode inferior to right clavicle, midclavicular line.

(6) Marriott MCL$_6$ lead:

    (a) Apply negative electrode inferior to right clavicle, midclavicular line.

    (b) Apply positive electrode to fifth inter-

(5) This is used frequently for patients with median sternotomy incisions and for telemetry monitoring. A tall QRS complex, ST and T wave changes, and left ventricular ectopy and right bundle branch block can be identified.

(6) This lead system offers the feasibility of switching from MCL$_1$ to MCL$_6$ by moving only the positive electrode.

ACTION   **RATIONALE**

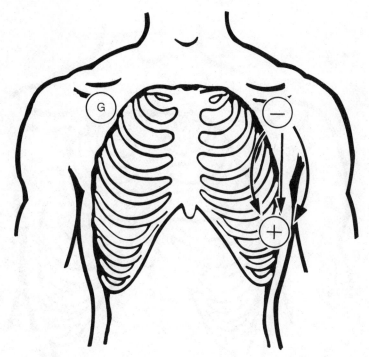

Figure 20. Modified chest Lead VI.

        costal space, midclavicular line.

    (c) Apply ground electrode inferior to left clavicle, midclavicular line.

B. Five-lead system (Fig. 21):

    (1) Apply right arm (RA) electrode inferior to right clavicle, midclavicular line.

    (2) Apply left arm (LA) electrode inferior to left clavicle, midclavicular line.

    (3) Apply right leg (RL) electrode on sixth intercostal space, right midclavicular line.

    (4) Apply left leg (LL) electrode on sixth intercostal space, left midclavicular line.

    (5) Apply chest (V) electrode on select chest sites V_1, V_2, V_3, V_4, V_5, or V_6 position.

B. The five-lead system facilitates rapid ECG monitoring from select sites. It should not be used as a complete 12-lead ECG for diagnostic purposes.

ACTION   **RATIONALE**

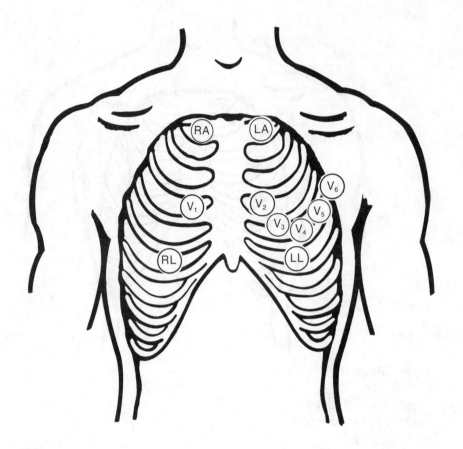

Figure 21.   Five-lead system.

(a) Place V electrode in
an insulating material
if not used on
patient's chest.

(6)   Activate ECG lead selector
for desired lead; record.

4.   Examine ECG recording; verify
quality of R wave.

5.   Set rate alarms.
6.   Label recording for the lead system
selected.
7.   Enter into computerized dysrhythmia system as directed by
manufacturer.

(a) This maintains elec-
trical patient isolation.

4.   The R wave should be approximately
twice the height of the wave form
components to assure proper ECG
triggering.

PRECAUTIONS

1. Check that alarms are always on.
2. Provide defibrillator, emergency cart, and medications for immediate use as necessary.
3. Follow electrical safety guidelines.
4. Check tension on ECG electrode wires, which may contribute to lead wire fractures.
5. Integrate monitoring with observation and care of the cardiac patient. Monitoring is one tool among many.

RELATED CARE

1. Perform continuous ECG monitor surveillance; provide prompt nursing intervention as necessary.
2. Check quality of pregelled disposable electrodes. Since quality and adhesion characteristics vary, a mixture of brands should not be used. Also, always check the disc after opening for sufficient moist gel; loss of ECG gel or paste will cause baseline instability and motion artifact.
3. Change nondisposable electrodes daily, using thorough site cleansing and applying fresh ECG gel. If there is excessive perspiration, tincture of benzoin applied onto electrode adhesive sites may help to maintain an adhesive bond.
4. Assess skin integrity every 24 hours; rotate electrode sites. Skin allergy or sensitivity is a potential problem with adhesive bonding.
5. Maintain a good ECG monitor recording with a good QRS signal voltage, a stable clear baseline, and the absence of artifact or distortion (Fig. 22).
6. Check for potential source of false alarm triggering.
   A. High rate alarm may be due to:
      (1) Excessive gain, causing the T wave to be "sensed" by the monitor as well as the R wave, thus doubling the rate.
      (2) Excessive muscle artifact, caused by patient movement.
      (3) Insufficient increase in high rate alarm setting above the patient's own rate.
   B. Low rate alarm may be due to:
      (1) Insufficient gain setting.
      (2) Presence of a wandering baseline, with not all signals being sensed.
      (3) Decrease of R wave signal on a particular lead, caused by axis shift.
      (4) Insufficient decrease in low rate alarm setting below the patient's own rate.

Figure 22. Good quality QRS signal, stable clear baseline, absence of artifact.

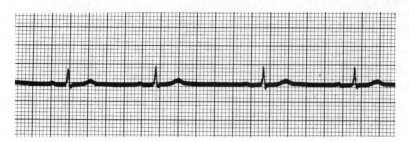

Figure 23. Low voltage signal.

C.   Other causes of false alarm triggering may be due to a loose lead, dried electrode gel, patient movement, muscle tremor due to shivering or seizure, damaged cable or leads, and/or AC interference.

7.   Identify alterations in ECG monitor recordings.

A.   Low voltage signal (Fig. 23):

(1)   Potential causes:

(a)   Low gain setting on the ECG monitor.

(b)   Poor electrode contact and/or disconnected electrode.

(c)   Disconnected or broken lead wire.

(d)   Loose cable connection from the monitor.

(e)   Loss of amplitude of QRS signal.

(2)   Significance: Will trigger false low rate alarm.

(3)   Intervention:

(a)   Check connections of lead wires and cable.

(b)   Reapply electrode as required.

(c)   Increase the gain.

(d)   Trouble-shoot for specific lead problem.

B.   Excessive artifact (Fig. 24):

(1)   Potential causes:

(a)   Patient movement.

(b)   Dry or loose electrode.

(c)   Intermittent electrical interference.

(2)   Significance:

(a)   Excessive artifact may cause irregular oscillations on the ECG trace.

(b)   May allow dysrhythmias to go unnoticed.

(c)   May trigger the false high rate alarm.

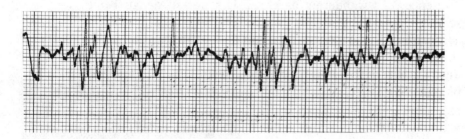

Figure 24.   Excessive artifact.

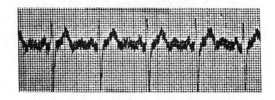

Figure 25. Electrical interference.

      (3) Intervention:
          (a) Check electrode contact.
          (b) Reposition electrodes to an area with less skeletal muscle.
          (c) Check lead wires for stress on patient movement.

C. Electrical interference (Fig. 25):
      (1) Potential causes:
          (a) Improper electrical equipment grounding.
          (b) X-ray or diathermy equipment in operation.
          (c) Exposed broken lead wires or cables.
      (2) Significance: ECG trace may be distorted by the production of 60 cycle per second artifact.
      (3) Intervention:
          (a) Presents a potential hazard to the patient.
          (b) The source may be isolated by disconnecting pieces of electrical equipment surrounding the patient one at a time, while checking for the elimination of the problem.

D. Wandering ECG baseline (Fig. 26):
      (1) Potential causes:
          (a) Poor electrode contact and/or too much gel.
          (b) Tension on electrode and lead wires.
          (c) Movement of the cable with respiration.
      (2) Significance:
          (a) Provides a tracing difficult to interpret for rhythm.
          (b) May trigger alarms, since not all beats will be sensed by the monitor.
      (3) Intervention:
          (a) Check tension on lead wires and cable.
          (b) Reposition the patient cable to the side of the chest or wherever there is the least movement.
          (c) Replace electrodes as required.

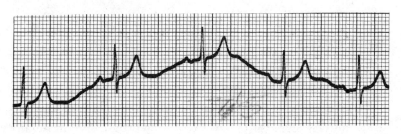

Figure 26. Wandering baseline.

E. Poor quality ECG recordings in select leads:
    (1) Intervention: Isolate cause to select ECG lead; correct.

Poor ECG Recording in:	*Potential Source*
Leads I, II, III	RL electrode/lead wire
Leads II, III	LL electrode/lead wire
Leads I, II	RA electrode/lead wire
Leads I, III	LA electrode/lead wire
Lead V	Replace

COMPLICATIONS

Dysrhythmias	Electromicroshock	Equipment
Cardiac arrest	Altered Skin In-tegrity	malfunction

SUPPLIERS

Abbott	Hewlett-Packard
American Optical	Lexington
Datascope	Midwest Analog and Digital
Electrodyne	Siemens
Electronics-for-Medicine	Telemed

REFERENCES

Andreoli, K.G., Fowkes, V.H., Zipes, D.P., Wallace, A.G.: Comprehensive Cardiac Care. St. Louis, C. V. Mosby, 1975, pp. 76–103.

Frost, D., et al.: Evaluation of a computerized arrhythmia alarm system. Am.J. Cardiol., *39*:583, 1977.

Huetgren, H.N., et al.: Clinical evaluation on a new computerized monitoring system. Heart Lung, *4*:241, 1975.

Moore, E.: Proper use of electrodes essential for successful monitoring. Hosp. Top. *47*:536, 1975.

Pinneo, R.: Cardiac monitoring. Nurs. Clin. North Am. *7*:411, 1972.

TELEMETRY

OBJECTIVE

To maintain continuous ECG monitoring utilizing a select lead-to-transmitter system for patients requiring progressive ambulatory activity and freedom from lead-to-monitor cable attachment.

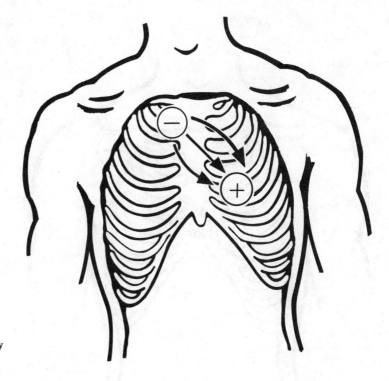

Figure 27. Lead II. Telemetry monitoring.

SPECIAL EQUIPMENT

Telemetry unit	Patient cable	Alcohol prep pads
Battery	ECG electrodes	

METHOD

ACTION	RATIONALE
1. Prepare display control console.	1. This enters patient into system for continuous ECG surveillance.

2. Apply electrodes to patient's chest for desired lead system.
A. Lead II (Fig. 27):
   (1) Apply negative electrode to first intercostal space, right of sternal border.
   (2) Apply positive electrode at fourth intercostal space, left of midclavicular line.
B. MCL₁ (Fig. 28):
   (1) Apply negative electrode left of midclavicular line, below clavicle.	

ACTION   RATIONALE

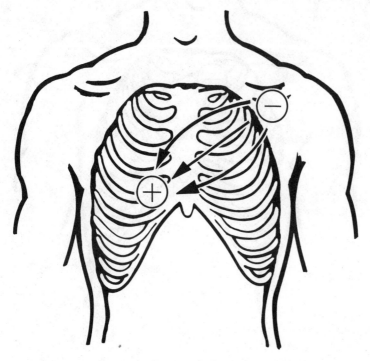

Figure 28. Modified chest Lead
I. Telemetry monitoring.

    (2)   Apply positive electrode at
          fourth intercostal space,
          right of sternal border.
3. Place battery in telemetry unit;
    check battery position for positive
    (+) and negative (−) poles.
4. Place ECG cable from telemetry
    unit to corresponding ECG elec-
    trodes for desired lead system.
5. Check ECG pattern on display con-
    trol oscilloscope; set rate alarms.

PRECAUTIONS

1. Check for proper ECG electrode placement and security.
2. Monitor patient's activity location for prompt intervention should
   dysrhythmias occur.
3. Provide defibrillator, emergency cart, and medications for immediate
   use as necessary.

RELATED CARE

1. Observe for dysrhythmias; provide appropriate nursing intervention.

2. Protect transmitter from direct trauma by securing in a gown pocket or in a pouch around the neck, or on a belt designed with a pocket.
3. Change battery for telemetry unit as necessary, utilizing indicator light.
4. Reposition ECG electrodes and check skin integrity every 24 hours.

COMPLICATIONS

Dysrhythmias   Altered skin in-   Equipment mal-
                         tegrity   functions

REFERENCES

Beaumont, E.: ECG telemetry. Nursing '74, *4*:27, 1974.
DeBusk, R.F.: The role of ambulatory monitoring in post-infarction patients. Heart Lung, *4*:536, 1975.

CARDIOVERSION

Martha Spence, R.N., M. N.

OVERVIEW

Cardioversion is an elective therapy to terminate tachydysrhythmias by delivering a synchronized direct current charge. This charge simultaneously depolarizes the entire myocardium, thereby interrupting re-entry circuits and establishing electrical homogeneity. As a result, the sinoatrial node resumes control of the rhythm. Synchronization with the QRS complex permits timing the electrical discharge so that it appears outside the vulnerable period of the T wave of the ECG.

Cardioversion is often effective in terminating atrial tachycardia, atrial flutter, atrial fibrillation, and ventricular tachycardia. Dysrhythmias associated with digitalis toxicity should not be cardioverted electrically because of the possibility of initiating complex ventricular ectopic rhythms after cardioversion. Digitalis is usually discontinued for 2 or more days prior to elective cardioversion, depending upon the specific glycoside preparation being used. Premedication with antiarrhythmic drugs is a common practice for ensuring maintenance of postconversion rhythms.

OBJECTIVE

To convert select supraventricular and ventricular tachydysrhythmias to sinus rhythm.

SPECIAL EQUIPMENT

Cardioverter/defibrillator capable of delivering a synchronized shock
Paddles: anterior-posterior or transverse
ECG monitor and recorder
Conductive medium, or saline gauze pads
Oxygen therapy equipment
Airway
Resuscitator bag
Emergency pacing equipment
Emergency cart and medications

METHOD

ACTION	RATIONALE
1. Obtain a 12-lead ECG.	1. Documentation of the precardioversion rhythm provides a baseline to be

ACTION	RATIONALE
	compared with that of postcardioversion ECG.
2. Secure patient's intravenous line.	2. This provides an access route for administration of medications and/or anesthetic.
3. Place patient in supine position.	3. The supine position facilitates a clear ECG recording, proper placement of paddles, easier access for resuscitation support, and greater relaxation with limb support.
4. Administer oxygen as prescribed *prior* to cardioversion; discontinue at the moment of cardioversion.	4. Unless contraindicated, oxygen therapy 5 to 10 min. before cardioversion promotes myocardial oxygenation. In the presence of electrical arcing, oxygen may support combustion.
5. Assess patient, including vital signs, cardiac rhythm, peripheral pulses, and mentation level.	5. This data will serve as a baseline for postcardioversion evaluation.
6. Remove dentures.	6. This reduces the risk of airway obstruction.
7. Prepare cardioversion equipment.	
A. Attach the patient to the ECG monitor, selecting a lead with a distinct tall R wave and a T wave of small magnitude or in a direction opposite to the R wave.	A. The synchronizer times the electrical current to be delivered only on the patient's R wave. Improper synchronization can lead to discharge on the T wave and result in ventricular fibrillation.
(1) Check monitor for artifact; change leads if artifact is present.	(1) Proper electrode placement and contact is critical, since artifact could result in the electrical current being delivered at an improper time during the cardiac cycle.
B. Plug grounded equipment into electrical outlet.	B. Proper grounding will prevent current leaks, microshocks, and/or accidental electrocution.
C. Turn power switch on several minutes prior to use.	C. Most equipment requires a warm-up period.
D. Turn synchronizer switch on.	D. In the synchronizing mode, the machine will sense an R wave and discharge the preset electrical current. Without activating the synchronizing mode, discharge occurs at the instant the

ACTION	RATIONALE
	paddle buttons are depressed, regardless of the phase of the cardiac cycle.

E. Test for synchronization.
   (1) Use manual synchronization button to determine the proper timing of the electrical charge.
   (2) Observe that charge release appears on the downslope of the R wave or within the S wave.
	E. This will ensure proper synchronization of charge to QRS and charge release outside of vulnerable period.

8. Administer medication as ordered.	8. Electrical shocks vary from being uncomfortable to being painful, depending upon the patient and the voltage used.
9. Prepare paddles by applying conductive medium to metal surface of paddles or moist saline pads to chest.	9. Conductive medium reduces resistance of skin to current flow. Adequate coverage of metal surfaces will prevent skin burns and allow for optimal current flow to the myocardium. Excess conducting medium contributes to skin burns or electrical arcing.

10. Charge cardioversion machine to prescribed voltage.
  A. Check that power switch is on and synchronizer mode is activated.
  B. Turn selector dial to the prescribed number of watt-seconds.
	B. The current level is prescribed by the physician according to the patient's body weight, ECG rhythm, and precardioversion medication(s). Initially, a low watt-seconds selection is normally used (50 to 100 watt-seconds); this is then increased in increments of 50 to 100 watt-seconds. Many dysrhythmias will convert with low voltages. The larger the voltage the more tissue trauma and the greater the discomfort to the patient.

C. Activate charge button.	
11. Place paddles firmly into position	11. Firm pressure establishes good con-

ACTION	**RATIONALE**

ANTERIOR-POSTERIOR

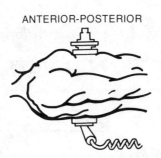

TRANSVERSE

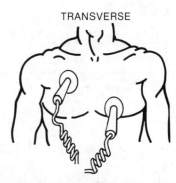

Figure 29. Placement of paddles on chest.

against the chest, using approximately 25 to 30 lb. of pressure (Fig. 29).

A. Transverse position:
   (1) Place one paddle at second intercostal space, right of sternum.
   (2) Place second paddle at fifth intercostal space, midclavicular line, left of sternum.

B. Anterior-posterior position:
   (1) Place one paddle at anterior-precordial area.
   (2) Place second paddle at posterior-intrascapular area.

12. Assess ECG rhythm on monitor.

13. Activate ECG recorder.

14. Check for synchronization indicator superimposed on the patient's R wave as presented on the ECG oscilloscope.

15. Stand clear of bed and give command to stand clear.

16. Depress discharge buttons on the two paddles simultaneously; continue keeping both firmly depressed until the electrical current is delivered.

---

tact. Current should flow across axis of cardiac muscle mass, regardless of paddle position used.

B. Anterior-posterior position may decrease amount of current required.

12. ECG rhythm may change prior to cardioversion.

13. Documentation during all phases of cardioversion assists with post-cardioversion assessment.

14. This ensures proper synchronization.

15. Electrical current follows the path of least resistance; this measure reduces risk of accidental micro- or macroshock.

16. Premature release of discharge buttons may result in failure of the machine to discharge energy.

ACTION   RATIONALE

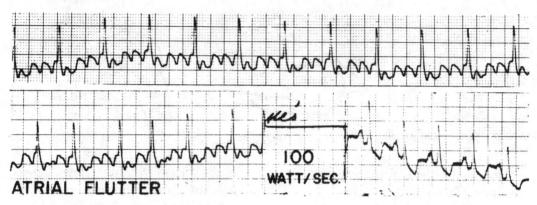

Figure 30.   Cardioversion of atrial flutter.

17. Assess ECG rhythm to ascertain postcardioversion ECG rhythm (Figs. 30 and 31).

18. Repeat method as prescribed to terminate tachydysrhythmia.

17. Cardioversion may convert original ECG rhythm, have no effect, or produce a lethal dysrhythmia.

18. Repeated cardioversion therapy is given by increasing current in increments of 50 to 100 watt-seconds and separating each attempt by approximately 3 minutes.

19. Perform postcardioversion care.

A. Assess the patient, peripheral pulses, and level of consciousness; auscultate lungs; monitor vital signs every 15 minutes times 4, then every hour, and then every 4 hours until stable.

A. Sedation may contribute to respiratory depression. Two postcardioversion complications are dysrhythmias and pulmonary edema.

B. Obtain a 12-lead ECG.

B. This data assists in assessing for myocardial damage.

C. Monitor the patient's ECG rhythm continuously for at least 2 hours.

D. Administer oxygen as prescribed.

D. Systemic arterial oxygen may be reduced, owing to unconsciousness and altered airway.

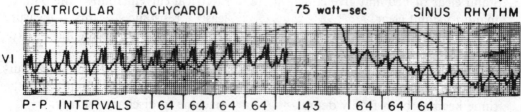

Figure 31.   Cardioversion of ventricular tachycardia.

ACTION	RATIONALE

E. Assess chest wall for presence
of burns.

F. Support patient and reorient
as necessary.

PRECAUTIONS

1. Be sure that cardioversion is performed in a setting where resuscitation and respiratory support are immediately available.
2. Check that equipment being used is properly grounded to prevent current leakage.
3. Determine serum potassium levels prior to cardioversion. Hypokalemia enhances electrical instability and thus may increase postconversion dysrhythmias.
4. Determine digitalis level, if time permits. Defer cardioversion if digitalis toxicity is suspected because of risk of lethal dysrhythmias. Set initial energy level at 5 watt-sec. and, if this low energy level results in frequent PVC's, do not proceed with cardioversion.
5. Assess for acid/base imbalances and hypoxia prior to cardioversion by a baseline blood gas determination.
6. Observe for respiratory depression due to premedication.
7. Turn off synchronizer if ventricular fibrillation occurs. Since there are no R waves in ventricular fibrillation, the unit will fail to discharge in the synchronized mode.

RELATED CARE

1. Keep patient on nothing by mouth for 6 to 12 hours prior to cardioversion.
2. Obtain signed consent according to hospital policy.
3. Prepare lidocaine, atropine, isoproterenol drip, and lidocaine drip for immediate use prior to cardioversion.
4. Check potential causes for failure to convert:
    A. Faulty equipment or frayed wires.
    B. Debris on paddles.
    C. Nonsynchronized mode.
    D. Artifact interference.
    E. Battery failure, if unit is portable.
5. Document sequence of therapy, including voltage delivered with each attempt and postcardioversion ECG rhythm.

COMPLICATIONS

Cardiac arrest
Respiratory depression or
    arrest
Dysrhythmias
Pulmonary edema

Pulmonary or systemic emboli
Hypotension
Skin burns
Equipment malfunction

REFERENCES

Andreoli, K.G., et al.: Comprehensive Cardiac Care, 3rd ed. St. Louis, C. V. Mosby, 1975, pp. 282–285.

Chung, E.: Cardiac Emergency Care. Philadelphia, Lea and Febiger, 1975, pp. 141–165.

Stephenson, H.: Cardiac Arrest and Resuscitation. St. Louis, C. V. Mosby, 1974, pp. 77–86.

Vinsant, M., et al.: A Commonsense Approach to Coronary Care. St. Louis, C. V. Mosby, 1975, pp. 199–203.

DEFIBRILLATION

Martha Spence, R.N., M.N.

OVERVIEW

Defibrillation is an emergency therapy whereby a nonsynchronized direct current charge is delivered to the myocardium in order to terminate ventricular fibrillation. Complete depolarization of the myocardium simultaneously disrupts all electrical circuits responsible for ventricular fibrillation, allowing the sinoatrial node or another potential pacemaker to regain control of the heart rhythm. The charge is delivered via metal paddles, either to the external chest wall or directly to the myocardium during cardiac surgery.

Careful assessment of the clinical state of the patient and ECG patterns is necessary pre- and postdefibrillation. Cardiopulmonary support measures and pharmacologic therapy are integral components of treatment. Success in patient survival depends upon early recognition and rapid treatment of lethal dysrhythmias.

OBJECTIVE

To terminate ventricular fibrillation immediately, facilitating the establishment of an effective cardiac rhythm.

SPECIAL EQUIPMENT

Defibrillator with external paddles/internal paddles (sterilized)
ECG monitor and recorder
Conductive medium or saline gauze pads
Emergency cart and medications

Oxygen therapy equipment
Airway
Resuscitator bag
Emergency pacing equipment
Emergency cart and medications

METHOD

ACTION	RATIONALE
1. Verify ventricular fibrillation by ECG; correlate with the clinical state of the patient.	1. Ventricular fibrillation may be mistaken for artifact on the ECG.
2. Prepare to defibrillate.	2. Assess the situation. If a second per-

ACTION	RATIONALE
	son is getting the defibrillator, establish an airway and begin ventilation and external cardiac massage.
A. Plug grounded defibrillator into electrical outlet, if necessary.	
B. Turn power on.	
C. Prepare defibrillator paddles. Options: (1) Cover entire metal surface of paddles with conductive medium. (2) Place moist saline gauze pads in desired position on chest.	C. Conductive medium on entire metal surface of paddles and moist saline gauze pads on chest reduce resistance of skin to current flow, prevent skin burns, and allow for optimal current flow to the myocardium.
D. Dial 350 to 400 watt-seconds for an adult.	D. High current levels are generally needed to convert ventricular fibrillation.
E. Activate charge button.	E. This will charge unit with electrical current.
F. Assess that defibrillation unit is in the nonsynchronized mode.	F. In the synchronized mode the machine will not fire owing to the absence of R waves in ventricular fibrillation.

G. Place paddles firmly into position against the chest, using approximately 25 to 30 lb. pressure (see Fig. 29 for illustration of transverse and anterior-posterior positions).
 (1) Transverse position:
    (a) Place one paddle at second intercostal space, right of sternum.
    (b) Place the second paddle at fifth intercostal space, midclavicular line, left of sternum.
 (2) Anterior-posterior position:
    (a) Place one paddle at anterior-precordial area.
    (b) Place the second pad-
	G. Firm pressure establishes good contact. Current should flow across axis of cardiac muscle mass, regardless of paddle position used.
	
	 (2) Anterior-posterior position may decrease amount of current required.

ACTION	RATIONALE

dle at posterior-intra-
scapular area.

3. Stand clear of bed; give command to stand clear prior to defibrillation. Visibly check to see that personnel are standing away from bed.

3. Electrical current follows the path of least resistance. This measure reduces the risk of accidental micro- or macroshock.

4. Recheck ECG rhythm on monitor to ascertain ventricular fibrillation.

4. ECG rhythm may change prior to defibrillation.

5. Depress the discharge buttons on the two paddles simultaneously; continue keeping both firmly depressed until the electrical current is delivered.

5. Premature release of the discharge buttons may result in failure of the machine to discharge energy.

6. Determine effects of defibrillation by checking the postdefibrillation ECG rhythm (Fig. 32).
   A. Prepare paddles and defibrillator for immediate reuse if ventricular fibrillation persists.
   B. Continue cardiopulmonary resuscitation during preparation of equipment.
   C. Assess patient status and precipating factors to prevent further decompensation of the patient.

7. Postdefibrillation care:
   A. Assess the patient, peripheral pulses, and level of consciousness; auscultate lungs, monitor vital signs every 15 minutes times 4, then every hour, and then every 4 hours until stable.

   A. This facilitates baseline data after medical emergency.

   B. Monitor ECG rhythm.

   B. This allows detection of recurrent warning and/or lethal dysrhythmias.

   C. Establish patent IV line.

   C. This may be needed to administer medications.

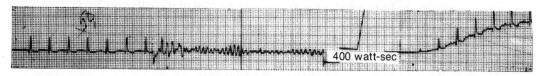

Figure 32. Defibrillation of pacer-induced ventricular fibrillation.

ACTION	RATIONALE

D. Administer prescribed medications.
  (1) Check that IV bolus antidysrhythmic medications are followed with an IV drip to maintain a therapeutic level.
  (2) Observe effect of medications by patient assessment and ECG monitoring.	

E. Administer oxygen.	E. Cardiac arrest constitutes an extreme case of hypoventilation and leads to severe hypoxemia.
F. Obtain a 12-lead ECG.	F. This data assists in assessing the myocardial damage and ECG rhythm.
G. Assess chest wall for presence of burns. Consult with the physician regarding treatment if burns are present.	G. Burns are a common complication of defibrillation. Steroid- or lanolin-based creams may be prescribed.

PRECAUTIONS

1. Check that all equipment is properly grounded to prevent current leakage.
2. Disconnect temporary pacemaker and other electrical equipment. Defibrillation may result in damage to the equipment.
3. Avoid soaking gauze pads or excessive conductive gel on paddles to prevent arcing of current with decreased flow to patient.

RELATED CARE

1. Support patient and family as necessary after defibrillation.
2. Clear defibrillator of remaining electrical current immediately; never set charged defibrillator paddles down. Prepare equipment for future use.
3. Support patient with cardiopulmonary resuscitation, as appropriate.
4. Document predefibrillation ECG rhythm, number of times defibrillation was attempted, voltage used with each attempt, postdefibrillation ECG rhythm, and multisubsystem status.
5. Check possible causes of failure to convert ventricular fibrillation.
   A. Defibrillator on synchronized rather than nonsynchronized mode.
   B. Debris on paddles, which impaired conductivity.
   C. Low amplitude fibrillatory waves, which can be associated with

long-standing ventricular fibrillation, acidosis, and hypoxia; this requires cardiopulmonary resuscitative measures prior to defibrillation.
   D.   Frayed wires and faulty equipment.
6.   Recognize the following differences for internal defibrillation.
   A.   Use sterile internal defibrillation paddles.
   B.   Use sterile, saline-moistened gauze pads between the myocardium and defibrillation paddles.
   C.   Charge defibrillator to prescribed voltage; a significantly lower (15 to 30 watts-sec.) energy level is used.
7.   Recognize the following changes for pacemaker defibrillation:
   A.   Turn off temporary external pacemaker.
   B.   Avoid placing defibrillator paddles over permanent pulse generator or electrode (see Fig. 33 for correct placement).

COMPLICATIONS

Dysrhythmias   Pulmonary edema
Cardiac arrest   Pulmonary or systemic emboli
Respiratory arrest   Equipment malfunction
Neurologic impairment   Death
Altered skin integrity

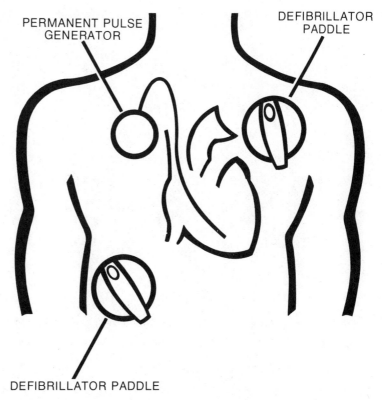

Figure 33.   Placement of defibrillator paddles on patient with a permanent pulse generator.

REFERENCES

Andreoli, K.G., et al.: Comprehensive Cardiac Care, 3rd ed. St. Louis, C. V. Mosby, 1975, pp. 285–286.

Chung, E.: Cardiac Emergency Care. Philadelphia, Lea and Febiger, 1975, pp. 141–165.

Stephenson, H.: Cardiac Arrest and Resuscitation. St. Louis, C. V. Mosby, 1974, pp. 336–366.

Vinsant, M., et al.: A Commonsense Approach to Coronary Care. St. Louis, C. V. Mosby, 1975, pp. 199–203.

VASCULAR INVASIVE TECHNIQUES

Karen M. Miller, R.N., M. S. N.

OVERVIEW

Venipuncture and arterial puncture are the two most common vascular invasive techniques used by the critical care nurse. Securing and maintaining a patent venous route is of high priority for the critically ill patient or the patient who is a *high* risk for dysrhythmias or a medical emergency. A single arterial puncture is performed selectively to obtain an arterial blood sample for immediate gas analysis in such instances as cardiopulmonary arrest, suspected altered respiratory function, and/or monitoring of oxygen therapy.

INSTRUMENTATION

Combination disposable catheter needles are widely used in the care of the critically ill; they are available in various lengths and lumen sizes. A *catheter-over-the-needle* set consists of an external catheter and internal needle, with the bevel point extending beyond the catheter tip (Fig. 34). The needle serves as a stylus during the venipuncture, after which it is withdrawn and discarded. A primed IV administration set is connected directly to the adapter. A *catheter-through-the-needle* set consists of a catheter enclosed within a needle and catheter guard sleeve (Fig. 35). Following a successful venipuncture, the catheter is threaded into the vein, the stylus removed, and a primed IV administration set connected directly to the adapter. This catheter set requires the needle to be withdrawn and protectively secured externally, utilizing the needle bevel cover and proper connection at the adapter point. Disposable arterial puncture kits with various gauges and lengths of needles, plastic or glass syringes, and multiple syringe sizes are available; these prepackaged kits are especially useful in critical care units and/or emergency carts for cardiopulmonary arrest situations.

This section presents methods for performing a venipuncture, using two types of indwelling catheters, and for performing a single arterial puncture.

VENIPUNCTURE

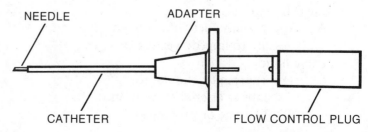

NEEDLE ADAPTER

Figure 34. Components of the catheter-over-the-needle type insertion set.

CATHETER FLOW CONTROL PLUG

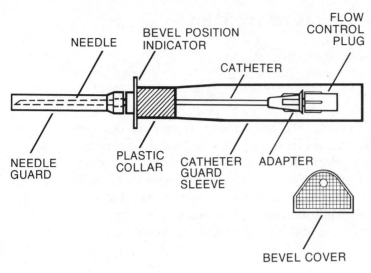

Figure 35.   Components of the catheter-through-the-needle type insertion set.

OBJECTIVES

1. To provide a route for administration of intravenous fluid, medication, blood, and blood components.
2. To provide nutritional supplement and hydration for individuals unable to obtain them by other means.

SPECIAL EQUIPMENT

Intravenous fluid

Intravenous administration set

Infusion needle (catheter-over-the-needle or catheter-through-the-needle)

Tourniquet

Depilatory or razor

Sterile gauze dressings

Povidone-iodine ointment

Povidone-iodine prep pads or swabs

Alcohol prep pads

Tape

Arm board

METHOD

ACTION	RATIONALE

1. Determine appropriate venipuncture site (Fig. 36):
A. Apply tourniquet with enough pressure to impede venous circulation.
   (1) Tourniquet should not impede arterial circulation.
   (2) Extreme or prolonged	

ACTION   **RATIONALE**

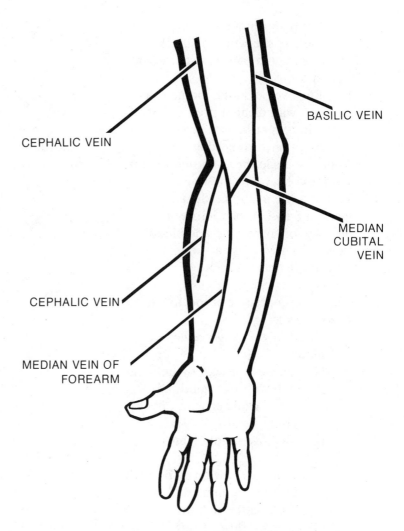

CEPHALIC VEIN

BASILIC VEIN

MEDIAN
CUBITAL
VEIN

CEPHALIC VEIN

MEDIAN VEIN OF
FOREARM

Figure 36. Anatomic sites for venipuncture.

pressure may make the
vein become tortuous.

(3) Minimal pressure is required for sclerosed veins;
in these cases a tourni-
quet may make venipunc-
ture even more difficult.

B. Select site for venipuncture.

C. Release tourniquet.

2. Prepare selected site for venipuncture.

A. Remove hair with depilatory or
razor as needed to facilitate
placement or removal of tape.

ACTION	RATIONALE

B. Apply tourniquet.

C. Cleanse site with povidone-iodine prep pad or swab; allow to dry.

D. Remove povidone-iodine solution with alcohol prep pad if vein cannot be visualized.

3. Puncture skin with needle at a 45-degree angle; bevel should be upward and lateral to the vein.

    3. This causes the least amount of discomfort for the patient.

4. Reduce angle of the needle and insert 1/8 to 1/4 inch into vein; observe for free retrograde blood flow, which will appear in catheter as needle enters the vein.

5. Release tourniquet.

6. Follow appropriate method for infusion needle.

   A. Catheter-over-the-needle technique:

     (1) Stabilize needle by holding hub with one hand; advance catheter with opposite hand.

          (1) Stabilization of the needle prevents posterior puncturing of the vein.

     (2) Remove needle from catheter.

     (3) Connect previously primed IV fluid administration set to catheter hub.

     (4) Initiate flow of intravenous fluid; assess for signs of local edema.

          (4) If the catheter has punctured the vein completely, fluid will infuse into surrounding tissue, as evidenced by edema.

     (5) Secure catheter with tape.

   B. Catheter-through-the-needle technique:

     (1) Stabilize needle by holding hub; advance catheter by applying pressure at base of catheter in plastic sleeve.

          (1) It is preferable to thread the catheter until catheter and hub of the needle are engaged. The catheter should be advanced a minimum of 4 inches; when the catheter cannot be advanced at least 4 inches the needle and

ACTION	RATIONALE
	catheter must be removed simultaneously and a new site located.
(2) Engage needle hub into catheter hub.	(2) If catheter is inserted at least 4 inches but less than the full length of the catheter, it is necessary to pull needle back until it engages the catheter hub.
(3) Apply slight pressure above puncture site with one hand; use opposite hand to withdraw needle from vein until 1½ inches of the catheter is exposed.	(3) The application of pressure should eliminate excessive bleeding or trauma.
(4) Remove catheter guard sleeve, holding catheter hub securely.	(4) Holding catheter hub securely prevents accidental catheter removal.
(5) Remove flow control plug and stylet.	
(6) Connect previously primed IV fluid administration set to catheter hub.	
(7) Initiate flow of intravenous fluid.	
(8) Apply needle guard securely over tip of needle.	(8) The guard will protect the catheter from being pierced by the needle inadvertently. Needle and catheter should lie firmly in the groove of the needle guard before it is closed. If the catheter is not in the groove, infusion will cease when the guard is closed.

(9) Secure with tape.

7. Apply povidone-iodine ointment at catheter insertion site; secure with gauze dressings and tape.

8. Adjust intravenous fluid infusion rate.

PRECAUTIONS

1. Select the type of infusion needle with the following considerations:

     A. Type of solution—fluids with higher viscosity may require a larger bore needle.

     B. Location of the vein.

     C. Phlebitis related to antibiotic infusion is less likely to result if larger deeper veins are used.

2. Select the vein with the following considerations:
   A. Activity/flexibility needed by the patient.
   B. Hand orientation of the patient (right or left handed).
   C. Condition of the vein.
   D. Type of solution or medication for which the infusion is required.
   E. Anticipated duration of therapy.
3. Observe care when shaving site selected; razor shaving can produce microabrasions of skin, with resultant bacterial access and growth.
4. Monitor length of time catheter is in place; maximum recommended duration is 72 hours.

RELATED CARE

1. Use a sterile catheter for each venipuncture.
2. Label dressing with type of infusion needle and gauge, date, and time of insertion.
3. Perform site care with povidone-iodine ointment and sterile gauze dressings every 24 hours (see the method for "Short Venous Indwelling Catheter Site Care").
4. Maintain catheter patency.
5. Monitor intravenous fluid infusion rate.

COMPLICATIONS

Thrombus formation	Tissue sloughing related to local fluid infiltration	Nerve injuries
Phlebitis		
Hematoma	Local or systemic infection	

SUPPLIERS

Abbott
Argyle
Becton-Dickinson
Deseret
Sorenson

REFERENCES

Berry, P.R., and Wallis, W.E.: Venipuncture nerve injuries. Lancet, *1*:1236–1237, 1977.

Hamlyn, A.N.: Venipuncture nerve injuries. Lancet *2*:39, 1977.

Nursing Procedure Manual. St. Luke's Hospital, Milwaukee, WI, October, 1977, Procedure No. 12.

ARTERIAL PUNCTURE

OBJECTIVES

1. To obtain a blood specimen for analysis of arterial pH, oxygen tension (Po_2), carbon dioxide tension (Pco_2) oxygen saturation, and acid-base balance.
2. To assist in diagnosis and treatment of hypoxic states, oxygen therapy, respiratory failure, and continuous ventilatory assistance.

SPECIAL EQUIPMENT

Arterial blood gas kit (disposable)
   One 5-ml. glass syringe with rubber cap and stopper
   One 22-gauge × 1″ needle (short bevel)
   One 20-gauge × 1½″ needle
   Two sterile gauze pads
   Two alcohol prep pads
   One adhesive bandage
   One patient label
   One sterile field
   One plastic bag or container with sufficient ice for cooling blood sample en route to laboratory
   One 1-ml. ampule sodium heparin
Povidone-iodine prep swabs
Local anesthetic (optional)
One 1-ml. syringe with 25-gauge needle
Laboratory requisition

METHOD

ACTION	RATIONALE
1. Instruct patient regarding method,	1. Instruction alleviates hyperventilation

ACTION	RATIONALE

purpose, and patient responsibilities.

2.   Select site.

A.   Radial artery (Fig. 37):

(1)   Use as first choice, except in the case of multiple radial artery punctures, hematoma, occlusion of ulnar artery, history of circulatory impairment to extremity, or cardiac arrest.

(2)   Perform the Allen test (see "Related Care").

that, when present, might alter arterial blood gas values.

(1)   The radial artery is a small artery; however, it is easily stabilized as it passes over a bone groove, located at the wrist. The percutaneous puncture and pressure control are enhanced by this anatomic landmark.

(2)   Collateral circulation to hand is provided by ulnar artery; the Allen test assesses for ulnar artery patency.

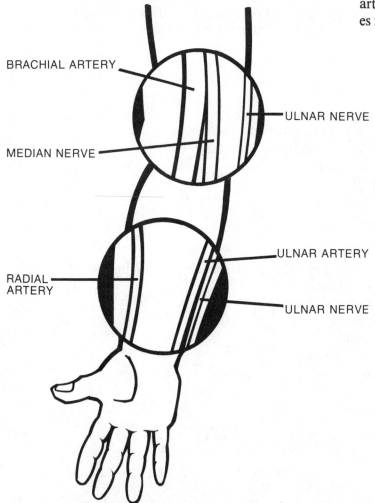

Figure 37.   Anatomic landmarks for radial and brachial arterial punctures.

ACTION	RATIONALE

B. Brachial artery (Fig. 37):
    (1) Use as second choice, except in the case of poor pulsation due to shock, obesity, or sclerotic vessel.

    (1) The brachial artery is larger than the radial artery. Pressure control after percutaneous puncture is enhanced by its proximity to bone if entry point is approximately 1½″ above antecubital fossa.

C. Femoral artery (Fig. 38):
    (1) Use as third choice, except in the case of cardiac arrest or altered perfusion to upper extremity arteries.

    (1) The femoral artery is a large artery; however, there is no collateral circulation available if it is injured. Because the femoral artery is located in close proximity to the femoral vein, there is potential risk for false pH,

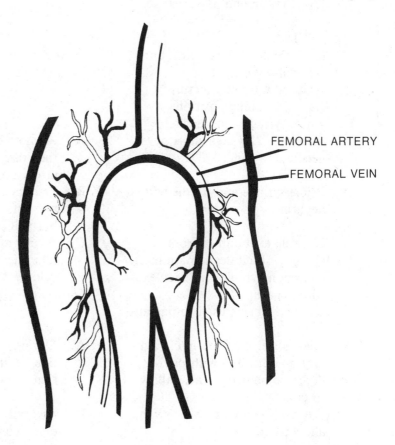

FEMORAL ARTERY

FEMORAL VEIN

Figure 38. Anatomic landmarks for femoral arterial puncture.

ACTION	RATIONALE
	Po_2, and Pco_2 values owing to venous blood contamination, arteriovenous fistulas, or hemorrhage/hematomas, since bleeding is more difficult to control.

3. Position patient.
   A. Radial arterial puncture:
      (1) Use semirecumbent position.
      (2) Elevate and dorsiflex wrist slightly, using a small pillow.
      (3) Rotate patient's hand until pulse is palpable.
   B. Brachial arterial puncture:
      (1) Use semirecumbent position.
      (2) Elevate and hyperextend arm, supporting with pillow.
      (3) Rotate patient's arm until pulse is palpable.
   C. Femoral arterial puncture:
      (1) Use supine position.

4. Heparinize syringe and needle.

A. Assemble 22-gauge short bevel needle on syringe.	A. A short bevel needle diminishes the risk of overshooting the artery during entry.
B. Prime syringe and needle with heparin.	B. Priming the syringe with heparin prevents specimen coagulation, but will not alter the blood pH.
C. Eject all air bubbles from syringe; fill all dead space in collection syringe and needle with heparin.	C. All air must be ejected to maintain accuracy of blood gas values.

5. Prep site and fingers used to palpate site.

A. Cleanse selected site in circular motion outwards with povidone-iodine prep swabs; allow to dry.	A. Drying of povidone-iodine solution reduces risk of local infection or systemic sepsis.
B. Cleanse site with alcohol swab; allow to dry.	B. Alcohol removes povidone-iodine coloring from site and thereby increases visibility. Puncturing through a moist

ACTION

RATIONALE

alcohol-prepared site can increase pain.

6. Locally anesthetize site (optional).
   A. Use 1-ml. syringe with 25-gauge needle and xylocaine 1%.
   B. Aspirate prior to injecting xylocaine to ascertain that a blood vessel has not been entered.
   C. Inject intradermally and then with full infiltration around artery, using approximately 0.2 to 0.3 ml. for an adult.
7. Perform percutaneous puncture of select artery.
   A. Ascertain pulsating artery.
   B. Stabilize artery by pulling skin taught and bracketing the area of maximum pulsation with fingertips of free hand.
   C. Puncture skin slowly, holding syringe like a pencil; advance needle slowly with bevel upward at approximately a 45- to 90-degree angle to the artery (Fig. 39).

   D. Observe syringe for flashback.

C. A slow gradual thrust will promote arterial entry without passing directly through it. Enter at angle comfortable for stabilizing your hand. Certainty of position matters more than entry angle.

D. Pulsation of blood into the syringe verifies that the artery has been punctured.

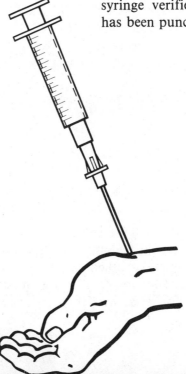

Figure 39. Radial arterial puncture.

ACTION	RATIONALE
E. If puncture is unsuccessful, withdraw needle to skin level, angle slightly toward artery, and readvance.	
8. Obtain a 3- to 5-ml. specimen.	8. This amount allows for rechecking and additional studies, if necessary.
9. Withdraw needle while stabilizing barrel of syringe.	9. This prevents inadvertent aspiration of air during withdrawal.
10. Apply firm continuous pressure to arterial puncture site for 5 minutes, or until bleeding stops. A. Apply firm pressure for 10 minutes if the patient has a history of coagulation problems.	10. Hematomas following an arterial puncture can cause circulatory impedance, discomfort, or predispose to infection.
11. Protect blood sample.	
A. Hold syringe upright; express air bubbles rapidly.	A. Air bubbles may alter laboratory test results.
B. Seal needle immediately, using rubber stopper or cap.	B. Specimen must be kept airtight to prevent alteration of test results.
C. Immerse blood sample in enough ice for transport to laboratory.	C. The use of ice reduces temperature of the sample to below 4° C and slows the metabolism of oxygen. A delay longer than 2 min. alters values.
D. Label specimen; complete appropriate laboratory requisition. Note the percentage of O_2 therapy, if applicable, the temperature, especially if elevated; and the time specimen was drawn.	
E. Expedite immediate laboratory services.	E. No test results for any specimen, even if chilled, can be accepted as reliable if sample is tested 15 to 30 min. after arterial puncture.

PRECAUTIONS

1. When possible, avoid femoral arterial punctures in patients with a history of aortofemoral synthetic grafts.
2. Check for medication allergies if local anesthetic is utilized.
3. Alternate sites for serial arterial blood gas punctures.

RELATED CARE

1. Consider arterial line placement to facilitate obtaining serial arterial blood gas samples.
2. Perform Allen test prior to radial artery puncture.

   A. Instruct patient to form a tight fist (or, if unresponsive, raise arm above heart level for several seconds) to force blood from hand.

   B. Apply direct pressure on radial and ulnar arteries to obstruct arterial blood flow to hand while patient opens and closes fist rapidly several times.

   C. Instruct patient to open hand (or, if unresponsive, keep arm above heart level) with radial artery remaining compressed.

   D. Examine palmar surface for an erythematous blush or pallor within 15 seconds. An erythematous blush indicates ulnar artery patency and is interpreted as a positive Allen's test. Pallor indicates occlusion of the ulnar artery and is interpreted as a negative Allen's test; with a negative Allen's test the radial arterial puncture should be avoided.

3. Monitor aftercare of arterial puncture site.

   A. Maintain continuous firm pressure on puncture site for 5 to 10 minutes after needle withdrawal; length of time varies with patient's age, health, medical history, and anticoagulation therapy.

   B. Check site for delayed hematoma formation and circulation to extremity every 5 minutes times 6. Circulatory impairment can occur for various reasons. A medical history of arteriosclerosis increases the risk of thrombosis, especially in the femoral artery. Large or small arterial occlusions due to thrombosis, intramural hemorrhage, or emboli may produce symptoms such as cold extremities, absence of pulses, or petechiae. In this event, protect the extremity from future punctures at the same site. Also, local edema not attributed to local anesthesia injection usually indicates internal hemorrhage that can be controlled by direct compression.

4. Assess results of arterial blood gas tests.
5. Document temperature of patient, oxygen percentage and method of delivery, site of arterial puncture, ease of puncture, time length of applied pressure, site assessment, and serial circulation assessment after arterial puncture.

COMPLICATIONS

False values	Arterial spasm
Intraluminal clotting	Thrombosis
Hematoma	Nerve injury
Hemorrhage	Arteriovenous fistulas
Impaired circulation to	Pulmonary embolism

extremity   Altered skin integrity
Infection (local or systemic)

SUPPLIERS

Argyle
Bard Parker
Travenol

REFERENCES

Bedford, R.F., and Wollman, H.: Complication of percutaneous radial-artery cannulation: An objective prospective study in man. Anesthesiology, *38*:228–236, 1973.

Wade, J.F.: Respiratory Nursing Care: Physiology and Technique. St. Louis, C. V. Mosby, 1973, pp. 64–69.

Critical Care Procedure Manual. St. Joseph's Hospital, Milwaukee, WI, 1978.

HEMODYNAMIC MONITORING

Karen C. Johnson, R.N., M.S., CCRN, and
Lani Moskowitz Strom, R.N., M.S., C.E.T.

OVERVIEW

Hemodynamic monitoring includes both invasive and noninvasive assessment techniques, and ranges from simple measurement using a blood pressure cuff to measure intracardiac pressures directly. Pressure measurement is critical for patient assessment; modern biomedical engineering has produced sophisticated equipment to monitor pressure continuously at the bedside. This is invaluable when caring for the critically ill patient in whom changes can occur rapidly.

Manifestations of Altered Hemodynamics. Signs and symptoms can vary from those of cardiac dysfunction, leading to pulmonary and/or systemic congestion with rales, pulmonary edema, increased jugular venous distention, and peripheral edema, to those of acute cardiovascular collapse and profound shock. These symptoms include weakness, pallor, confusion, cold clammy skin, diminished to absent pulses, cardiac dysrhythmias, low arterial blood pressure, and decreased cardiac output. Also, new murmurs, rubs, and extra heart sounds may develop.

Fluid Challenge. Further evaluation of left ventricular performance can be obtained by altering therapy according to pressure measurements; this is known as fluid challenge. Fluid volume expansion causes an increase in myocardial end-diastolic fiber length. According to the Starling principle, this increases the force of ventricular contraction. In uncomplicated hypovolemia fluids may be pushed until adequate *central venous pressure* (CVP) and *pulmonary artery wedge pressures* (PAWP) are reached, returning the patient to a normal volemic state. If the CVP and PAWP rise with the fluid challenge but the patient remains hypotensive, then the possibility of heart failure must be considered.

Preload and Afterload. Preload may be defined briefly as end-diastolic fiber length (PAWP). Afterload is the resistance to ventricular ejection (aortic pressure). Cardiac function may be improved by increasing preload to increase the length of fiber stretch, thereby increasing myocardial contractility, and decreasing afterload, thereby increasing cardiac output. There are both mechanical and pharmaceutical agents which accomplish this. A common method is to administer Dopamine to increase preload while simultaneously titrating Nipride to decrease afterload. This careful balance of vasotonic agents may assist the failing heart.

Assessment of Altered Hemodynamics. Multiple hemodynamic parameters are used in subsystem assessment of the critically ill patient. Physiologic monitoring can include measurement of central venous, pulmonary artery, pulmonary artery wedge, left atrial, and arterial pressures, and cardiac output determination.

Central Venous Pressure.   The CVP indicates the pressure in the right atrium; this directly reflects right ventricular diastolic pressure, or the ability of the right side of the heart to pump blood. In patients with normal cardiac reserve and normal pulmonary vascular resistance, the CVP can be valuable for assessing the dynamic interrelationships between cardiac action, vascular tone, and blood volume. CVP is not an accurate index of left ventricular function and may, indeed, be one of the last parameters to change. However, it is a valuable diagnostic tool for many patients in whom fluid status is of concern. Fluid replacement or restriction can be prescribed more judiciously on the basis of the CVP findings. A normal CVP ranges from 5 to 10 cm. of water or 6 to 12 mm. Hg.

Pulmonary Artery Wedge Pressure.   The flow-directed pulmonary artery catheter makes possible indirect measurements of left-sided heart pressures at the bedside (Fig. 40). A small balloon at the end of the catheter becomes buoyant when inflated, and passes through the cardiac chambers in the direction of blood flow. Thus, when the catheter is inserted into a large intrathoracic vein, it passes into the right atrium, through the tricuspid valve

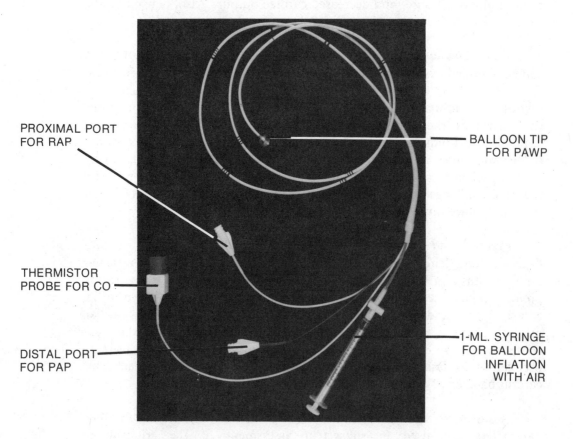

Figure 40.   Pulmonary artery catheter.

into the right ventricle, and through the pulmonary valve into the pulmonary artery (PA), where it finally wedges itself in a smaller lumen of the pulmonary artery (Fig. 41). The opening of the catheter beyond the inflated balloon reflects pressures distal to the pulmonary artery—that is, the passive run-off of pulmonary venous blood into the left atrium. This pulmonary artery wedge pressure (PAWP), then, measures left ventricular function indirectly, since the mean PAWP (PAWP) and left atrial pressure (LAP) closely approximate left ventricular end-diastolic pressure (LVEDP) in patients with normal left ventricular and mitral valve function. When the balloon is deflated, the catheter measures pressures from the pulmonary artery directly.

Pulmonary artery catheters are available in multiple sizes and with assorted features. These include a single-lumen catheter for PAP, a double-lumen catheter for PAP and PAWP, a triple-lumen catheter for PAP, PAWP, and CVP, a quadrilumen catheter for PAP, PAWP and CVP, and a thermistor probe for cardiac output studies. In addition, some catheters feature a pacing electrode.

Left Atrial Pressure.   This is measured by a left atrial catheter which is inserted by the surgeon during cardiac surgery and connected to a pressure transducer system. Mean left atrial pressure (LAP) closely reflects left ventricular end-diastolic pressure in patients with normal left ventricular and

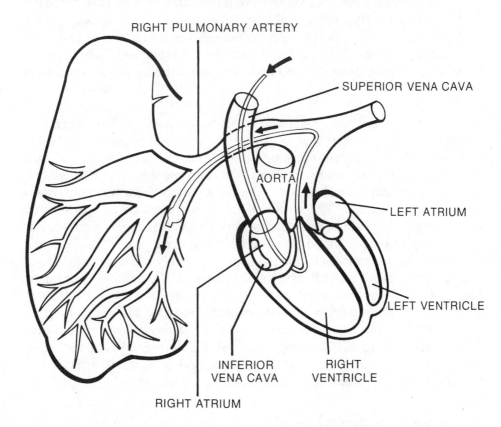

Figure 41.   Pulmonary artery catheter and balloon inflation.

mitral valve function. Patients with LAP monitoring are potential risks for air emboli; security of all connections must be checked closely and frequently.

Cardiac Output.   This is the product of heart rate times stroke volume, in liters per minute. Normal resting cardiac output is about 4 to 8 liters per minute. Unless an intracardiac shunt is present, the cardiac output of both the right and left ventricles is essentially the same. Monitoring cardiac output is important in assessment of cardiac status and the patient's response to therapy. A low resting cardiac output may be due to poor ventricular filling from hypovolemia, valvular stenosis, or poor ventricular emptying, as in aortic stenosis. The usual cause is myocardial dysfunction. A high cardiac output may be caused by hypermetabolic states such as hyperthyroidism or by anxiety. Cardiac output may be increased by increasing preload and decreasing afterload. There are three basic methods for measuring cardiac output—the method based upon the Fick principle, the indicator-dilution method, and the thermodilution technique.

5 L/min
5000 ml/min
80 strokes/min
$$\frac{5000}{80} = 62.5 \text{ ml/stroke}$$

Techniques of Hemodynamic Monitoring.   Arterial pressure monitoring may be obtained by continuous pressure monitoring, intermittent and automatic indirect techniques, or cuff pressure technique.

Direct Monitoring.   In direct arterial monitoring, the arterial wave form should be sharp, with a rapid upstroke (anacrotic limb), clear systolic peak, definite dicrotic notch, and definite end-diastolic component. The recorded wave forms may be delayed from the corresponding electrical event of the cardiac cycle due to the recording pressure delay of events when using a long catheter.

Automated Systems.   Automatic blood pressure measurements are generally programmed so that the frequency of blood pressure determinations may be selected; determinations may be made as often as every minute or as infrequently as every 8½ minutes. On many models, once a determination is completed, the values are given on a digital display(s) until a new determination is made. The results of the most recent determinations are then shown on the face of the blood pressure unit. Equipment varies according to the automatic blood pressure device utilized. Some have external transducers or microphones; others may include only the automated blood pressure apparatus, an ordinary blood pressure cuff, and two pneumatic hoses between the cuff and blood pressure machine. Many different automatic blood pressure monitoring models are being utilized to measure arterial blood pressure noninvasively with or without heart rate. Some models record Korotkoff's sounds electronically during automatic inflation and deflation of the cuff; others use ultrasound to measure arterial wall movement during automatic cuff deflation and inflation.

Pressure transducer systems for bedside utilization can be of the single or multiple type, continuous or intermittent, with various modifications. Basic components to a pressure monitoring system can include: (1) a transducer, which detects the physiologic event; (2) an amplifier, which increases the magnitude of the signal from the transducer; and (3) a recorder, meter, and/or oscilloscope, which displays the resultant signal.

Transduction is the conversion of one form of energy into another. Physiologic transducers can convert such parameters as pressure, temperature, or sound into a usable electrical signal which can then be displayed on a bedside oscilloscope. Pressure is transmitted to the transducer diaphragm through a fluid-filled column. It is important that the transducer be positioned at the level of the cardiac chamber in which the catheter is placed. If the transducer is located lower than the heart level, the force of hydrostatic pressure onto the transducer will result in a false high pressure reading. Conversely, if the transducer is positioned above the level of the heart, the combination of hydrostatic and gravitational forces will result in a false low pressure reading. Positioning the air-fluid interface of the transducer to the midaxillary line and fourth intercostal space approximates heart level most accurately for correct pressure monitoring. The pressure transducer system is closed, air-free, and contains an infusion/flushing component.

The entire pressure system should be kept simple and compact in order to eliminate signal distortion from artifact. Catheters and tubing should be short and of a firm substance for high pressure monitoring. Use of stopcocks and adapters should be minimized to reduce potential sources for air leaks and/or clot formation which, in turn, could distort the signal.

Amplifiers contained within the monitor may simply amplify or may process, filter, and amplify the electrical signals sent from the transducer. These signals are converted to the standard measurement for pressure, millimeters of mercury, and are displayed on the meters or digital component of the bedside pressure module. The pressure wave form can be displayed on a device such as an oscilloscope or chart recorder. These are mandatory for viewing the pressure wave form as a function of time.

Precautions. The same electrical equipment that is invaluable in critical care monitoring and resuscitation also may be a potential risk to the patient; the most hazardous is ventricular fibrillation. Respect of electrical and safety monitoring guidelines is crucial. (See section on "Safety," pp. 454–460). A defibrillator, emergency cart, and medications must be readily accessible.

This section will present methods for pressure transducer systems, select hemodynamic pressure monitoring, and automatic blood pressure measurements.

SINGLE PRESSURE TRANSDUCER SYSTEM _____

OBJECTIVE

To monitor one pressure continuously using a single pressure system (Fig. 42).

SPECIAL EQUIPMENT

Pressure transducer (sterile)
Monitor capable of one pressure reading
Transducer mount
Transducer holder
IV pole
Transducer dome (sterile, disposable)
Normal saline (0.9% soldium chloride) IV solution (bag)
Sodium heparin for normal saline IV solution: 1 unit per ml. of fluid (or as ordered by physician)

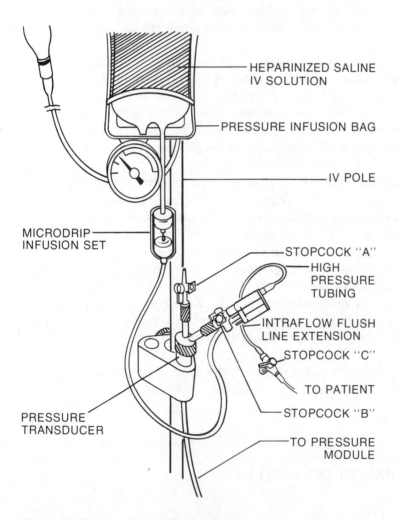

HEPARINIZED SALINE
IV SOLUTION

PRESSURE INFUSION BAG

IV POLE

MICRODRIP
INFUSION SET

STOPCOCK "A"

HIGH
PRESSURE
TUBING

INTRAFLOW FLUSH
LINE EXTENSION

STOPCOCK "C"

TO PATIENT

STOPCOCK "B"

PRESSURE
TRANSDUCER

TO PRESSURE
MODULE

Figure 42.   Single pressure transducer system.

Inflatable pressure cuff
Intraflow (sterile)
Solution administration set
High pressure tubing (approximately 2 feet)
Sterile water to prime transducer
Three three-way stopcocks
Three protective stopcock caps
One 10-ml. syringe

For single pressure system with direct patient mounting, substitute:
Transducer (sterile)
Pressure monitor tubing (6 inches)
Transducer mounting clip
Inflatable pressure cuff (for arterial only)

METHOD

ACTION	RATIONALE
1. Prepare transducer dome. 　A. Remove protective dome from transducer. 　B. Hold the transducer level and place several drops of sterile water on the diaphragm. 　C. Screw on the sterile disposable transducer dome.	 B. Use sterile water since saline solution may cause rust.
2. Mount transducer on IV pole.	
3. Connect transducer to pressure monitor; allow 5 to 10 minutes as a warm-up period.	3. This ensures accurate transducer calibration.
4. Prepare heparinized normal saline IV solution. 　A. Add 1 unit of heparin per ml. of normal saline IV solution, or as prescribed by physician. 　B. Connect IV administration sets with clamps off to IV port and medication port of heparinized normal saline IV solution.	 A. Heparinized normal saline IV solution prevents clotting and embolic complications.
5. Attach pressure cuff over heparinized normal saline IV solution bag; inflate to approximately 300 mm. Hg.	5. Pressure should be above the systolic pressure of the patient to ensure the forward and continuous IV solution flush at a rate of approximately 2 to 3 ml. per hour.
6. Attach sterile stopcocks to each port	

ACTION   **RATIONALE**

of the transducer dome and patient side of intraflow.

A. Identify stopcock at 90° angle port of transducer dome as stopcock A.

B. Identify stopcock at 45° angle port of transducer dome as stopcock B.

C. Identify stopcock at patient side of intraflow as stopcock C.

7. Prime transducer dome:

A. Attach 10-ml. syringe filled with sterile normal saline solution to side port of stopcock B.

B. Open stopcock A to transducer and air.

C. Open stopcock B to transducer and prefilled syringe.

D. Prime transducer, flushing with prefilled syringe.

E. Close stopcock A to transducer.

8. Prime IV administration set and intraflow:

A. Close stopcock C to intraflow.

B. Attach IV administration tubing to long line of intraflow.

C. Open IV clamp; flush all air from IV administration set and intraflow by pulling on intraflow flush line extension (red tail).

9. Attach Intraflow to transducer (options).

A. Direct connection to transducer:

(1) Attach intraflow to stopcock B with intraflow flush line extension pointing towards transducer.

(2) Connect high pressure tubing to patient port of intraflow using stopcock C between high pressure line and patient catheter.

(2) Do not use tubing longer than 4 feet; increased length adversely affects the system frequency response.

RATIONALE

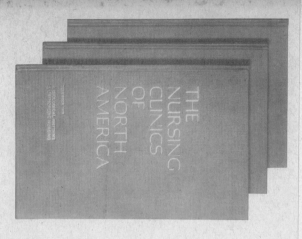

(4) Do not use tubing longer than 4 feet; increased length adversely affects the system frequency response.

bubbles trapped within system dampen pressure tracing, posing tential risk for air emboli.

ed to transducer, and stopcock C opened to intraflow and patient catheter.

B. Prime intraflow or high pressure tubing by pulling intraflow flush line extension with stopcock A closed to transducer, and stopcock B opened to intraflow or high pressure tubing and syringe.

11. Using single pressure transducer system with direct patient mounting:

A. Attach primed intravenous tubing system to intraflow (see steps 4 and 5 above).

B. Connect sterile transducer to transducer mounting clip; turn power on; allow 10 to 15 minutes as a warm-up period.

B. This ensures accurate calibration.

C. Attach three-way stopcock to male end of intraflow; close to intraflow.

ACTION	RATIONALE
D. Prime intraflow by pulling intraflow flush line extension.	
E. Attach primed transducer with sterile dome to female end of intraflow.	E. Air bubbles trapped within system may dampen pressure tracing and pose a potential risk for air emboli.
F. Position transducer to level of patient's right atrium; secure with transducer mounting clip.	F. This will ensure accuracy of pressure determinations.
G. Connect pressure monitoring tubing to stopcock of intraflow; prime tubing.	
H. Attach pressure monitoring tubing to stopcock at patient's catheter.	

12. Balance the transducer.
   A. Select appropriate ranges on monitor pressure module.
   B. Close stopcock B to transducer.
   C. Open stopcock A to transducer and air.
   D. Balance to zero reading according to manufacturer's instructions.
   E. Proceed with calibration or leave open to air if transducer will not be connected directly to patient for a time, or close stopcock A to transducer and open stopcock B to transducer and patient system.

   D. Transducer must be adjusted to zero at room air conditions for proper balancing.
   E. Leaving the transducer open to air while waiting for an indefinite period of time prevents pressure build-up and inaccurate readings.

13. Calibrate according to range selected.
   A. Balance to zero.
   B. Adjust calibration dial to correct number that has been preassigned for selected ranges.
   C. Close stopcock A to transducer.
   D. Open stopcock B to transducer and intraflow or high pressure tubing.

13. This involves checking the output of the transducer against a known value; not all transducers require calibration.

14. Cover all open ports of the intraflow and stopcocks with sterile caps.

14. This reduces the risk of infection.

15. Rebalance and recalibrate 30 min-

15. This ensures proper calibration.

ACTION	RATIONALE

utes after connecting system to patient and leveling to right atrial
position.

PRECAUTIONS:

1. Maintain sterile technique throughout preparation of system.
2. Disconnect transducer from patient during defibrillation or cardioversion to prevent damage to the transducer.
3. Check for accurate readings; rebalance and recalibrate as necessary. Be sure that fluid-air interface is at the level of the patient's right atrium during pressure system connection.
4. Check that all connections are secure and dome is free from cracks.
5. Ascertain that all stopcocks are in the proper position.
6. Free all tubing and cables from potential pressure or kinking points.
7. Respect electrical safety guidelines for invasive monitoring; see also the method for "Safety."
8. Maintain 300 mm. Hg pressure in inflatable pressure cuff during pressure monitoring.
9. Set alarm limits.
10. Control for artifact by minimizing the number of electrical items in use, patient movement, and/or faulty transducers. Transducers that have been dropped, cleaned improperly, and/or exposed to even minimal diaphragm surface scratching are potential sources of erroneous readings or equipment artifact.

RELATED CARE:

1. Follow disposable dome package instructions, some domes do not require the use of sterile water during preparation.
2. Flush system manually during transient blood pressure elevations.
3. Check trace position or correct range pressure curve when pressure curve is positioned off the oscilloscope.
4. Change single pressure system every 24 hours.

COMPLICATIONS

Hemorrhage	Air emboli	Electromicroshock
Sepsis	Tubing separation	Equipment malfunction

REFERENCES

Hewlett Packard Company: Guide to Physiological Pressure Monitoring. Waltham, MA., Hewlett Packard, 1977, pp. 8–15 and 45–63.

Horovitz, J.L., and Leterman, A.: Postoperative monitoring following critical trauma. Heart Lung, *4*:270, 1975.

Schroeder, J.S., and Daily, E.K.: Techniques in Bedside Hemodynamic Monitoring. St. Louis, C. V. Mosby, 1976, pp. 79–87.

MULTIPLE PRESSURE TRANSDUCER SYSTEM

OBJECTIVE

To monitor two or more pressures using a multiple pressure system or modified single transducer systems (Fig. 43).

SPECIAL EQUIPMENT

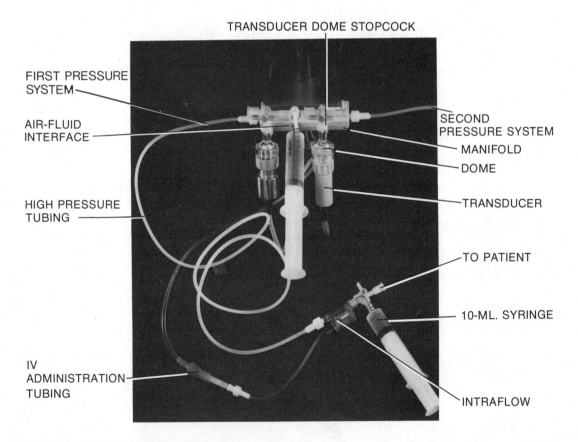

Figure 43.   Multiple pressure transducer system set-up.

Multiple Pressure System
    Pressure transducer (sterile; one for each pressure being monitored)
    Monitor capable of two or more pressures
    Manifold
    Manifold mount
    IV pole
    Transducer dome (sterile, disposable; one for each transducer)
    Normal saline (0.9% sodium chloride) IV solution (bag)
    Sodium heparin for normal saline IV solution:
      1 unit per ml. of fluid (or as ordered by physician)
    Inflatable pressure cuff
    Intraflow (one for each pressure being monitored)
    Solution administration set (one for each intraflow)
    High pressure tubing (approximately 2 feet; one for each pressure
      being monitored)
    Sterile water to prime transducer
    Three-way stopcocks (approximately two for each intraflow)
    Protective stopcock caps (approximately two for each pressure
      system)
    10-ml. syringe
Single Pressure System with Separate Transducers
    See the method for "Single Pressure Transducer System" and
    double, triple, etc., the equipment listed.
Single Pressure System with One Transducer for Two Pressures
    See the method for "Single Pressure Transducer System"
      and double the following:
        Intraflow
        High pressure tubing

METHOD

ACTION	RATIONALE
Multiple Pressure System	
1. Prepare transducer domes.	
A. Remove protective dome from transducer.	
B. Hold the transducer level and place several drops of sterile water on the diaphragm.	B. Use sterile water since saline solution may cause rust.
C. Screw on the sterile disposable transducer dome.	
2. Mount manifold on IV pole, using manifold holder; secure transducers.	
3. Connect transducers to pressure monitor; allow 5 to 10 minutes as a warm-up period.	3. This ensures accurate transducer calibration.

ACTION	RATIONALE
4. Prepare heparinized normal saline IV solution.	
A. Add 1 unit of heparin per ml. of normal saline IV solution, or as prescribed by physician.	A. Heparinized normal saline IV solution prevents clotting and embolic complications.
B. Connect IV administration sets, with clamps off, to IV port and medication port of heparinized normal saline IV solution (see Fig. 44).	
5. Attach pressure cuff over heparinized normal saline IV solution bag; inflate to approximately 300 mm. Hg.	5. Pressure should be greater than the systolic pressure of the patient to ensure the forward and continuous IV solution flush at approximately 2 to 3 ml. per hour.
6. Prime IV administration sets, intra-	

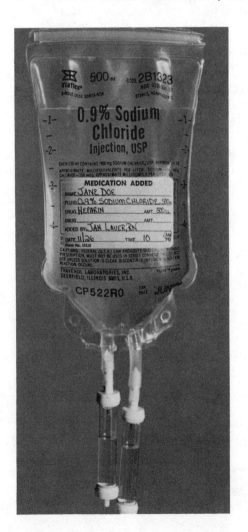

Figure 44. Multiple pressure monitoring using one flush/continuous infusion for two pressures.

ACTION	RATIONALE

flows, high pressure tubings, and transducers.

A. Attach stopcock to patient port of intraflow; close stopcock to intraflow.

B. Connect prepared intraflow to high pressure tubing at transducer port of intraflow.

C. Attach IV administration tubing to long line port of intraflow.

D. Connect male end of high pressure tubing from each prepared system to side ports of manifold.

E. Attach 10-ml. sterile syringe to middle port of manifold.

F. Open manifold stopcocks to syringe and one preassembled system at side port of manifold.

G. Open IV clamp; flush preassembled system free from all air by pulling on intraflow flush line extension (red tail).

H. Observe and control filling of syringe.

I. Check that all air has been removed from system: IV tubing, intraflow, and high pressure tubing.

      I. This ensures accurate pressure determinations and reduces risk of air emboli.

J. Close manifold stopcock to primed system; prepare to prime transducer.

      J. The closed system approach reduces the risk of contamination and infection.

K. Connect three-way stopcock to exposed port of each transducer dome; open stopcock to transducer and air.

L. Open manifold stopcocks from syringe to transducer.

M. Flush transducer using prefilled syringe; check that all air bubbles have been eliminated from dome.

N. Close transducer stopcock to

ACTION	RATIONALE
air; close manifold stopcock to transducer.	
O. Repeat steps A through N for each pressure system.	
7. Balance each transducer.	
A. Select appropriate ranges on monitor pressure module for each system.	
B. Close manifold stopcocks to syringe and patient system.	
C. Open transducer stopcock to transducer and air.	
D. Balance to zero reading according to manufacturer's instructions.	D. Transducer must be adjusted to a zero reading at room temperature for proper balancing.
E. Proceed with calibration, or leave open to air if transducer will not be connected directly to patient for an indefinite time, or close transducer stopcock to air and open manifold stopcocks to transducer and patient systems for use.	E. Leaving the transducer open to air while waiting for an indefinite time prevents pressure build-up and inaccurate readings.
8. Calibrate each transducer.	8. This involves checking the output of the transducer against a known value; not all transducers require calibration.
A. Balance to zero.	
B. Adjust calibration dial to correct number that has been pre-assigned for selected ranges.	
C. Close transducer stopcock to air.	
D. Open manifold stopcocks to transducer and patient system.	
9. Cover all open ports of the intraflows and stopcocks with sterile caps.	9. This reduces the risk of infection.
10. Rebalance and recalibrate 30 minutes after connecting multiple pressure systems to the patient and leveling to right atrial position.	10. This ensures proper calibration.

Single Pressure System with Separate Transducers

1. Although this method increases the

ACTION	RATIONALE

amount of bedside equipment, it is useful for staff competent in the use of the single pressure monitoring system. Follow all steps in the method for the "Single Pressure Transducer System" for multiple pressures desired.

Single Pressure System with One Transducer for Two Pressures

1. This method modifies the single pressure system by using one transducer for two pressures. Follow all steps in the method for the "Single Pressure Transducer System" with the following exceptions:

    A. Prepare second pressure system by connecting IV administration set into medication port of heparinized normal saline IV solution. Attach IV administration tubing to long line port of intraflow. Connect stopcock to patient port of intraflow and close stopcock to intraflow. Connect high pressure tubing to transducer port of intraflow. Prime system.

    B. Connect primed system to a prebalanced and precalibrated single pressure transducer system set-up by attaching the high pressure tubing to the 90° angle stopcock port on the transducer dome.

    C. Obtain pressure readings by turning the stopcocks on the transducer dome to "on" position for one line and "off" to the other; then reverse to obtain the second pressure reading.

    D. Ascertain that the stopcock is turned to the "on" position for the pressure to be monitored continuously; the second pres-

1. One pressure can be monitored continuously while the other is monitored intermittently.

ACTION	RATIONALE

sure can only be read by turning off one pressure intermittently while reading the second
pressure.

PRECAUTIONS

1. Maintain sterile technique throughout preparation of system.
2. Disconnect transducer from patient during defibrillation or cardiover-
    sion to prevent damage to the transducer.
3. Check for accurate readings; rebalance and recalibrate as necessary. Be
    sure that fluid-air interface is at the level of the patient's right atrium
    during pressure system connection.
4. Check that all connections are secure and dome is free from cracks.
5. Ascertain that all stopcocks are in the proper position.
6. Free all tubing and cables from potential pressure or kinking points.
7. Respect electrical safety guidelines for invasive monitoring; see the
    method for "Safety."
8. Maintain 300 mm. Hg pressure in inflatable pressure cuff during pres-
    sure monitoring.
9. Set alarm limits.
10. Control for artifact by minimizing the number of electrical items in use,
    patient movement, and/or faulty transducers. Transducers that have
    been dropped, cleaned improperly, and/or exposed to even minimal
    diaphragm surface scratching are potential sources of erroneous read-
    ings or equipment artifact.

RELATED CARE

1. Follow disposable dome package instructions; some domes do not re-
    quire the use of sterile water during preparation.
2. Flush system manually during transient blood pressure elevations.
3. Check trace position or correct range pressure curve when pressure curve
    is positioned off the oscilloscope.
4. Change multiple pressure system every 24 hours.

COMPLICATIONS

Hemorrhage	Air emboli	Electromicroshock
Sepsis	Tubing separation	Equipment mal- function

REFERENCES

Hewlett Packard Company: Guide to Physiological Pressure Monitoring. Waltham, Mass., Hewlett Packard, 1977, pp. 45–63.

Horovitz, J.L., and Leterman, A.: Postoperative monitoring following critical trauma. Heart Lung, *4*:270, 1975.

Schroeder, J.S., and Daily, E.K.: Techniques in Bedside Hemodynamic Monitoring. St. Louis, C. V. Mosby, 1976, pp. 79–87.

CENTRAL VENOUS PRESSURE

OBJECTIVES

1. To obtain intermittent or continuous central venous pressure (CVP) to assist in assessing the hemodynamic profile and/or clinical evaluation of a patient.
2. To assess fluid replacement for select patients, such as the postoperative patient, the patient who is actively bleeding, or the patient in whom volume status is questioned.
3. To obtain frequent blood samples without discomfort to the patient.

SPECIAL EQUIPMENT

For Continuous Pressure Monitoring
   Single or multiple pressure transducer system set-up
   ECG and pressure monitor and recorder
   Central venous line
   One 10-ml. sterile syringe
For Intermittent Readings with a Water Manometer
   CVP manometer
   Three-way stopcock
   Central venous catheter
   IV solution (as prescribed)
   IV administration set

METHOD

ACTION	RATIONALE
For Continuous Pressure Monitoring 1. Prepare a pressurized monitoring system. See the methods for the "Single Pressure Transducer	

ACTION	RATIONALE

System" or "Multiple Pressure Transducer System."

2. Connect pressure monitoring system to indwelling CVP catheter.
   A. Attach CVP catheter to intraflow stopcock; close stopcock to intraflow and CVP catheter.
   B. Attach syringe to intraflow stopcock; open stopcock to CVP catheter and syringe. Aspirate CVP catheter until blood returns into syringe; reinfuse.
   C. Open intraflow stopcock to intraflow and syringe; pull intraflow flush line extension until blood is removed from stopcock.
   D. Open stopcock to intraflow and CVP catheter; flush using intraflow flush line extension.

3. Level the air-fluid interface of the transducer with the patient's right atrium.
   A. Use the 90° angle port of the transducer dome stopcock as the air-fluid interface.
   B. Use midaxillary line, fourth intercostal space, as a landmark for the patient's right atrium.

3. Pressures reflect pressure changes or a movable diaphragm through a fluid-filled column. A transducer lower than heart level will reflect false high pressures because of hydrostatic and gravitational forces. Conversely, a transducer higher than heart level heart will reflect a false low pressure.

4. Rebalance and recalibrate the transducer (see the methods for the "Single Pressure Transducer System" or "Multiple Pressure Transducer System").

4. Variations in room temperature and withdrawal of blood may cause the transducer to drift; recalibration will ensure accuracy.

5. Monitor CVP pressure.
   A. Place monitor pressure selector on "venous."
   B. Check wave form (Fig. 45). CVP or right atrial (RA) wave forms show an *a, c,* and *v* wave with an *x* and *y* descent. Atrial contraction produces the *a* wave. Closing of the tricuspid valve produces the *c* wave.

ACTION   **RATIONALE**

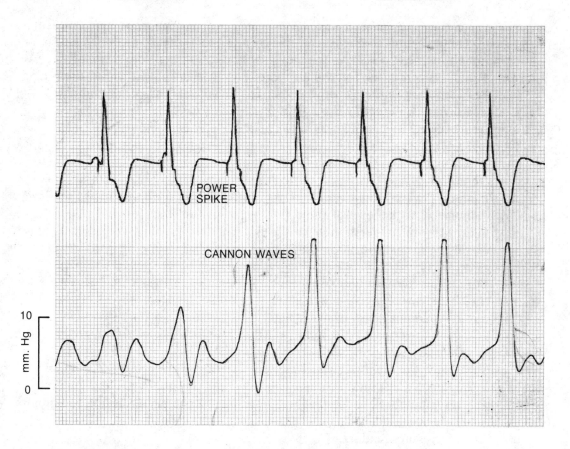

Figure 45. Central venous pressure; normal is 1 to 6 mm. Hg. The wave forms are delayed from the electrodynamic components due to the time factor when recording pressure events through a long catheter.
Note: Cannon waves occur as a result of atrial contraction against a closed tricuspid valve.

Pressure changes in the RA produce the *v* wave. Normal valve for CVP is 1 to 6 mm. Hg.

For Intermittent Readings with a Water Manometer

1. Prepare CVP equipment.
    A. Connect IV administration set to prescribed IV solution. Normal saline solutions are recommended; however, these may be contraindicated in certain patients.
    B. Connect CVP manometer to IV solution administration set.
    C. Use a connecting tubing be-   C. This may be necessary for ease

ACTION	RATIONALE
tween the CVP catheter and CVP manometer tubing (optional).	of patient movement, measurement, etc.
D. Prime system; check that all air has been removed.	D. Air entrapped within the tubing poses a risk of air emboli.
2. Connect air-free CVP catheter to prepared system.	
3. Obtain CVP reading.	
A. Check patency of CVP catheter.	
B. Position the zero line of the manometer at the level of the midaxillary line, fourth intercostal space; mark location on skin.	B. This best approximates the level of the RA.
C. Fill manometer (see Fig. 46).	
(1) Turn three-way stopcock on manometer on to manometer and IV administration set.	
(2) Allow the manometer to fill with IV solution to approximately 10 to 20 cm. H$_2$O above the anticipated pressure reading.	(2) Preventing the manometer from overfilling minimizes the possibility of contamination.

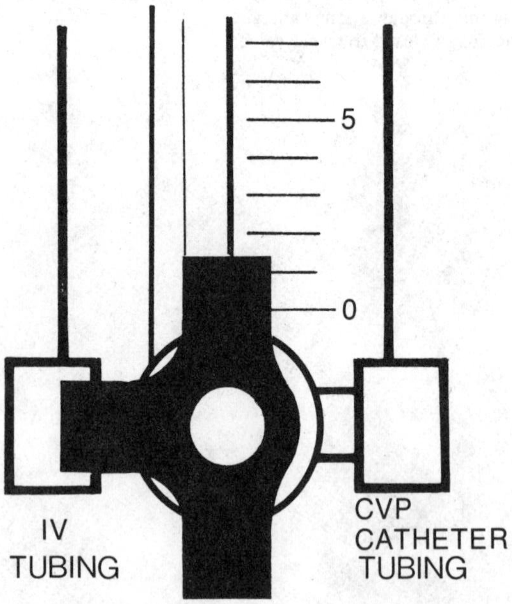

Figure 46. Position for filling CVP manometer.

ACTION

RATIONALE

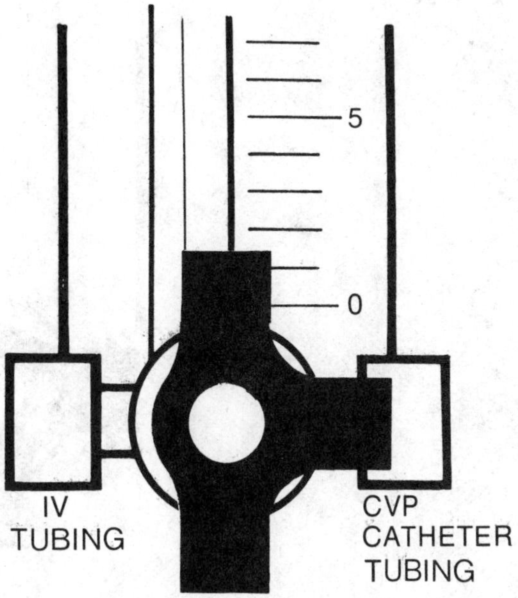

D. Establish fluid flow for CVP (Fig. 47).
  (1) Turn three-way stopcock on manometer on to manometer and CVP catheter.

Figure 47. Position for CVP measurement.

  (2) Observe the falling fluid column in the manometer; check for respiratory fluctuations in the fluid column.

  (2) For accuracy, there must be a free fall of fluid, pulsations with each heartbeat, and fluctuation of approximately 1 cm. H_2O with each respiration. Respiratory fluctuations reflect changes in intrathoracic pressures during the respiratory cycle.

E. Identify CVP measurement when the fluid level stops falling. Normal value of CVP is 3 to 15 cm. H_2O.

4. Resume IV infusion to patient; check for prescribed infusion rate and CVP line patency (Fig. 48).

PRECAUTIONS

1. Maintain patency of CVP line; aspirate before irrigating.
2. Monitor CVP line for absence of air and/or clots, and check that all connections are secure.
3. See also the precautions for the "Single Pressure Transducer System" or "Multiple Pressure Transducer System Set-Up."

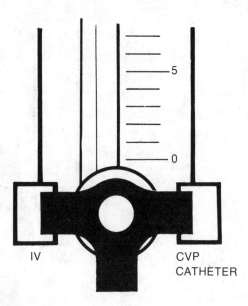

5

0

IV   CVP
                      CATHETER

Figure 48.   Position for IV fluid administration.

RELATED CARE

1. Facilitate preinsertion responsibilities.
    A. Maintain aseptic technique.
    B. Place patient in Trendelenburg position during subclavian CVP insertion approach to prevent air emboli and facilitate gravitational filling of vessel.
    C. Choose proper length of catheter, depending upon insertion site.
2. Facilitate postinsertion responsibilities.
    A. Order chest x-ray to confirm catheter position and to rule out a pneumothorax.
    B. Perform dressing change and site assessment. (See the method for "Invasive Site Care—Long Venous and Arterial Indwelling Catheter Site Care," pp. 407–413.)
    C. Obtain CVP measurement from same zero reference point to ensure continuity and validity of data.
    D. Monitor CVP hourly, or as ordered by the physician. Observe for significant changes, CVP line obstruction, or potential sources for emboli.
    E. Change system every 24 hours.
    F. Recheck calibration of the transducer every 4 hours.
    G. See related care for the "Single Pressure Transducer System" or "Multiple Pressure Transducer System."
    H. Respect electrical safety guidelines.

    I.   Maintain continuity in pressure readings and observe changes in pressure trends. Pressures taken with the patient on a ventilator will reflect false high pressure readings due to positive intrathoracic pressures. Read the pressures consistently on or off the ventilator, and document them.

    J.   Observe ECG for right ventricular dysrhythmias or left bundle branch block, indicating CVP catheter positioning in the right ventricle.

3.   Obtain blood samples.

    A.   Attach sterile syringe to CVP stopcock; open to CVP catheter and syringe.

    B.   Aspirate slowly; amount will vary according to length of CVP line.

    C.   Turn stopcock to halfway position to close to all ports; remove syringe and attach syringe for blood sample. Open to CVP catheter and syringe; obtain blood sample. Close to halfway position and remove syringe.

    D.   Connect sterile syringe; open stopcock to syringe and IV fluid administration set. Clear stopcock and port of blood. Open stopcock to IV fluid administration and CVP catheter; resume infusion to clear line.

    E.   Connect protective cap to stopcock; check prescribed fluid rate.

4.   Remove CVP line.

    A.   Expose site; culture as necessary.

    B.   Clean incision with povidone-iodine prep swabs.

    C.   Remove catheter slowly, noting ease of withdrawal and effect on patient.

    D.   Check CVP catheter length; culture tip.

    E.   Apply pressure to site until bleeding is controlled.

    F.   Apply povidone-iodine ointment to site and secure sterile occlusive pressure dressing for 24 hours.

    G.   Observe site for hematoma or delayed bleeding.

    H.   Facilitate suture removal after 72 hours.

COMPLICATIONS

Pulmonary emboli	Nonpatent CVP line
Phlebitis	Fluid overload
Vein trauma	Air emboli
Pneumothorax	Altered skin integrity
Infection (local and/or systemic)	Inaccurate pressures
Malposition of catheter into jugular system	Equipment malfunction
Dysrhythmias	Electromicroshock

REFERENCES

Hewlett Packard Company: Guide to Physiological Monitoring. Waltham, MA., Hewlett Packard, 1977, pp. 24–27.
Schroeder, J.S., and Daily, E.K. Techniques in Bedside Hemodynamic Monitoring. St. Louis, C. V. Mosby, 1976, pp. 65–73.

PULMONARY ARTERY PRESSURE _____

OBJECTIVES

1. To assess the left ventricular end-diastolic pressure indirectly when mitral valve function is normal.
2. To determine precisely the hemodynamic response of the patient to fluid therapy, medication, or other treatment.
3. To obtain accurate central vascular pressures in the presence of low cardiac output.
4. To obtain mixed venous blood samples.
5. To measure cardiac output directly or indirectly.

SPECIAL EQUIPMENT

Single or Multiple pressure transducer system monitor
Recorder
Pulmonary artery catheter (single lumen, double lumen, triple lumen, quadruple lumen)
10-ml. syringe
1-ml. syringe
Sterile basin containing normal saline solution.
Fluoroscopy table and equipment, if ordered
Defibrillator
Emergency cart and medications
Povidone-iodine ointment
Sterile occlusive dressing
Sterile gauze pads
Pressure dressing

METHOD

ACTION	RATIONALE
1. Obtain vital signs and ECG recording.	1. These serve as baseline data.

ACTION	RATIONALE
2. Check security and position of ECG electrodes.	
3. Prepare a pressurized monitoring system. See the methods for the "Single Pressure Transducer System" or "Multiple Pressure Transducer System."	
A. Balance transducer.	
B. Calibrate.	
4. Level air-fluid interface of the transducer with the patient's right atrium.	4. Pressures reflect pressure changes or a movable diaphragm through a fluid-filled column. A transducer lower than heart level will reflect false high pressures with the addition of hydrostatic and gravitational forces. Conversely, a transducer higher than heart level reflects false low pressures.
A. Use 90° angle port of the transducer dome stopcock as the air-fluid interface.	
B. Use midaxillary line, fourth intercostal space, as a landmark for the patient's right atrium.	
5. Monitor patient's response during PA catheter insertion.	
A. Perform site care; drape.	
B. Test PA catheter balloon for air leaks by submerging into a sterile basin of normal saline solution while inflating the balloon with 1.0 to 1.5 ml. of air.	
C. Attach a primed and calibrated monitoring system to PA and RA ports; prime catheter lumens.	
D. Antecubital site is anesthetized and cutdown is performed by physician. PA catheter is advanced until the RA wave form appears on the monitor.	
(1) Instruct patient to cough; observe wave form for RA pressure and fluctuation.	(1) Coughing produces fluctuation in RA wave.

ACTION	RATIONALE
(2) Inflate PA balloon with 1.0 ml. of air to enhance passage to PA.	
(a) Observe ECG for PVC's during RV passage.	(a) Ventricular irritability may occur during catheter passage.
(b) Ready lidocaine bolus.	
E. Observe wave forms; record pressures:	
(1) Right atrial pressure (RAP) (Fig. 49). RAP has *a, c,* and *v* waves and an *x* and *y* descent. The *a* wave represents atrial systole; the *c* wave represents closure of the semilunar valve; the *v* wave represents ventricular systole. The *x* descent follows atrial systole; the *y* descent represents A-V opening.	(1) Elevated $\overline{RAP}$ may indicate volume overload, RV failure, tricuspid stenosis or regurgitation, pulmonary hypertension, LV failure, or constrictive pericarditis.

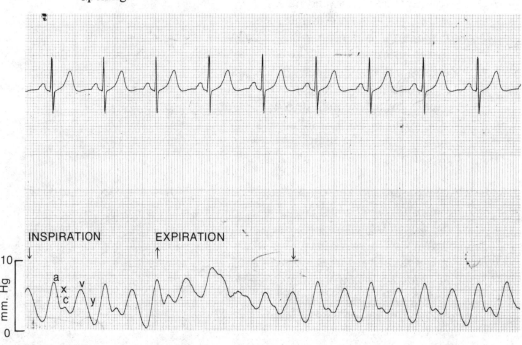

Figure 49.   Right atrial pressure; normal RAP = 1 to 6 mm. Hg. The wave forms are delayed from the electrodynamic components due to the time factor when recording pressure events through a long catheter.

ACTION

RATIONALE

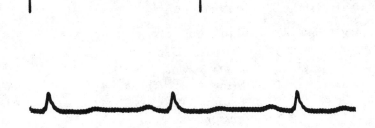

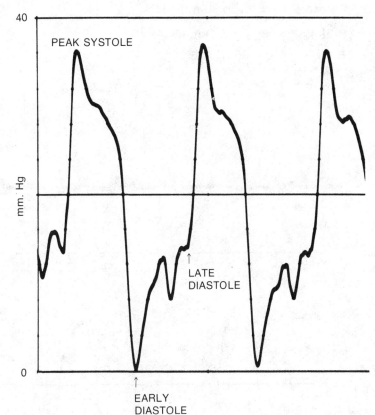

Figure 50. Right ventricular pressure; normal RAP = (20-30)/(0-5) mm. Hg. The wave forms are delayed from electrodynamic components due to the time factor when recording pressure events through a long catheter.

$\overline{\text{RAP}}$ = 1 to 6 mm. Hg

(2) Right ventricular pressure (RVP) (Fig. 50). RVP has three components: peak systolic pressure, early diastole, and late diastole. Ventricular end-diastolic pressure is read in late diastole.

(2) Elevated RVP may indicate pulmonary hypertension, RV failure, constrictive pericarditis, chronic congestive heart failure, ventricular septal defect or hypoxemia.

ACTION	RATIONALE

RVP systolic = 20 to 30 mm. Hg

RVP diastolic = 0 to 5 mm. Hg

(3) Pulmonary artery pressure (PAP) (Fig. 51). PAP has three features: peak systolic pressure, dicrotic notch (pulmonary valve closure), and diastole.

(3) Elevated PAP may indicate left-to-right shunt, LV failure, mitral stenosis or pulmonary hypertension.

PAP systolic   = 20 to 30 mm. Hg

PAP diastole = 0 to 10 mm. Hg

$\overline{\text{PAP}}$ = 20 mm. Hg

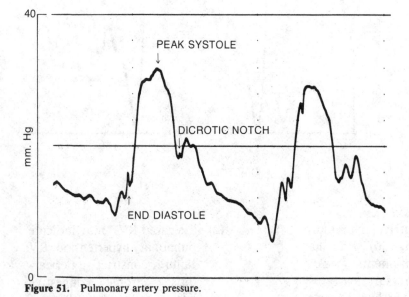

Figure 51.   Pulmonary artery pressure.

$$\frac{\text{Normal}}{\text{PAP}} = \frac{\text{PAP}}{20 \text{ mm. Hg}} = \frac{20\text{-}30}{0\text{-}10} \text{ mm. Hg}$$

The wave forms are delayed from electrodynamic components due to the time factor when recording pressure events through a long catheter.

ACTION	RATIONALE
(4) Pulmonary artery wedge pressure (PAWP) (Fig. 52). $\overline{PAWP}$ has an *a, c,* and *v* wave. The *a* wave occurs during atrial systole; it is absent in atrial fibrillation. The *c* wave represents close of the A-V valves. The *v* wave is high during systolic regurgitation.	(4) Elevated $\overline{PAWP}$ may indicate LV failure, mitral insufficiency, or mitral stenosis.

$\overline{PAWP}$ = 4 to 12 mm. Hg

F. Deflate balloon by removing syringe from balloon stopcock; allow balloon to deflate passively. Ensure deflation by proper PA tracing.	F. Aspirating balloon manually may cause premature balloon rupture. A balloon left inflated can cause pressure ischemia and necrosis of segments of the PA.

6. Wedge balloon.
    A. Rebalance and recalibrate transducer.
    B. Ascertain that balloon is deflated.

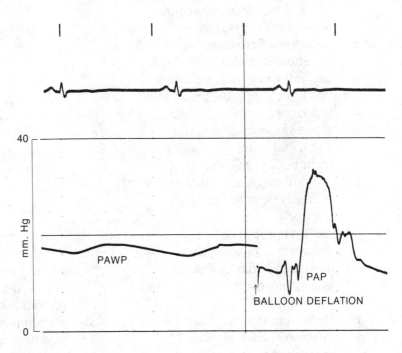

Figure 52. Pulmonary artery wedge pressure.

ACTION	RATIONALE
C. Inflate slowly with 0.8 to 1.5 ml. air; make sure that wedge is tracing on recorder.	C. Inflate slowly to prevent over-inflation or balloon rupture.
D. Deflate balloon; leave syringe in place.	
7. Obtain blood sample of mixed venous blood by aspirating from distal port with balloon deflated.	7. Balloon must be deflated; aspiration with balloon inflated may cause sample to become partially contaminated with arterial blood, and not be a mixed venous sample.
A. Attach a 10-ml. sterile syringe to intraflow stopcock.	
B. Open intraflow stopcock to syringe and distal port; aspirate to clear line and ascertain purity of sample.	B. Amount of blood aspirated will vary due to tubing and catheter length. It is critical to obtain a pure sample.
C. Close stopcock to the halfway position; remove syringe and maintain sterile technique.	
D. Attach blood sample syringe to intraflow stopcock; open intraflow stopcock to syringe and distal port; aspirate blood sample.	
E. Turn intraflow stopcock to halfway position and remove blood sample syringe.	
F. Attach sterile syringe; open intraflow stopcock to syringe and intraflow; pull intraflow flush line extension until blood is removed from stopcock.	
G. Open stopcock to intraflow and distal port; flush using intraflow flush line extension.	
H. Discard syringe; replace sterile protective cap to intraflow stopcock.	
8. Monitor PAP and PWP.	
A. Integrate data with hemodynamic profile and clinical assessment of patient.	A. Insolated and absolute levels are not as important as *trend alterations* and the *effects of these alterations on the patient.*
B. Make sure that no other IV infusion is administered through the PA line.	B. Pulmonary extravasation is a potential risk.

ACTION	RATIONALE
C. Obtain chest x-ray to ascertain catheter position.	
D. Assess circulation to extremity.	
9. Prepare for removal of PA line.	
A. Close intraflow stopcocks to patient on all ports; open transducer stopcock to air; disconnect transducer from monitor.	A. These safety measures to protect the patient and transducer.
B. Assess circulation to extremity prior to removal.	
C. Obtain vital signs.	C. These serve as baseline data.
D. Monitor patient while physician removes catheter.	
(1) Observe for dysrhythmias.	
(2) Anticipate that balloon will be inflated with approximately 0.3 to 0.5 ml. of air until the catheter has been withdrawn to the RA position.	(2) This prevents ventricular trauma to the chordae tendineae and valves.
E. Apply firm pressure until bleeding stops; apply povidone-iodine ointment and sterile occlusive dressing.	
F. Perform circulation assessment to extremity and site inspection every 5 minutes times 2; then every 15 minutes times 2; remove pressure dressing in 8 hours postbleeding at site.	

PRECAUTIONS

1. See also the precautions for the "Single Pressure Transducer System" or "Multiple Pressure Transducer System."
2. Set alarms at all times, approximately 20 mm. above and below the pressure readings.
3. Monitor entire system for absence of air and/or clots and check security of all connections.
4. Observe PAP wave form for potential of catheter slipping into RV. Notify physician *immediately* due to risk of ventricular irritability and/or trauma.
5. Check for catheter wedge position. Move the patient's arm, have patient cough and deep breathe, and reposition patient. Notify the physician *immediately* if unable to dislodge a wedged catheter.

6. Use PAP line with caution for obtaining blood samples; monitor IV infusions, since pulmonary extravasation is a potential risk.
7. Ready defibrillator, emergency cart, and medications during insertion and removal of catheter.
8. Respect electrical safety guidelines.

RELATED CARE

1. Record pressures hourly or as ordered by the physician; monitor continuously. Observe for significant changes or potential sources of emboli.
2. Perform site care. See the method for "Invasive Site Care—Long Venous and Arterial Indwelling Catheter Site Care."
3. Change pressure transducer system every 24 hours.
4. Recheck calibration every 4 hours.
5. See related care for the "Single Pressure Transducer System" or "Multiple Pressure Transducer System."
6. Assess circulation to extremity every 2 to 4 hours.
7. Monitor PAWP every 2 to 4 hours; check integrity of balloon by using correct amount of air for balloon inflation and feeling for resistance during inflation. Keep syringe attached to catheter with correct amount of air.

COMPLICATIONS

Air emboli
Thromboembolism
Cardiac arrest
Dysrhythmias
Catheter displacement/dislodgment
Infection
Electromicroshock
Altered skin integrity
Inaccurate pressures
Equipment malfunction
Hemothorax

Cardiac tamponade
Loss of balloon integrity
Balloon rupture
Lung ischemia
Pulmonary artery rupture
Pulmonary extravasation, hemorrhage, or infarction
Altered circulation to extremities
Frank hemorrhage
Altered hemodynamics

SUPPLIERS OF PULMONARY ARTERY CATHETERS

American Catheter Company
Electrocatheter Company
Swan Ganz—Edwards Laboratories

REFERENCES

Hewlett Packard Company: Guide to Physiological Monitoring. Waltham, MA., Hewlett Packard, 1977, pp. 28–34.

Schroeder, J.S., and Daily, E.K.: Techniques in Bedside Hemodynamic Monitoring. St. Louis, C. V. Mosby, 1976, pp. 73–90.

ARTERIAL PRESSURE

OBJECTIVES

1. To provide accurate, continuous, and objective data regarding a patient's altered hemodynamic status due to *high risk* for dysrhythmias, excessive vasoconstriction, low cardiac output, and/or unstable condition.
2. To obtain continuous blood pressure readings during the administration of potent vasoactive and vasodilating medications so as to measure the trends and effects of therapeutic interventions.
3. To obtain frequent blood gas determinations without discomfort to the patient and without disturbing the steady state.

SPECIAL EQUIPMENT

Single or multiple pressure transducer system
ECG and pressure monitor and recorder
Arterial line
10-ml. sterile syringe

METHOD

ACTION	RATIONALE
1. Prepare a pressurized monitoring system. See the methods for the "Single Pressure Transducer System" or "Multiple Pressure Transducer System."	
2. Connect pressure monitoring system to indwelling arterial line.	
A. Attach arterial line to intraflow stopcock; close stopcock to intraflow and arterial line.	

ACTION	RATIONALE
B. Attach syringe to intraflow stopcock; open stopcock to arterial line and syringe. Aspirate arterial line until blood returns into syringe; reinfuse.	
C. Open intraflow stopcock to intraflow and syringe; pull intraflow flush line extension until blood is removed from stopcock.	
D. Open stopcock to intraflow and arterial line; flush using intraflow flush line extension.	
3. Level the air-fluid interface of the transducer with the patient's right atrium.	3. Pressures reflect pressure changes on a movable diaphragm through a fluid-filled column. A transducer lower than heart level will reflect false high pressures with the addition of hydrostatic and gravitational forces. Conversely, a transducer higher than heart level will reflect false low pressures.
A. Use the 90° angle port of the transducer dome stopcock as the air-fluid interface.	
B. Use midaxillary line, fourth intercostal space, as a landmark for the patient's right atrium.	
4. Rebalance and recalibrate the transducer. (See the methods for the "Single Pressure Transducer System" or "Multiple Pressure Transducer System.")	4. Variations in room temperature and withdrawal of blood may cause the transducer to drift; recalibration will ensure accuracy.
5. Monitor arterial pressure.	
A. Place monitor pressure selector on "systolic," "diastolic," or "mean"; read meter or digital display reading.	A. Changes in systolic, diastolic, and/or mean arterial pressures require select assessment respective of trending and effect on patient.
B. Check wave form (Fig. 53). Appearance of the arterial wave form is important data. Normal arterial pressure is 120/80, with a mean of 83 mm. Hg.	B. Location of the dicrotic notch should be one-third or greater the height of the systolic peak or suspect reduced cardiac output. A delay in the rapid rising anacrotic limb suggests a de-

ACTION

RATIONALE

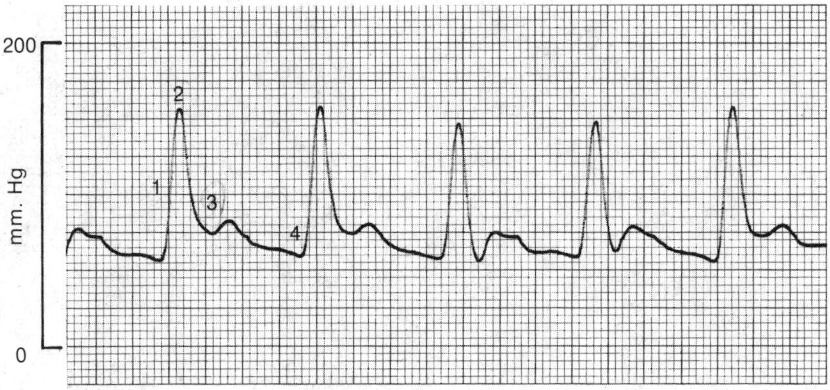

Figure 53. Arterial pressure tracing. *1,* Anacrotic limb; *2,* systolic peak; *3,* dicrotic notch (Note: low due to hypovolemic status); *4,* diastolic pressure.

crease in myocardial contractility, aortic stenosis, or dampened pressure movement secondary to catheter position or clot formation.

C. Check wave form for various physiologic effects (Fig. 54).

C. Variations in arterial curves are due to increases in tachypnea, hypotension, and/or irregular ventricular rates such as atrial fibrillation or PVC's.

D. Notify the physician of significant pressure changes.

E. Maintain patency of arterial line; control infusion rate of 3 to 4 ml. per hour.

E. This prevents the potential of emboli.

F. Integrate arterial pressure data with hemodynamic profile and clinical assessment of patient.

F. Isolated and absolute values are not as important as *trend alterations* and the *effects of these alterations on the patient.*

6. Obtain a blood sample.
   A. Attach 10-ml. sterile syringe to intraflow stopcock.
   B. Open intraflow stopcock to syringe and arterial catheter; aspirate to clear the line and check for purity of arterial sample.

B. Amount of blood aspirated will vary due to tubing and catheter length. It is critical to obtain a *pure* sample.

   C. Close stopcock to the halfway position; remove syringe and maintain sterile technique.
   D. Attach blood sample syringe to

ACTION   **RATIONALE**

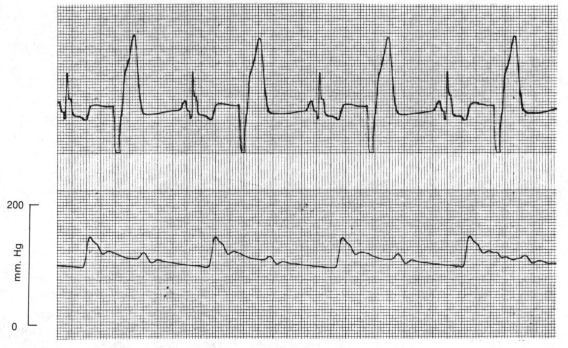

Figure 54. Arterial pressure tracing showing effect of bigeminy PVC's.

intraflow stopcock; open intraflow stopcock to syringe and arterial catheter; aspirate blood sample.

E. Turn intraflow stopcock to halfway position and remove arterial blood sample syringe.

F. Eject all air bubbles from arterial blood sample, cap immediately, and put on ice.

G. Attach sterile syringe; open intraflow stopcock to syringe and intraflow; pull intraflow flush line extension until blood is removed from stopcock and port.

H. Open stopcock to intraflow and arterial line; flush using intraflow flush line extension.

I. Discard syringe; replace sterile protective cap to intraflow stopcock.

7. Prepare for removal of arterial line.

A. Close intraflow stopcock to pa-

E. To prevent loss of blood from the system, the stopcock should be in a halfway position.

A. These are safety measures

ACTION	RATIONALE
tient; open transducer stopcock to air; disconnect transducer from monitor.	to protect the patient and transducer.
B. Expose arterial line site.	
C. Gently remove catheter from artery and place sterile gauze pads over the insertion site; apply direct pressure for a minimum of 5 minutes or until bleeding stops.	C. Direct pressure assists in sealing the puncture site; heparinized solution decreases clotting ability.
D. Apply povidone-iodine ointment, sterile gauze pads, and pressure dressing.	
E. Assess circulation to extremity.	
F. Assess circulation and dressing every 5 minutes times 2; then every 15 minutes times 2; remove pressure dressing in 8 hours postbleeding at site.	

PRECAUTIONS

1. See the precautions for the "Single Pressure Transducer System" or "Multiple Pressure Transducer System."
2. Set alarms at all times, approximately 20 mm. above and below the pressure readings.
3. Monitor arterial line for absence of air and/or clots and check security of all connections.
4. Maintain patency of arterial line; flush arterial lines after blood samples are drawn or tracing becomes dampened. Avoid excessive pressure when flushing or withdrawing samples from line; this prevents arteriospasms. If tracing dampens more often than every 30 minutes, suspect clotting and notify physician. Correct dampened pressure tracing by repositioning catheter, straightening extremity, and/or aspirating with a syringe; flush line slowly with heparinized saline solution.
5. Perform the Allen test prior to arterial line insertion.
6. Respect electrical safety guidelines.

RELATED CARE

1. Monitor arterial pressure hourly or as ordered by the physician. Observe for significant changes or potential sources of emboli.
2. Perform arterial line site care. See the method for "Invasive Site Care—Long Venous and Arterial Indwelling Catheter Site Care."

3. Change pressure transducer system set-up every 24 hours.
4. Recheck calibration every 4 hours.
5. See related care for the "Single Pressure Transducer System" or "Multiple Pressure Transducer System."
6. Assess circulation to extremity every 2 to 4 hours.

COMPLICATIONS

Air emboli
Thromboembolism
Altered hemodynamics
Dysrhythmias
Catheter displacement/
    dislodgment
Infection

Electromicroshock
Altered skin integrity
Inaccurate pressures
Equipment malfunction
Frank hemorrhage
Impaired circulation to extremities

REFERENCES

Hewlett Packard Company: Guide to Physiological Pressure Monitoring. Waltham, MA., Hewlett Packard, 1977, pp. 17–24.
Horovitz, J.L., and Leterman, A.: Postoperative monitoring following critical trauma. Heart Lung, 4:270, 1975.

LEFT ATRIAL PRESSURE

OBJECTIVES

1. To determine the left ventricular-end diastolic pressures indirectly when mitral valve function is normal.
2. To determine precisely the hemodynamic response of the central vascular system to fluid therapy, medication, or other treatment.
3. To obtain accurate and continuous central vascular pressures in the presence of low cardiac output.

SPECIAL EQUIPMENT

Single or multiple pressure transducer system
Monitor
Recorder
Left atrial line
Air filter
10-ml. sterile syringe

METHOD

ACTION	RATIONALE

1. Prepare a pressurized monitoring system with an air filter.
   A. Select the method for a "Single Pressure Transducer System" or "Multiple Pressure Transducer System."
   B. Attach air filter to pressurized monitoring line.
   C. Prime air filter using intraflow flush line extension (red tail).
   D. Check that entire pressure transducer system and line with air filter is free from air.
	
	 D. LA line offers a high risk for air emboli.

2. Connect pressure monitoring system to patient.
   A. Attach LA line to intraflow stopcock; close stopcock to intraflow and LA line.
   B. Attach syringe to intraflow stopcock; open stopcock to LA line and syringe. Aspirate LA line until blood returns into syringe; reinfuse.
   C. Open intraflow stopcock to intraflow and syringe; pull intraflow flush line extension until blood is removed from stopcock.
   D. Open stopcock to intraflow and LA line; flush using intraflow flush line extension.	

3. Level the air fluid interface of the transducer with the patient's right atrium.
   A. Use the 90° angle port of the transducer dome stopcock as the air-fluid interface.
   B. Use midaxillary line, fourth intercostal space, as a landmark for patient's right atrium.
	3. Pressures reflect pressure changes on a movable diaphragm through a fluid-filled column. A transducer lower than heart level will reflect false high pressures with the addition of hydrostatic and gravitational forces. Conversely, a transducer higher than the heart level reflects false low pressures.

4. Rebalance and recalibrate the transducer. (See the method for the	4. Variations in room temperature and withdrawal of blood may cause the

ACTION	**RATIONALE**
"Single Pressure Transducer System" or "Multiple Pressure Transducer System.")	transducer to drift; recalibration will ensure accuracy.
5. Monitor left atrial pressure (LAP).	
A. Place monitor pressure selector on "mean."	A. Pressure changes between systolic and diastolic are insignificant.
B. Check wave form and LAP (Fig. 55). Normal $\overline{LAP}$ is 4 to 12 mm. Hg.	B. Appearance of wave form is important in assessing left ventricular function and accuracy of displayed pressures. $\overline{LAP}$ is increased in pulmonary edema, left ventricular failure, mitral stenosis, and mitral insufficiency.

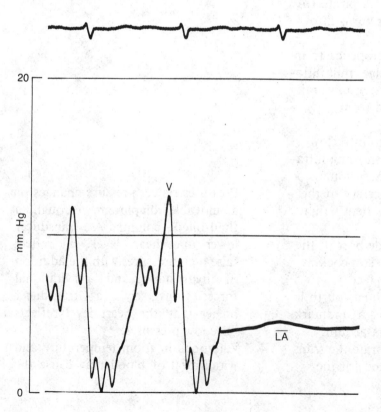

Figure 55. Left atrial pressure. The wave forms are delayed from the electrodynamic components due to the time factor when recording pressure events through a long catheter. Note the absence of a wave due to atrial fibrillation.

ACTION	RATIONALE
C. Notify the physician of significant pressure changes.	
D. Maintain patency of LA line; control infusion rate of 3 to 4 ml. per hour.	D. This prevents the potential of emboli.
E. Be sure that no other IV infusion is administered through LA line.	E. Constant entering of the closed system increases risk for air emboli and/or infection.
F. Integrate LAP data with hemodynamic profile and clinical assessment of the patient.	F. Isolated and absolute levels are not as important as *trend alterations* and the *effects of these alterations* on the patient.

6. Prepare for removal of LA line.

ACTION	RATIONALE
A. Close intraflow stopcock to patient; open transducer stopcock to air; disconnect transducer from monitor.	A. These safety measures protect the patient and transducer.
B. Don sterile gloves.	B. This reduces the risks of electro-microshock and infection.
C. Expose LA line site.	
D. Assess patient as physician removes LA line.	
E. Perform site care.	
F. Observe for increased bloody drainage at site and/or through chest tubes.	F. Cardiac tamponade is a potential complication.
G. Obtain chest x-ray 1 hour post-removal of LA line.	G. This measure assists in ruling out hemothorax or cardiac tamponade. In the absence of bleeding, the chest tube may be removed.

PRECAUTIONS

1. Maintain patency of LA line; do not irrigate or flush LA line manually.
2. Notify physician immediately if the system is nonfunctional or a good wave form is not obtained; anticipate removal of LA line.
3. Monitor LA line for absence of air and/or clots, and check security of all connections.
4. Use an air filter close to LA catheter insertion site to minimize the potential for air emboli.
5. See also the precautions for the "Single Pressure Transducer System" or "Multiple Pressure Transducer System."
6. Respect electrical safety guidelines.

RELATED CARE

1. Monitor the $\overline{\text{LAP}}$ hourly, or as ordered by the physician. Observe for significant changes, LA line obstruction, or potential sources for air emboli.
2. Perform LA line insertion site care. See the method for "Invasive Site Care—Long Venous and Arterial Indwelling Catheter Site Care."
3. Change pressure transducer system set-up every 24 hours.
4. Recheck calibration every 4 hours.
5. See related care for the "Single Pressure Transducer System" or "Multiple Pressure Transducer System."

COMPLICATIONS

Air emboli
Thromboembolism
Cardiac arrest
Dysrhythmias
Catheter displacement/dis-
    lodgment
Infection

Electromicroshock
Altered skin integrity
Inaccurate pressures
Equipment malfunction
Hemothorax
Cardiac tamponade

REFERENCES

Hewlett Packard Company: Guide to Physiological Monitoring. Waltham, MA, Hewlett Packard, 1977, p. 35.
Schroeder, J.S., and Daily, E.K.: Techniques in Bedside Hemodynamic Monitoring. St. Louis, C. V. Mosby, 1976, pp. 6 and 76.

CARDIAC OUTPUT

OBJECTIVES

1. To measure cardiac output indirectly in order to determine overall hemodynamic status and assess patient's response to therapy.
2. To provide data for determining the cardiac index, which is cardiac output per square meter of body surface area.

SPECIAL EQUIPMENT

Fick Method
  Two heparinized syringes
  Douglas bag for collection
    of expired gases

  Volume meter
  Gas analyzer
  Stopwatch

Nose clip
Mouthpiece

Indicator-Dilution Method
Densitometer
Dye injection/flush system
Optical dye
Thermodilution Method
Thermodilution catheter
1-ml. syringe for balloon
inflation
Thermodilution cardiac out-
put computer

Blood oxygen saturation
analyzer
Calculator

Arterial and venous catheter
lines
Recording apparatus

10- ml. sterile syringe
Iced normal saline IV solution
at known temperature
(between 0 and 5°C).

METHOD

ACTION	RATIONALE
1. Monitor patient during cardiac output determination.	
2. Select appropriate method. Normal cardiac output (CO) at rest is 4 to 8 liters per minute. Normal cardiac index (CI) at rest is 2.5 to 4.0 liters /min/m².	
A. Fick method. This method is based upon the principle of oxygen uptake per unit of blood as it flows through the lungs.	A. This method requires a stable patient and is respected for accuracy even in low cardiac output, shunts, or valvular insufficiency.
(1) Collect expired air sample.	
(a) Prepare and assess patient for an airtight system using nose clip, mouthpiece, and Douglas bag.	
(b) Turn three-way stopcock to facilitate expelling expired air while patient breathes with the system for approximately 2 to 5 minutes.	(b) This enhances patient adjustment to the breathing system and primes the total system with the patient's expired air.
(c) Turn three-way stopcock to facilitate collection of expired air	

ACTION	RATIONALE

from the patient into the Douglas bag while simultaneously starting the stopwatch.

    (d) Collect expired air for approximately 2 minutes; then obtain blood samples.

  (1) Collect a 10-ml. pure arterial blood sample slowly from arterial line.

  (2) Collect a 10-ml. pure venous blood sample slowly from pulmonary artery line.

    (e) Continue collection of expired air for 5 to 6 minutes.

    (f) Turn off stopcock to the Douglas bag.

    (g) Record time of collection stopped, using stopwatch.

    (h) Facilitate blood and gas analysis; calculate cardiac output using Fick formula:

(1) Controlled, slow withdrawal is important for a timed study.

(e) This varies with bag size and patient variables.

$$CO \ (ml/min) = \frac{O_2 \text{ consumption (ml/min)}}{\text{arterial } O_2 \text{ content (vol \%)} - \text{venous } O_2 \text{ content (vol \%)}}$$

B. Indicator-dilution method. This method utilizes a time-based dye concentration curve. A select amount of dye indicator is injected into the right atrium and concentrations are measured during arterial blood withdrawal.

  (1) Attach syringe containing known amount of dye to venous catheter.

  (2) Attach precalibrated recording densitometer to arterial catheter.

B. Utilizing a computer, the results are made known immediately. This method is not affected by oxygen administration.

ACTION	RATIONALE
(3) Simultaneously inject dye while steadily withdrawing an arterial sample through the densitometer.	(3) This records time-concentration curve as the dye passes through one circulation.
(4) Observe for dye reaction symptoms.	
(5) Remove syringe; flush IV lines and densitometer system.	(5) This prevents clot formation.
(6) Compute cardiac output from dye concentration curve. (a) Use computer. (b) Calculate mean concentrate in mg./liter.	
C. Thermodilution method. This method records a temperature-time curve.	C. It can be performed rapidly by one person. Inaccuracies may occur in low cardiac output, shunts, or valvular insufficiencies.
(1) Check that thermodilution catheter is positioned properly in the pulmonary artery and that balloon is deflated.	(1) There is a possibility of ventricular dysrhythmias due to current leakage if thermistor probe is in right ventricle and connected to computer.
(2) Attach pretested thermodilution catheter thermistor port to precalibrated thermodilution computer; allow 5 minutes warm-up time for computer (Fig. 56).	

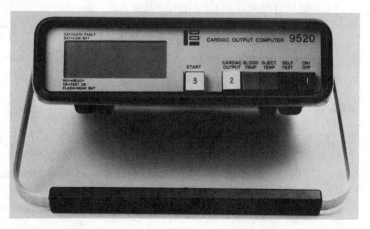

Figure 56. Thermodilution cardiac output computer. Courtesy of Edwards Laboratories.

ACTION	RATIONALE
(3) Take patient's temperature rectally; dial into computer.	
(4) Rapidly inject known quantity of known temperature (cold; temperature of the injectate must be between 0 and 5°C.) sterile normal saline IV solution through proximal port (right atrium) of thermodilution catheter. Follow specific computer instructions.	(4) The injectate must be completely infused within 10 seconds after removal from ice bath so as not to alter temperature. Thermistor located at distal end of catheter reads temperature change in pulmonary artery.
(5) Read cardiac output from computer.	(5) Computer calculates temperature change into cardiac output.
(6) Obtain average of three sequential thermodilution readings. Remove syringe from proximal port of thermal dilution catheter; resume IV infusion.	
(7) Disconnect thermodilution computer.	

3. Check IV infusion rate and assess patient status.

PRECAUTIONS

1. Maintain strict aseptic technique.
2. Follow electrical safety guidelines.
3. Observe for lethal dysrhythmias.
4. Check for proper position of the thermodilution catheter into pulmonary artery before connecting to computer.
5. Also see precautions for "Pulmonary Artery Pressure."

RELATED CARE

1. Fick method:
    A. Assess patient for hyperventilation, which can contribute to a false high reading of the respiratory quotient. Repeat the expired air collection.
    B. Determine if the patient has a health history of perforated ear-

drums, which can contribute to expired air leakage. Cover external auditory canal tightly.

2. Indicator dilution method:
   A. Monitor for variation in results due to dye recirculation, curve interpretation, and/or catheter position.
3. Thermodilution method:
   A. Monitor for curve distortion due to catheter malposition, temperature change of injectate, or time delay in injection technique.
4. Provide defibrillator, emergency cart, and medications for immediate use, as necessary.

COMPLICATIONS

Dysrhythmias	Air emboli
Cardiac arrest	Electrical micro- or macroshock
Dye reaction	Injection
Pulmonary emboli or infarction	Equipment malfunction

REFERENCES

Hewlett Packard Company: Guide to Physiological Pressure Monitoring. Waltham, MA, Hewlett Packard, 1977, pp. 28–34.
Schroeder, J.S., and Daily, E.K.: Techniques in Bedside Hemodynamic Monitoring. St. Louis, C. V. Mosby, 1976, pp. 107–128.

AUTOMATIC BLOOD PRESSURE MONITORING _____

OBJECTIVES

To monitor systolic, diastolic, and mean arterial pressures indirectly and noninvasively by automatic means.

SPECIAL EQUIPMENT

Automatic blood pressure monitoring device (equipment specific to model)

METHOD

ACTION	RATIONALE

1. Prepare automatic blood pressure monitoring equipment.
   A. Place blood pressure device on rigid surface.
   B. Insert plug into proper voltage outlet.
   C. Arrange pneumatic hoses for free air flow and tube patency.	

2. Wrap deflated cuff around selected extremity.	
3. Position patient's extremity at heart level and in such a way that external contact will be avoided.	
4. Turn on automatic blood pressure monitoring equipment; set alarm.	
5. Instruct patient to remain as motionless as possible during blood pressure readings. Cuff inflation will be felt; patient must remain motionless until cuff is deflated and blood pressure values recorded.	5. Excessive motion will cause altered readings.

PRECAUTIONS

1. Avoid attaching the blood pressure cuffs to an extremity being used for intravenous infusion; this will result in cutting off the infusion while the cuff is being inflated. If the intravenous catheter is inserted in a marginal position, the increased pressure during inflation may potentiate infiltration.
2. Provide adequate ventilation around equipment console; rear of machine should be unobstructed so that heat generated by internal components is allowed to escape through the rear panel.
3. Restrict fluid placement around equipment console area; this contributes to electrical safety precautions for the patient and helps to protect equipment.
4. Monitor the patient for excessive movement during a blood pressure determination to ensure accuracy of readings.

RELATED CARE

1. Check frequently for correct positioning of patient's arm to obtain accurate blood pressure readings.

2. Check for incorrect cuff connections, leaks in the system, kinks or obstructions in the system, or failure of the blood pressure device itself during an alarm alert.
3. Observe extremity for altered circulation and/or altered skin integrity; rotate extremity as needed.

COMPLICATIONS

Inaccurate blood pressure
  readings
Electrical shock

Altered skin integrity
Equipment malfunction

SUPPLIERS

Applied Medical Research
Roche
Omega
Physio Control

REFERENCES

Schroeder, J.S., and Daily, E.K. Techniques in Bedside Hemodynamic Monitoring. St. Louis, C. V. Mosby, 1976, p. 39.

Penny Ford, R.N., M.S., and
Rebecca Preston, R.N., B.S.N.

INTRA-AORTIC BALLOON PUMP MANAGEMENT

OVERVIEW

The intra-aortic balloon pump (IABP) is a form of temporary circulatory assistance which has been used in: (1) cardiogenic shock; (2) mechanical defects after myocardial infarction; (3) refractory cardiac ischemia; and (4) failure to wean from cardiopulmonary bypass. The balloon, mounted on a catheter, is usually threaded retrograde into the descending thoracic aorta through a femoral arteriotomy, and is connected to an external control console. The balloon is inflated and deflated with gas in synchrony with the mechanical events of the cardiac cycle. Balloon inflation occurs during diastole, with deflation occuring during systole. Typically, the R wave of the ECG is utilized as the triggering stimulus for synchronization of balloon and cardiac action.

The balloon catheter consists of a semiflexible tubing with a central gas lumen. The catheter is approximately 3 feet in length; the balloon is mounted on the distal 10 inches. The surface of both the balloon and catheter is antithrombogenic to minimize clot formation. Balloon capacity is variable, ranging from 15 to 40 ml. Balloon size is selected according to total body surface area and size of the femoral artery.

Two balloon designs are widely used at present. The first type has three segments, and is of a nonocclusive design (Fig. 57). Inflation of the middle segment occurs first, followed by inflation of the end segments. This inflation pattern produces omnidirectional blood flow during diastole,

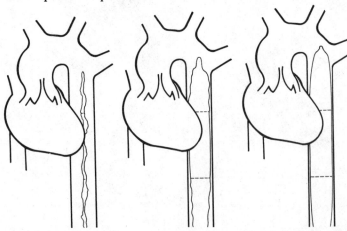

BALLOON DEFLATED   BALLOON INFLATING   BALLOON FULLY INFLATED

Figure 57. Trisegment omnidirectional balloon.

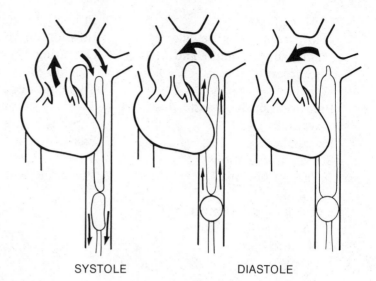

SYSTOLE   DIASTOLE

Figure 58.   Dual-chambered unidirectional intra-aortic balloon.

simultaneously improving retrograde flow into the coronary system and forward flow into the periphery. The second type has two chambers, a cylindrical proximal chamber and a spherical distal chamber (Fig. 58). The distal chamber inflates first and occludes the aorta, followed by inflation of the proximal chamber. This sequence favors retrograde blood flow into the coronary bed and is referred to as unidirectional flow.

The external control console performs three important functions. First, the ECG sensing circuitry within the unit permits synchronization of balloon and cardiac action. Second, the console contains the pneumatic controls which activate balloon inflation and deflation with either helium or carbon dioxide gas. Finally, automated alarms and safety features are incorporated into the design of all units. In the event of console malfunction or unsafe pumping conditions, the unit shuts down to a safe, inoperative mode with the balloon deflated. Patient transport during balloon pumping is made possible by switching the power source from wall current to battery power.

OBJECTIVES

1. To reduce cardiac work by decreasing the resistance to ventricular ejection.
2. To increase cardiac output by decreasing the resistance to ventricular emptying.
3. To improve coronary perfusion by elevating diastolic pressure.
4. To improve myocardial oxygenation by reducing oxygen demand and increasing oxygen supply.
5. To maintain systemic perfusion.

SPECIAL EQUIPMENT

IABP console   Defibrillator

IABP catheter
Fluoroscopic bed (if available)
Multichannel monitor and
   recorder
IV poles
Pressure transducers and flush
   systems
Pacemaker
Standby medications:
   Vasopressor mix
   Colloid
   Rheomacrodex infusion
   Local anesthetic bolus
   Heparin bolus

Intubation equipment
Infusion pump
Operating room light or head
   light
Two continuous suction outlets
Two oxygen outlets
Surgical instrument tray
Sterile dressing
Tape
Povidone iodine prep swab

METHOD

ACTION	RATIONALE
1. Prepare equipment in patient cubicle for easy access and patient safety.	1. Arrangement of cubicle and preparation of equipment must be meticulous prior to insertion. Omission of these steps can be catastrophic during insertion, when the cubicle is crowded and the draped patient is relatively inaccessible.
A. Prepare bedside ECG and pressure modules for accurate recording (see the methods for "Hemodynamic Monitoring").	
B. Plug in IABP console; turn on. Check gas supply and function of controls.	
C. Check function of additional equipment: suction, oxygen, operating room light, pacemaker.	
D. Prepare standby medications: vasopressor mix, colloid, Rheomacrodex infusion, local anesthetic bolus, heparin bolus.	
2. Establish ECG on bedside monitor upon admission of patient.	
3. Administer oxygen as prescribed.	
4. Record baseline vital signs, includ-	4. Preinsertion pulses are essential for

ACTION	RATIONALE
ing peripheral pulses, and 12-lead ECG.	evaluating any existing peripheral vascular disease that might preclude or complicate insertion and for comparison after insertion.
5. Assess hematologic profile.	5. Hematologic studies are important, since heparin may be administered during insertion and platelet reduction can occur during pumping. Blood must be available during insertion in the event of arterial trauma and bleeding.
6. Sedate the patient, as necessary.	
7. Establish ECG input to IABP console, either directly via patient cable or indirectly via the bedside monitor.	7. The ECG is the triggering stimulus for ballon activation.
A. Position patient electrodes to obtain ECG configuration with maximal R wave amplitude and minimal amplitude of all other waves and artifacts.	A. The sensing circuitry within the console utilizes wave amplitude as the primary criterion for R wave detection.
B. Select desired sweep speed.	
C. Using appropriate controls, ensure that the console is sensing the R wave consistently. Trigger light should flash once for each R wave.	C. Sensing of ECG components other than the R wave will disrupt balloon and cardiac synchrony.
8. Assist with the insertion of hemodynamic and intravenous catheters, as indicated.	
A. Connect radial artery catheter, preferably in left wrist, to pressure transducer and continuous flush system.	A. Balloon timing is adjusted utilizing the arterial trace. The left arm is preferred since the balloon is located distal to the left subclavian artery. Upward displacement of the catheter can readily be detected by damping of the left radial trace.
B. Connect pulmonary artery thermodilution catheter to pressure transducer and continuous flush system.	B. Accurate evaluation of left heart function and cardiac output is possible with this catheter.
C. Connect central line to a slow continuous infusion of 5% dextrose in water.	C. A central line must be kept available for the infusion of vasopressors. The right atrial lumen

ACTION	RATIONALE
	of the PA catheter may be used in an emergency. However, if cardiac output measurements are to be made vasopressors should not be infused in this lumen.
D. Connect peripheral angiocatheter to a slow continuous infusion of 5% dextrose in water.	D. A peripheral line should be kept available for the infusion of colloid, if necessary.
E. Connect transvenous pacing wire to pacemaker, on standby, unless otherwise indicated (optional).	
F. Connect urinary catheter to drainage system.	F. Urinary output is a sensitive index of cardiac output.
9. Administer broad spectrum antibiotic, as prescribed by physician.	9. Adequate tissue levels of antibiotic should be established.
10. Shave and prep both groins.	10. In the event that balloon passage is impossible via one femoral artery, insertion in the other groin may be necessitated.
11. Restrain the patient, as necessary.	
12. Ready standby medications.	
A. Attach vasopressor to central line via infusion pump.	
B. Place colloid and bolus medications near angiocatheter.	
13. Connect Rheomacrodex to angiocatheter and adjust infusion rate to 10 to 20 ml./hr. (optional).	13. This decreases platelet aggregation.
14. Mask, cap, and gown all persons in immediate area.	
15. Enclose "sterile" area and assist surgical team with preparation of operative field.	
A. Drape patient, maintaining access to lines.	
B. Provide suction for operative field.	
C. Position overhead light.	
D. Provide requested equipment: antibiotic flush, heparin flush, local anesthetic, balloon catheter.	
16. Ready IABP console for start-up.	
A. Turn power on.	

ACTION	RATIONALE
B. Check gas tank or pressure gauge.	
C. Zero and calibrate pressure channels, as needed.	
D. Make preliminary timing adjustments, using appropriate controls. Select trigger logic, if necessary.	
E. Select 1:1 pumping ratio.	
17. Note arterial systolic and diastolic pressures off balloon utilizing reference trace, if available.	
18. Monitor ECG, pressures, and clinical status throughout procedure. Notify physician of significant change or pain.	18. Acute back pain may signify aortic dissection, warranting immediate notification of physician. Angina must be controlled to prevent infarction during insertion.
19. Administer bolus of heparin approximately 3 minutes prior to arteriotomy (optional).	19. Despite the fact that the balloon surface is antithrombogenic, anticoagulation may be desirable.
20. Evacuate and purge gas lines.	
A. If safety chamber present:	
(1) Extend and attach securely to balloon.	
(2) Evacuate air from safety chamber and balloon with syringe.	
(3) Fill safety chamber with CO_2.	
(4) Secure connections.	
B. If safety chamber is not utilized:	
(1) Evacuate air from balloon during insertion by aspirating with syringe attached to balloon plug.	(1) Aspiration reduces the diameter of the balloon, facilitating passage through the femoral artery.
(2) Connect balloon plug to console once balloon is positioned in the aorta.	
(3) Purge gas lines with helium and fill balloon, using appropriate controls.	(3) Purging removes room air from balloon catheter, filling lines with gas.
21. Initiate ballon pumping at low volume.	
22. Adjust balloon timing using the ap-	22. Timing should be adjusted to achieve

ACTION	RATIONALE
propriate controls, visualizing the arterial trace (Fig. 59).	maximal diastolic augmentation and reduction of afterload. The end-diastolic pressure on the balloon should be equal to or 5-15 mm. less than diastolic pressure off the balloon.

23. Evaluate balloon function by observing safety chamber or balloon pressure configuration.
24. Increase balloon volume to full capacity.
25. Recheck balloon timing.
26. Turn console alarms on.
27. Assess peripheral pulses and record quality.
28. Apply sterile dressing, using sterile technique.
29. Arrange for a portable chest x-ray.

29. A chest x-ray is essential to verify balloon position if fluoroscopic bed is not used during insertion.

PRECAUTIONS

1. Protect balloon surface so that it does not come into contact with metal objects; perforation or damage to the antithrombogenic surface may result.
2. Never resterilize or reuse balloons; the integrity and performance of IABP balloons cannot be guaranteed under these circumstances.
3. Ensure that the IABP console senses the R wave of the ECG to maintain accurate synchronization of balloon action.
4. Establish two potential routes of ECG input to the ballon console due to the ECG dependence: one via a direct patient cable, and one indirectly via the bedside monitor.
5. Prepare emergency equipment and medications for the insertion.
6. Arrange for blood availability during insertion in the event of arterial trauma and/or hemorrhage.
7. Arrange for insertion of an arterial line prior to balloon insertion to ensure accurate balloon timing.
8. Timing should be adjusted by skilled personnel.

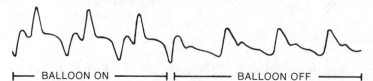

⊢— BALLOON ON ———⊣ ⊢——— BALLOON OFF ———⊣

Figure 59. Arterial trace with balloon on and off.

9. Avoid balloon deflation for more than 15 to 30 minutes. In the event of console malfunction, periodic quick inflation of the balloon with a 20-ml. syringe should prevent blood pooling, minimizing potential clot formation.
10. Notify physician of recurrent angina during balloon pumping, since more aggressive therapy may be indicated.
11. Avoid inducing ECG artifact during chest physical therapy.

RELATED CARE

1. Evaluate clinical and hemodynamic responses to balloon pumping every 15 to 60 minutes.
2. Assess quality of posterior tibial and dorsalis pedalis pulses in both extremities hourly; note skin temperature and color. Doppler flow technique may be necessary to detect weak pulses.
3. Evaluate balloon timing hourly, and adjust as needed.
4. Maintain quality ECG signals for balloon activation.
5. Evaluate hematologic status to detect abnormalities: thrombocytopenia; fall in hematocrit (usually secondary to excessive blood loss during insertion or blood sampling); inadequate or excessive anticoagulation.
6. Perform routine respiratory care with minor modifications of position; head of the bed should not be elevated over 45°, nor should the involved leg be flexed.
7. Maintain strict aseptic technique during dressing changes. Dressings should be occlusive and should be changed as necessary.
8. Continue antibiotic coverage for 24-48 hours after insertion.
9. Reduce the ratio of patient to balloon cycles (e.g., 1:1 to 1:8) during weaning, as prescribed by physician; monitor patient response closely.
10. Recreate the insertion environment during removal: organize equipment, reinstitute antibiotic coverage, turn IABP console off as ordered, aspirate or deflate balloon.
11. Evaluate peripheral pulses and patient tolerance after removal.
12. Check incision for bleeding 15 minutes after removal, then every 30 minutes times 2, then hourly for 24 hours.

COMPLICATIONS

Wound sepsis	Arterial trauma or dissection
Thrombocytopenia	Embolization of thrombi or
Thrombus formation on balloon surface or catheter	plaque
	Equipment malfunction

REFERENCES

Bregman, David: Clinical experience with a new cardiac assist device. J. Thorac. Cardiovasc. Surg. *62*:577–591, 1971.

Ford, Penny, and Weintraub, Ronald: Intra-Aortic Balloon Pumping Manual. Cambridge, MA, Artistocrat Press, 1974.
Massachusetts General 'Hospital: Concepts of Intra-Aortic Balloon Pumping: An Interdisciplinary Approach. Boston, AVCO, 1975, I-1 to X-9.

EXTERNAL PRESSURE CIRCULATORY ASSIST

Penny Ford, R.N., M.S., Rebecca Preston, R.N., B.S.N., and Patricia A. Yanul, R.N.

OVERVIEW

External counterpulsation is a noninvasive form of temporary circulatory assistance. During external counterpulsation, the legs are enclosed in water-filled sleeves encased in a pumping chamber. The pressure exerted on the extremities is varied in synchrony with the cardiac cycle, alternately compressing the legs during diastole and decompressing the legs during systole. Compression reduces the capacity of the peripheral vasculature, which displaces blood centrally and produces diastolic augmentation. Decompression during systole increases the peripheral vascular capacity, which displaces blood into the extremities and lowers central aortic pressure, thereby reducing afterload. The magnitude of afterload reduction is not as great with external counterpulsation as with intraaortic balloon pumping. Vasodilators may be infused during external pressure circulatory assist to reduce afterload further.

External pressure circulatory assist devices consist of a leg unit and control console. The leg unit functions as a pumping chamber; it is comprised of two parallel cylindrical leg cavities lined with plastic bladders (Fig. 60). The bladders are filled with water to obliterate the space between the unit and the legs. Consequently, the application of pressure to the water-filled bladders is transmitted directly to the legs. Contoured leg padding, referred to as *leg inserts*, can be applied to the legs to increase leg girth if there is excessive space between the legs and leg unit.

If negative pressure operation is desired, a pressure blanket must be placed over the leg unit and lower torso to produce an airtight pumping seal. Once the pressure blanket is sealed, pressure within the unit can be reduced to levels lower than atmospheric pressure. Negativity cannot be achieved within the unit without the negative pressure blanket.

The control console contains all the electronic and hydraulic controls. In addition, an oscilloscope and recorder with electrocardiographic and pressure modules are incorporated. The R wave of the ECG provides the triggering stimulus for counterpulsation. Visual markers on the oscilloscope indicate the timing of leg pressurization relative to the cardiac cycle. The timing and duration of leg pressurization are adjustable, as are the amplitudes of positive and negative pressure exerted. Both the ECG and arterial pressure tracings must be observed to adjust leg pressurization accurately. Water temperature is automatically maintained at approximately 95 °F. by the console when connected to wall current.

OBJECTIVES

1. To augment diastolic pressure, improving coronary and systemic perfusion.
2. To reduce afterload if negative pressure operation or vasodilator infusion is utilized.

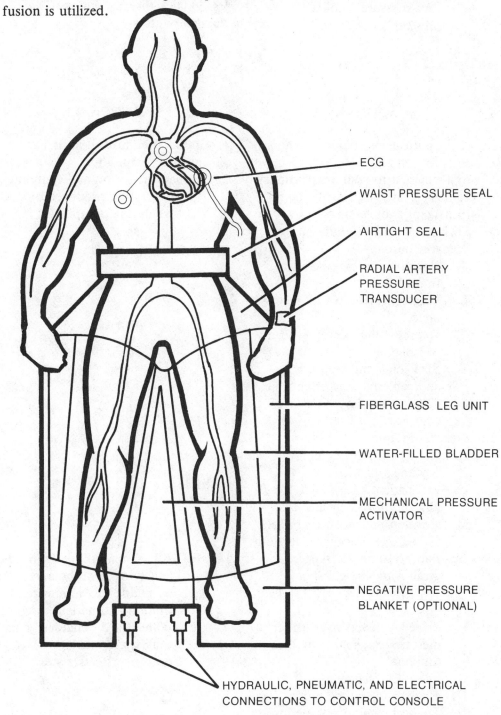

ECG

WAIST PRESSURE SEAL

AIRTIGHT SEAL

RADIAL ARTERY PRESSURE TRANSDUCER

FIBERGLASS LEG UNIT

WATER-FILLED BLADDER

MECHANICAL PRESSURE ACTIVATOR

NEGATIVE PRESSURE BLANKET (OPTIONAL)

HYDRAULIC, PNEUMATIC, AND ELECTRICAL CONNECTIONS TO CONTROL CONSOLE

Figure 60.   External pressure circulatory assist device.

SPECIAL EQUIPMENT

Leg unit
Control console, oscilloscope,
    recorder
Negative pressure blanket
    (optional)

Urinary catheter irrigant and
    clamp, if catheter is in place
Surgical sponges
Vasodilator therapy optional
Pajama pants

METHOD

ACTION	RATIONALE
1. Assist patient into pajama pants.	1. Pants minimize skin irritation and absorb perspiration.
2. Assist patient to void or, if urinary catheter is in place, instill 100 ml. of irrigant and clamp.	2. Urinary irrigation and clamping minimize irritation produced by catheter motion during pumping.
3. Position patient centrally on bed.	
4. Prepare console.	
A. Position control console at foot of bed.	
B. Plug console into wall receptacle.	
C. Depress "line power" to turn console on.	
D. Straighten and secure hoses and cables at rear of console.	
E. Check water level at rear of console.	
5. Prepare leg unit.	
A. Remove top of leg unit.	
B. Open leg bladders.	
C. Lift patient's legs; slide leg unit onto bed beneath legs.	
D. Position patient so that heels extend over bottom of leg unit.	
E. Pad heels, ankles, knees, and groin with surgical sponges.	E. All potential pressure points and bony protuberances should be padded to minimize skin irritation and patient discomfort.
F. Place leg inserts over legs to increase leg girth, if necessary (optional).	F. Water-filled bladder must fit snugly around legs to transmit pressure effectively.
G. Close leg bladders.	
H. Replace top of leg unit.	
I. Recheck position of leg inserts, if utilized.	

ACTION	RATIONALE
6. Secure negative pressure blanket over leg unit and lower torso if application of negative pressure is anticipated (optional).	6. Leg unit must have airtight seal to maintain negativity relative to atmospheric pressure.
7. Establish ECG input to console directly via patient cable or indirectly via monitor.	7. ECG is triggering stimulus for console operation.
A. Position electrodes on chest to obtain ECG configuration with maximal R wave amplitude and minimal amplitude of all other waves and pacing artifacts.	A. Console must sense R wave to synchronize leg pressurization with cardiac cycle correctly.
B. Connect cable or jack to console.	
C. Check quality of ECG and console sensing. Gain light should flash once for every R wave.	
8. Establish arterial pressure input to console via finger plethysmograph, transducer connected to arterial line, or arterial pressure module on monitor.	8. The arterial pressure signal is essential for accurate adjustment of timing.
A. Check quality of arterial tracing. Dicrotic notch must be visible.	A. The onset of diastolic augmentation produced by leg pressurization must coincide with the dicrotic notch. Plethysmograph should be attached to finger providing best trace and immobilized on a towel or arm board.
B. Zero and calibrate arterial pressure channel if recording is desired (optional).	
9. Position visual markers on ECG and arterial pressure wave forms, using appropriate controls.	9. Visual markers provide a safeguard to ensure that leg pressurization does not occur during systole. Markers must be adjusted prior to the application of pressure.
A. Adjust "phasing delay" control until visual marker on ECG coincides with end of T wave.	
B. Adjust "marker position" control until small arterial marker coincides with beginning of the systolic upstroke. The large	B. Small arterial marker must always coincide with the onset of systole to avoid pumping during systole. The timing of leg pres-

ACTION	RATIONALE
arterial marker, or applied pressure marker, should now coincide with the dicrotic notch.	surization is referenced from this marker to avoid systole.
10. Administer prescribed intravenous vasodilator therapy to maximize unloading (optional).	
11. Make preliminary console adjustments.	
A. Adjust duration of pressurization with "phasing duration" control; 0.20 second is recommended.	A. Duration of pressurization will depend upon length of cardiac cycle (i.e., R-R interval).
B. Adjust amplitude of positive pressure to approximately 50 mm. Hg.	B. Initial pressures should be low until synchronization and effect can be assessed.
C. Adjust amplitude of negative pressure to desired level; 25 mm. Hg. is recommended unless negative pressure operation with blanket is indicated.	
12. Depress "water control-fill" control to fill leg bladders with preheated water.	
A. Check water temperature manually in bladder as unit fills.	A. Temperature is automatically maintained at approximately 95°F. if unit remains plugged in; otherwise, 4 hours is required to warm water.
B. Check that bladder is filled manually once "water monitor-full" light appears. Bladder should be firmly in contact with legs.	
13. Turn motor on with "assist power" control.	
14. Inform patient that unit will begin to rock; offer ongoing reassurance and sedation, as necessary.	
15. Initiate pulsation with "assist pressure" control.	
16. Observe arterial pressure trace to insure that applied pressure marker and onset of diastolic augmentation coincide with dicrotic notch. Adjust	

ACTION	RATIONALE

"phasing delay" control, if necessary.

17. Gradually increase positive amplitude by 25 to 50 mm. Hg. every few seconds, until desired level of diastolic augmentation is achieved.

   A. Confirm amplitude control settings on chart recorder as pressure is increased.

   B. Once maximal level of diastolic augmentation is reached, reduce positive amplitude until augmentation is reduced, about 25%.

18. Check with patient regarding comfort and reduce pressure if excessive discomfort is noted.

19. Adjust phasing duration and delay, constantly observing ECG and arterial tracings.

   A. Adjust "phasing duration" control until maximal diastolic augmentation is observed on arterial trace; check ECG to insure that ECG marker does not extend beyond upstroke of P wave.

   B. Adjust "phasing delay" control until onset of diastolic augmentation coincides with the dicrotic notch.

      (1) Turn counterpulsation off momentarily to identify notch, if necessary.

      (2) Check ECG to insure that ECG marker does not begin before latter third of T wave.

20. Recheck positive amplitude to identify pressure producing best augmentation.

21. Adjust negative amplitude (optional).

22. Adjust vasodilator infusion (optional).

23. To discontinue pumping:

RATIONALE

17. Typically, pressures of 150 to 180 mm. Hg. usually achieve desired results and can be tolerated.

   A. Chart recorder provides written documentation of amplitude of applied pressure.

19. Adjustments are intended to maximize the effect of pressurization without encroaching upon systole.

ACTION	RATIONALE

A. Decrease pressure gradually by 25 mm. Hg. approximately every 30 seconds.

B. Empty water from bladder by depressing "water control-empty" prior to removal of leg unit.

PRECAUTIONS

1. Monitor position of the visual markers on the oscilloscope constantly; timing must be readjusted manually for any change in cycle length.
2. Avoid inadvertent pressurization during systole by improper control adjustment.
3. Protect leg bladders from sharp objects to avoid perforation.
4. Check water temperature manually during filling of bladders.
5. Turn off console power during defibrillation.
6. Discontinue pumping immediately in the following situations: angina, dysrhythmias, respiratory distress, excessive elevation of CVP or PAP.

RELATED CARE

1. Assess peripheral circulation prior to application of leg unit and hourly thereafter.
2. Interrupt pumping for 10 minutes every hour during long periods of prescribed pumping.
3. Monitor vital signs as patient's condition dictates, without interrupting pumping. Slight elevation of CVP and PAP may be noted due to increased right heart venous return.
4. Encourage foot exercises during pumping; leg exercises should be encouraged during pumping interruption periods.
5. Encourage voiding during pumping interruption periods, as necessary.
6. Elevate the head to 30° for patient comfort, as needed.
7. Provide sedation, as necessary.
8. Massage pressure areas during breaks.

COMPLICATIONS

Systemic embolization
Pulmonary embolization

Pulmonary edema
Patient discomfort

REFERENCES

Cardioassist, EPCA: Rationale for Application and Physiologic Response. Medical Innovations, Inc., Waltham, Mass., 1973, pp. 1–28.
Cardioassist—Operator's Manual. Cardioassist, Foxriver Grove, Illinois, 1972.

EXTERNAL COUNTERPRESSURE WITH G-SUIT ──────────

Penny Ford, R.N., M.S., and Rebecca Preston, R.N., B.S.N.

OVERVIEW

External compression of bleeding sites is recognized as an initial emergency maneuver for achieving hemostasis. Compression of intra-abdominal sites can be effected with the application of the external pressure suit, referred to as the G-suit or antigravity suit. External pressure also redistributes the vascular volume by shunting blood from vascular beds beneath the diaphragm proximally to maintain perfusion of vital organs. External counterpressure is indicated for: (1) temporary preoperative control of subdiaphragmatic bleeding due to ruptured abdominal aneurysms or massive trauma, until surgical correction can be undertaken; and (2) temporary postoperative control of intractable hemorrhage due to diffuse bleeding or coagulopathies, until clotting abnormalities are corrected.

The G-suit consists of a double-layered, clear plastic sheet. A space between the layers allows the sheet to be inflated with gas. The gas volume contained between the layers regulates pressure within the suit. A gas inflow tube and a gas outflow tube regulate gas volume and consequently pressure within the suit. The gas inflow tube is connected to an external source of noncombustible gas. The gas outflow tube is attached to a plastic chamber filled with fluid to a predesignated level; the fluid level in the column regulates the amount of pressure exerted by the G-suit.

The mechanism for pressure regulation with a fluid column is analogous to that utilized in a three-bottle chest tube drainage system (see p. 242). The fluid column exerts a given amount of resistance or pressure to gas outflow from the G-suit. When the pressure within the suit exceeds the amount of resistance offered by the water column, gas is forced through the fluid and bubbling is observed. The bubbling releases excess pressure within the system, maintaining pressure at the designated level.

OBJECTIVES

1. To minimize blood loss from intra-abdominal bleeding sites.
2. To redistribute intravascular volume proximally, maintaining perfusion of vital organs during hypotensive episodes.

SPECIAL EQUIPMENT

> Lanolin
> G-suit
> Rope (if lacing is required)
> Bath blanket
> Source of noncombustible gas (e.g., compressed air or nitrogen)
> Bottle of distilled water
> Ampule of methylene blue (if colored solution is preferred for visualization)
> 50-ml. barrel-tipped syringe
> Extension tubing and adapter for gas source
> Surgical pads (nonsterile)
> Gauze roll

METHOD

ACTION	RATIONALE
1. Apply lanolin to body surface.	1. Lanolin protects skin, minimizing irritation.
2. Spread G-suit on bed with arrow in center of mattress and hook side down. Smooth bath blanket over surface of suit.	2. Blanket absorbs perspiration and minimizes blistering of skin.
3. Position patient so upper edge of G-suit lies beneath the xiphoid, with the arrow centered between the legs.	3. Compression of the thorax above the xiphoid will compromise ventilation. Suit must be centered with equal lengths of material on each side to facilitate closure.
4. Place surgical pads between knees and under coccyx; secure with gauze roll if necessary.	4. Padding minimizes pressure necrosis during compression.
5. Straighten all drainage tubes and position them to insure unimpeded flow.	
6. Wrap both ends of the blanket around patient and smooth blanket.	6. Blanket should be as wrinkle-free as possible to prevent skin breakdown.
7. Wrap free edges of suit securely around patient and close securely from bottom to top with rope or Velcro adhesive; maintain even pressure along length of suit.	
8. Suspend plastic fluid chamber over side of bed. Markings on chamber indicate pressure equivalent in mm.	8. Fluid column functions as a pressure manometer reflecting the pressure in the suit.

ACTION	RATIONALE

Hg. The recommended pressure is 20 to 30 mm. Hg.; 40 mm. Hg. is not considered safe.

9. Add methylene blue to distilled water.

10. Fill fluid chamber to designated pressure level with barrel syringe.

11. Connect gas inflow tubing to source of noncombustible gas.

    11. Oxygen must *never* be used. The use of flammable gas is an unacceptable fire hazard.

12. Adjust gas flow until constant gentle bubbling is observed in fluid column.

PRECAUTIONS

1. Never use combustible gas due to fire hazard.
2. Avoid perforation of suit with sharp objects.
3. Pad all bony prominences and potential pressure points to minimize skin breakdown.
4. Never position G-suit above the level of the xiphoid to minimize interference with ventilation.
5. Avoid sudden deflation of the G-suit to prevent abrupt alteration in vascular volume and pressure.
6. Prevent kinking of the gas inflow and outflow tubes to maintain designated pressure.

RELATED CARE

1. Monitor vital signs every 30 minutes to evaluate hemodynamic responses.
2. Assess peripheral circulatory status every 30 minutes to detect alterations in circulation.
3. Check arterial blood gas levels within 15 to 30 minutes of application of the G-suit, and as needed thereafter, to detect altered pulmonary status.
4. If ventilated, closely monitor ventilator function, especially inspiratory pressure and expired volume, to detect changes in lung compliance.
5. If extubated observe closely for signs of respiratory distress.
6. Check level of fluid in column hourly to maintain designated pressure; replace evaporated fluid as needed.
7. Use a portable tank of noncombustible gas during transport. Never use oxygen; never clamp. Pressure control must be precise.
8. Reduce pressure gradually prior to removal of G-suit—approximately 5 mm. Hg every ½ hour, or as ordered. Appropriate amount of fluid can be removed from pressure chamber through bottom drainage port.

COMPLICATIONS

Atelectasis secondary to reduced vital capacity
Pneumonia with immobilization
Pulmonary edema with redistribution of fluid
Skin necrosis and blistering
Thromboembolic complications

REFERENCES

Burdick, J.F., Warshaw, A.L., and Abbott, W.M.: External counterpressure to control postoperative intra-abdominal hemorrhage. Am. J. Surg., *129*:369–373, 1975.

TEMPORARY PACEMAKER MANAGEMENT

Betty Norris, R.N., M.S.N.

OVERVIEW

Pacemaker therapy improves cardiac output by restoring a more normal heart rate. The patient's need for temporary and/or permanent pacing is determined by the underlying condition. Indications may include: (1) AV blocks; (2) bifascicular or trifascicular blocks; (3) bradycardia—sinus bradycardia, junctional rhythm, sinoatrial block, carotid sinus sensitivity produced by drug therapy; (4) supraventricular rhythms unresponsive to medical therapy; (5) supraventricular rhythms with slow ventricular response; (6) sick sinus syndrome; (7) asystole; (8) ventricular dysrhythmias unresponsive to other therapy; (9) prophylactic measures during open heart surgery and following a myocardial infarction; (10) pacing-induced ischemia as a diagnostic test; and (11) pacing studies for sick sinus syndrome to determine sinoatrial recovery time. The critical care nurse contributes to multidimensional aspects of pacemaker therapy. The methods presented in this section are offered to provide a greater perspective for pacemaker responsibilities.

INSTRUMENTATION

Regardless of the model, external temporary pacing units share basic components (Fig. 61).

Pulse Generator. This is the external battery-operated source which initiates electrical activity and controls the rate and intensity of each energy discharge. Its clear plastic cover enables the dials to be seen and protects the dial controls.

On-Off Lever. This controls the power component for activating the pulse generator. A safety lock protects against accidental termination of pacing. It requires two steps to turn off the pacemaker: (1) depress small button; (2) slide lever across top of the depressed button.

Mode Dial. Options include modalities for fixed rate pacing or demand pacing. The fixed rate, or asynchronous, mode disregards electrical impulses and fires continuously at a predetermined discharge. Fixed rate pacing is obtained by turning the mode dial to the maximum counterclockwise position. The demand, or synchronous, mode fires only after awaiting a signal through the exploring electrode. It is normally noncompetitive to the patient's electrical impulse. Demand pacing is obtained by adjusting the mode dial to the maximum clockwise position and/or adjusting the same dial as the sensitivity control for the R wave signal.

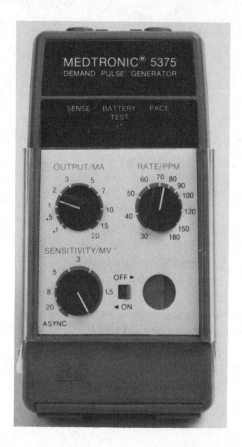

Figure 61.   Temporary external pacemaker. Courtesy of Medtronic, Inc., Minneapolis, Minn.

Rate Dial.   The rate dial regulates beats per minute. Atrial pacing requires higher rate options than those usually needed for ventricular pacing.

Ma or Output Dial.   This regulates the amount of energy delivered to the distal electrode. It is reported in milliamperes (ma.); it ranges from 0.1 to 20 ma.

Sense/Pace Indicator.   Each time an R wave is sensed the dial moves to the "sense" position or a light flashes, depending upon the pacemaker model. Each time the pacemaker fires the dial moves to the "pace" position or a light flashes. This component is utilized to check for battery depletion by observing the amount of deflection on the indicator dial or the light intensity.

Connector Terminals.   The pacing electrodes to the temporary external pacemaker are usually connected at the top of the pacing unit; connector terminals are identified as positive (+) and negative (−). The mechanism for securing the pacing electrode terminals varies with different models.

Battery Cartridge.   A small compartment on the lower portion of the pacing unit protects the battery. Newer models eliminate the need for tools in battery removal.

Temporary pacing systems are used for atrial and/or ventricular pacing, with provisions for variable rates of pacing and flexibility for continuous, synchronous, or demand modes. The pacing catheter is either bipolar or unipolar. The bipolar pacing catheter includes both positive and negative electrodes, positioned approximately 1 cm. apart. The unipolar electrode is the negative electrode and requires an indifferent, externally positioned electrode.

EMERGENCY INSERTION OF A TEMPORARY PACING ELECTRODE (ASSISTING WITH) _____

OBJECTIVES

1. To institute temporary pacing promptly when fluoroscopy is not immediately available.
2. To determine output threshold and sensitivity threshold, using an external temporary pacemaker.

SPECIAL EQUIPMENT

Select pacing electrode
External temporary pacemaker
Cable
Sterile towels
Masks
Sterile gown
Local anesthetic
Povidone-iodine prep solution
Suture with needle

ECG monitor and recorder
Defibrillator
Emergency cart and medications
For site care:
  Sterile gauze pads
  Povidone-iodine prep swabs
  Rubber glove
  Tape

METHOD

ACTION	RATIONALE
1. Connect patient to ECG monitor; monitor ECG recording continuously.	
2. Mask, gown, and glove all persons in immediate area.	
3. Prep selected site with povidone-iodine solution; drape with sterile towels.	

ACTION	**RATIONALE**
A. Transvenous approach may include use of the jugular, subclavian, antecubital, or femoral veins.	
B. Transthoracic approach is through the chest wall to the heart.	B. This approach is often used during advanced life support therapy.
4. Anesthetize the area locally.	
5. Prepare external temporary pacemaker.	
A. Set the ma. on 6.	
B. Turn rate control to 10 beats per minute above patient's rate.	B. The rate set above patient's rate will suppress the patient's natural pacemaking site.
C. Turn sensitivity dial fully clockwise.	
6. Monitor patient while pacing electrode is inserted by a physician.	
A. Transvenous method:	
(1) A percutaneous puncture to the vein is performed.	
(a) The needle is removed and pacing electrode is passed through cannula.	
(b) Pacing electrode is positioned in right ventricle.	
(2) Connect pacing electrode to external temporary pacemaker, positive to positive and negative to negative.	
(3) Turn on external temporary pacemaker.	
(4) Adjust rate and ma. appropriately for effective capture.	
(a) Capture is indicated by a ventricular response after each pacemaker impulse.	
B. Balloon-tipped pacing electrode method:	
(1) Follow all preceding steps through 6-(2).	

ACTION	RATIONALE
(2) Balloon inflation occurs when pacing electrode is in vena cava.	(2) The air-inflated balloon allows blood flow to carry the catheter tip into desired position in right ventricle.
(3) Turn on external temporary pacemaker when pacing electrode is in the heart.	
(4) Observe ECG monitor.	(4) The ECG pattern is distinctive when the pacing electrode is in the vena cava, right atrium, and right ventricle.
(a) Assess ECG rhythm for small inverted P waves.	(a) This depicts pacing electrode in vena cava.
(b) Assess ECG rhythm for tall biphasic P waves.	(b) This depicts pacing electrode in right atrium.
(c) Assess ECG rhythm for large QRS complexes and progressively smaller P waves.	(c) This depicts pacing electrode in right ventricle.
(d) Assess ECG rhythm for elevated ST segments.	(d) This depicts pacing electrode wedged against endocardial wall of right ventricle.
(5) Capture is indicated by a ventricular response after each pacemaker impulse.	
(6) Deflate balloon.	
C. Transthoracic method:	
(1) A transthoracic puncture is made into the myocardium.	
(a) Needle and obturator are inserted transthoracically into ventricle through fourth intercostal space.	
(b) Inner obturator is removed; pacing stylet is inserted through needle.	
(2) Secure stylet by taping or suturing.	

ACTION	RATIONALE
(3) Attach stylet to external temporary pacemaker using connecting adapter.	
(a) Insert proximal end of stylet into adapter and tighten both locks.	
(b) Connect distal lead to negative pole of external temporary pacemaker and proximal lead to positive pole of external temporary pacemaker.	
(4) Turn on external temporary pacemaker.	
(5) Adjust rate and ma. appropriately for effective capture and pacing.	
(a) Capture is indicated by a ventricular response after each pacemaker impulse.	
7. Determine stimulation threshold.	
A. Gradually decrease output until 1:1 capture is lost.	
B. Gradually increase output until 1:1 capture is regained; this is the stimulation threshold. Acceptable stimulation threshold is 1.0 ma. or less for most endocardial leads.	B. If threshold exceeds these values, lead should be repositioned and procedure repeated.
8. Determine sensitivity threshold.	
A. Turn rate to 10 beats per minute less than patient's rate.	A. The sense/pace indicator should deflect to sense zone as it senses R waves.
B. Turn the sensitivity control counterclockwise slowly (from the fully clockwise position) until pacemaker begins to fire; this is the sensitivity threshold. Adequate threshold is in the 6 millivolt range.	B. The sense/pace indicator will deflect to the pace zone as it begins not to sense the R waves. A low sensitivity threshold is indication for repositioning.
9. Set external temporary pacemaker at desired rate, set output at ma. of 3 to 5 increments above threshold,	9. P or T wave sensing may require sensitivity to be decreased.

ACTION	RATIONALE
and set sensitivity in maximum clockwise position unless there is P or T wave sensing.	
10. Secure electrode wire at site of insertion by suturing or taping.	10. This prevents dislodgment of the electrode catheter.
11. Perform site care.	
A. Cleanse pacing electrode insertion site with povidone-iodine prep swabs, using sterile technique; apply sterile dry dressing.	A. A thoroughly dry dressing provides protective measure of safety insulation.
B. Check insulation; exposed electrode wire should be insulated in a rubber glove.	
C. Maintain skin integrity by placing sterile gauze pads under rubber glove.	
D. Increase safety protection by placing gauze pads over rubber glove, and sealing with tape.	D. Padding on top of glove prevents displacement or accidental removal or dislodgment of electrode during tape removal.
E. Label dressing "Pacing wire" and "date."	

PRECAUTIONS

1. Provide a defibrillator, emergency cart, and medications for immediate use. Pacemaker stimuli may inadvertently be delivered in vulnerable period during checking of threshold, causing lethal dysrhythmias.
2. Follow electrical safety guidelines for patients with pacemakers.
3. Observe monitor carefully during threshold checking. Do not be distracted.
4. Monitor ma. setting; too low may cause no capture and dangerously slow rhythms; too high may cause irritability and lead to ventricular dysrhythmias.
5. Monitor sensitivity setting; too high may cause sensing of P or T wave, resulting in failure to pace at appropriate times; too low will cause fixed rate pacing with the possibility of the pacing stimulus being delivered during the vulnerable period of the cardiac cycle, leading to lethal dysrhythmias.

RELATED CARE

1. Obtain chest x-ray postinsertion to validate position of pacing electrode.

ACTION	RATIONALE

2. Perform site care daily; check external pacing electrode wire position, insulation, and security of catheter terminals within pacemaker connectors.
3. Check pacemaker dressings for dryness; change immediately if damp or wet.
4. Check threshold profile daily; verify that pacemaker system is functioning properly.
5. Monitor patient's temperature every 4 hours.

COMPLICATIONS

Competitive dysrhythmias
Lethal ventricular dysrhythmias
Cardiac arrest
Cardiac perforation
Catheter electrode displacement or fracture

Pneumothroax
Thrombophlebitis
Infection
Electromicroshock
Equipment malfunction

REFERENCES

Baptist Medical Center-Montclair: Nursing Policy and Procedure Manual. Birmingham, Ala., Baptist Medical Center-Montclair, 1979.

Hoechst Pharmaceutical, Inc.: Cardiac Pacemaking: Directions in Cardiovascular Medicine. Somerville, N.J.: Hoechst Pharmaceutical, 1974, pp. 5–40.

Javiar, B.P., et al.: Temporary cardiac pacing: Technique and indications. Chest, 59:498, 1971.

Medtronic, Inc.: External Pacemaker. Minneapolis, Medtronic, 1976.

Meester, S.G., Bank, V.S., and Helfant, R.H.: Transfemoral pacing with balloon-tipped catheters. J.A.M.A. 225:712, 1973.

INITIATING TEMPORARY EPICARDIAL PACING _____

OBJECTIVES

1. To facilitate emergency electrical stimulation of the heart, using an epicardial electrode that has been temporarily inserted into the atrial and/or ventricular myocardium.
2. To control dysrhythmias.
3. To improve cardiac output.

SPECIAL EQUIPMENT

ECG monitor and recorder
External temporary pacemaker
Steel needle or indifferent elec-
  trode
Patient cable
Rubber gloves
Defibrillator

Emergency cart and medica-
  tions
For site care:
  Sterile gauze pads
  Povidone-iodine prep swabs
  Rubber glove
  Tape

METHOD

ACTION	RATIONALE
1. Obtain ECG recording.	1. This serves as baseline data.
2. Don rubber gloves.	
3. Expose pacing electrode.	
4. Select appropriate method.	
A. Bipolar ventricular pacing:	
(1) Connect ventricular pacing wire to negative pole of external temporary pacemaker.	(1) The electrode which is connected to the negative pole determines the type of pacing.
(2) Connect atrial wire to positive pole of external temporary pacemaker.	(2) In the bipolar system the current is between the electrodes.
B. Unipolar ventricular pacing:	
(1) Connect ventricular pacing wire to negative pole of external temporary pacemaker.	(1) The electrode which is connected to the negative pole determines the type of pacing.
(2) Insert a steel needle or indifferent electrode subcutaneously usually in the upper abdomen.	(2) This serves as indifferent electrode.
(3) Connect needle or electrode to positive pole of external temporary pacemaker.	
C. Bipolar atrial pacing:	
(1) Connect the two atrial wires to positive and negative poles of external temporary pacemaker.	(1) Atrial pacing is fixed rate pacing. The electrode which is connected to the negative pole determines the type of pacing.
D. Unipolar atrial pacing:	

ACTION	RATIONALE
(1) Connect an atrial wire to the negative pole of external temporary pacemaker.	(1) The electrode which is connected to the negative pole determines the type of pacing.
(2) Connect a subcutaneously inserted indifferent electrode or steel needle to the positive pole of external temporary pacemaker.	
5. Set prescribed rate; set sensitivity mode and ma. at lowest settings.	5. It is dangerous to alter the rate in a fixed mode, since pacer spike may fall in the vulnerable period.
A. Use asynchronous (fixed) mode for atrial pacing.	A. Use of demand mode may result in failure to sense or capture.
B. Use asynchronous (fixed) or synchronous (demand) mode for ventricular pacing.	
6. Turn on the external temporary pacemaker; observe ECG monitor.	
7. Gradually increase ma. until complete capture is reached.	7. The myocardium requires time to adjust; turning the pacemaker on and off suddenly may be dangerous to cardiac electrodynamics.
A. Capture is indicated by a ventricular response after each pacemaker impulse.	
B. Increase ma. 3 to 5 increments above stimulation threshold.	
C. Note that atrial pacing requires a setting four to five times greater than that used for ventricular pacing.	
8. Secure ECG recording.	
9. Protect all exposed connections in rubber; secure with dressing.	

PRECAUTIONS

1. Provide defibrillator, emergency cart, and medications for immediate use.
2. Protect connector sites from potential current leakage and moisture.
3. Wear rubber gloves when working with conductive ends of pacing wires.
4. Follow electrical safety guidelines for patients with pacemakers.
5. Protect epicardial electrodes not in use.

6. Observe for pacemaker stimulation of the heart during the repolarization period (T wave); this may cause lethal dysrhythmias.
7. Monitor ma. setting: too low may cause failure to capture and a bradycardia may continue; too high may cause irritability, leading to lethal dysrhythmias.
8. Monitor sensitivity setting: too high may cause sensing of P or T wave, resulting in failure to pace at appropriate times; too low will cause fixed rate pacing with the possibility of pacing stimulus being delivered during the vulnerable period of the cardiac cycle, leading to lethal dysrhythmias.
9. A patient with an epicardial electrode should have the site identified at all times and special equipment at the bedside for rapid emergency intervention.

RELATED CARE

1. Ensure that pacing system is functioning properly; check that connections are secure and properly protected from potential sources of current leakage every 8 hours.
2. Perform pacing electrode site care daily or as needed if dressings become moist.
   A. Cleanse pacing electrode insertion site with povidone-iodine prep swabs, using sterile technique.
   B. Check insulation: exposed electrode wire should be insulated in a rubber glove.
   C. Maintain skin integrity by placing sterile gauze pads under rubber glove.
   D. Increase safety protection by placing gauze pads over rubber glove and sealing with tape.
3. Assess ECG recording for appropriate pacing and sensing.
4. Assess threshold profile daily.

COMPLICATIONS

Lethal dysrhythmias
Competitive dysrhythmias
Cardiac arrest
Infection

Dislodgment of pacing wire
Electromicroshock
Equipment malfunction

REFERENCES

Baptist Medical Center-Montclair: Nursing Policy and Procedure Manual. Birmingham, Ala., Baptist Medical Center-Montclair, 1979.
Preston, T.A.: A comparison of bipolar and unipolar stimulation electrodes. Impulse, Sept., 1976.

CONVERSION FROM BIPOLAR TO UNIPOLAR SYSTEM WITH TEMPORARY PACING _____

OBJECTIVE

To enhance the pacemaker's ability to sense electrical activity of the heart by increasing the distance between the electrodes, thereby increasing the electrical potential.

SPECIAL EQUIPMENT

ECG monitor and recorder
Small gauge steel needle and/
  or indifferent electrode
Patient cable
Rubber gloves
Defibrillator
Povidone-iodine prep solu-
  tion

Emergency cart and medica-
  tions
For site care:
  Sterile gauze pads
  Povidone-iodine prep
    swabs
  Rubber glove
  Tape

METHOD

ACTION	RATIONALE
1. Obtain ECG recording.	1. This provides baseline data.
2. Turn off external temporary pacemaker.	
3. Prep select site on abdomen with povidone-iodine; insert steel needle subcutaneously and secure.	
4. Don rubber gloves.	4. These prevent possibility of transmitting electrical current to myocardium.
5. Disconnect external temporary pacemaker from pacing electrode at terminals.	
6. Attach negative (black) alligator clip of patient cable to bipolar connectors pin for distal tip electrode.	
7. Attach positive (red) alligator clip to steel needle placed subcutaneously in abdomen.	7. The needle becomes the indifferent electrode, thus increasing the distance between electrodes; it increases the electrical potential and makes it easier for the pacemaker to sense the heart's activity.

ACTION	RATIONALE

8. Connect patient cable to external temporary pacemaker, negative to negative and positive to positive.
9. Turn sensitivity dial fully clockwise; check that rate dial is set at desired rate and output is set at 6 to 10 ma.
10. Turn on external temporary pacemaker; observe monitor.
11. Obtain ECG recording.
12. Secure alligator clips with dressing.
13. Protect all exposed connections in rubber; secure with dressing.

PRECAUTIONS

1. Provide defibrillator, emergency cart, and medications for immediate use.
2. Wear rubber gloves when handling connector tips of pacing catheter electrode.
3. Follow electrical safety guidelines for patients with pacemakers.
4. Observe for lethal dysrhythmias which may occur when the pacemaker fails to sense the patient's own heart beat. The pacemaker may stimulate the heart during the repolarization period (T wave).
5. Decrease ma. if the muscle around the steel needle has a noticeable twitch with each paced beat, but continue to maintain capture of the heart.
6. Securely cover both the exposed end of the metal needle and the metal connector of the pacing catheter electrode with rubber in order to protect the electrical pathway to the heart.

RELATED CARE

1. Note appropriate pacing and sensing on ECG monitor.
2. Check that all connections are secure every 8 hours.
3. Check for pacemaker firing felt by the patient.

COMPLICATIONS

Lethal dysrhythmias	Electromicroshock
Cardiac arrest	Equipment malfunction

REFERENCES

Baptist Medical Center-Montclair: Nursing Policy and Procedure Manual. Birmingham, Ala., Baptist Medical Center-Montclair, 1979.
Medtronic, Inc.: External Pacemaker. Minneapolis, Medtronic, 1976.
Peterson, C.R.: Temporary Pacing: Indications, Techniques and Troubleshooting. Minneapolis, Medtronic, no date.

ATRIAL ECG WITH TEMPORARY ATRIAL PACING ELECTRODE

OBJECTIVE

To improve diagnostic accuracy of supraventricular dysrhythmias.

SPECIAL EQUIPMENT

12-Lead ECG recorder or modified bedside ECG monitoring equipment, select cables, and bedside strip chart recorder
Rubber gloves
Defibrillator

Emergency cart and medications
For site care:
  Sterile gauze pads
  Povidone-iodine prep swab
  Rubber gloves
  Tape

METHOD

ACTION	RATIONALE
1. Don rubber gloves.	
2. Expose atrial pacing electrode.	
3. Select appropriate method.	
A. Bipolar system:	
(1) Connect one atrial electrode to RA connector and the other atrial electrode to LA connector on 12-lead recorder.	
(2) Place lower limb leads on ankles.	
(3) Turn lead selector to lead I.	
B. Unipolar system:	

ACTION	RATIONALE
(1) Connect one atrial electrode to RA connector and the other atrial electrode to LA connector on 12-lead recorder.	
(2) Place lower limb leads on ankles.	
(3) Turn lead selector to lead II or III.	(3) Left leg serves as indifferent electrode.
C. Alternative unipolar system:	
(1) Connect atrial wire to chest lead on 12-lead recorder.	
(2) Connect all limb leads.	
(3) Turn lead selector to V_1.	

4. Obtain ECG recording.
5. Secure atrial electrode as found prior to atrial ECG recording.

PRECAUTIONS

1. Follow electrical safety guidelines for patients with temporary pacing electrodes.
2. Provide defibrillator, emergency cart, and medications for immediate use.
3. Observe for dysrhythmias.

RELATED CARE

Perform site care postatrial ECG; protect all exposed connections.

COMPLICATIONS

Lethal dysrhythmias
Cardiac arrest

Electromicroshock
Equipment malfunction

REFERENCES

Maclean, W.A.H., et al.: Use of Cardiac Electrodes in Diagnosis and Treatment of Tachyarrhythmias. Birmingham, Ala., Department of Medicine, University of Alabama.

Mantle, J.A., et al.: A multipurpose catheter for electrophysiologic and hemodynamic monitoring plus atrial pacing. Chest, 72:285–290, 1977.

OVERDRIVE ATRIAL PACING

OBJECTIVE

To provide overdrive suppression of tachydysrhythmias.

SPECIAL EQUIPMENT

External atrial temporary pacemaker

ECG monitor or 12-lead ECG recorder

Defibrillator

Emergency cart and medications

For site care:
  Sterile gauze pads
  Povidone-iodine prep swabs
  Rubber glove
  Tape

METHOD

ACTION	RATIONALE
1. Obtain initial ECG recording.	1. This provides baseline data.
2. Confirm that electrode is in right atrium by an atrial electrogram (AEG) tracing and/or fluoroscopy.	2. Accidental high rate stimulation of right ventricle could induce lethal dysrhythmias.
3. Prepare atrial external temporary pacemaker.	
A. Connect lead connector tips to terminals.	
(1) Connect positive to positive, negative to negative.	
(2) An interconnecting cable is sometimes used between atrial pacemaker and electrode.	
(3) Adjust "rate" dial and "output" to desired setting on atrial pacemaker.	
4. Turn on external atrial temporary pacemaker, observing pacing activity on ECG monitor.	
A. Heart rate is increased.	
B. Observe for atrial pacing capture.	
C. Obtain ECG recording.	

ACTION	RATIONALE

5. Select prescribed method to achieve suppression of tachydysrhythmias.
   A. Terminate atrial pacing abruptly.

                                              A. Abrupt cessation allows for SA node to assume pacemaking role.

   B. Slow atrial pacing to an acceptable rate.

6. Obtain ECG recording.

7. Complete postcare.
   A. Perform site care if pacing electrode is removed.
   B. Secure and insulate pacing electrode, perform site care, and check for dry dressing when:
      (1) Pacing electrode is left in place and pacemaker unit is disconnected.
      (2) Pacing unit is turned off but remains connected.

8. Monitor patient's response to therapy.

PRECAUTIONS

1. Follow electrical safety guidelines for patients with pacemakers.
2. Provide defibrillator, emergency cart, and medications for immediate use.
3. Observe for dysrhythmias.

RELATED CARE

1. Perform site care daily; check external pacing electrode wire position, insulation, and security of catheter terminals within pacemaker connectors.

COMPLICATIONS

Dysrhythmias
Cardiac arrest
Electromicroshock

Altered skin integrity
Equipment malfunction

REFERENCES

Cohen, H.C., and Arbel, E.R. Tachycardias and electrical pacing. Med. Clin. North Am., *60*:343–367, 1976.

Medtronic, Inc.: External Atrial Pacing Pulse Generator. Minneapolis, Medtronic 1976.

ASSESSING TEMPORARY PACEMAKER FUNCTION

OBJECTIVE

To provide a systematic method of assessing temporary pacemaker function, and to offer potential solutions.

SPECIAL EQUIPMENT

ECG recorder
Defibrillator

Emergency cart and medications

METHOD

ACTION	RATIONALE
1. Determine proper functioning of rate, current output, open circuit voltage pulse duration, and sensitivity. The function of a temporary or permanent pulse generator may be checked by using a specific pacing systems analyzer. (See the method for "Assessing Select Parameters of a Permanent Pacing System.")	
2. Check pacemaker's performance using "sense-pace" indicator.	
A. Note whether indicator needle is deflected to the right of center.	A. This indicates that a pacing stimulus has been delivered.
B. Note whether indicator needle is deflected to the left of center.	B. This indicates that an R wave has been sensed, thus inhibiting the pacemaker output for one cycle.
C. Note if there is absence of de-	C. This indicates approaching bat-

ACTION	RATIONALE
flection (or only slight deflection).	tery depletion. This forewarning occurs before pacemaker output characteristics are significantly affected.
D. Note if there are erratic deflections (or quivering about center).	D. This indicates external interference strong enough to inhibit the pacemaker output temporarily.
3. Perform pacemaker battery assessment.	
A. Turn on pacemaker and observe deflection on the "sense-pace" indicator.	A. No deflection (or only slight deflection) indicates that the battery is nearing depletion. This forewarning occurs before pacemaker output characteristics are significantly affected.
B. Facilitate battery replacement and enter in battery log record as required by hospital policy.	
C. Check battery for shelf-life expiration date prior to inserting into pacemaker; label appropriately.	C. Close monitoring of battery shelf-life expiration date is important for emergency life support equipment.
4. Check for failure to sense. This is illustrated by competitive pacing complexes (Fig. 62).	
A. Check connection site.	A. Poor connection of positive or indifferent pole may result in failure to sense.
B. Check that "pace/sense" needle deflects to right, showing pacing.	
C. Turn sensitivity dial to fully clockwise position and deter-	C. Sensitivity threshold can change with time.

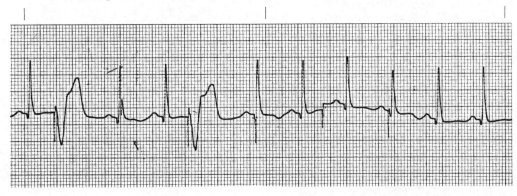

Figure 62. Example of failure to sense.

ACTION	RATIONALE
mine sensitivity threshold.	
D. Convert from bipolar to unipolar system (the method for "Conversion from Bipolar to Unipolar System with Temporary Pacing").	D. The unipolar system increases distance between the electrode and, in turn, increases ability to sense heart activity.
E. Provide defibrillator for immediate use.	E. Pacing spikes that occur in the vulnerable period can cause ventricular fibrillation.
F. Increase pacing rate above patient's heart rate to determine if pacemaker is operational when functioning in standby mode.	

5. Check for failure to pace. This is recognized by absence of pacing artifact on ECG recording at appropriate intervals (Figs. 63 and 64).

ACTION	RATIONALE
A. Check lead connector sites.	A. Poor connections may cause loss of pacing.
B. Check for battery depletion; change battery if indicated or change external pacemaker unit.	B. Battery depletion signals vary with different brands.
C. Check for ungrounded equipment as potential interfering electrical field.	C. Electrical interference may cause demand mode to function improperly and result in erratic deflections or no deflection of "sense/pace" indicator.

6. Check for failure to capture. This is recognized by presence of pacing artifact without an accompanying QRS complex (Fig. 65).

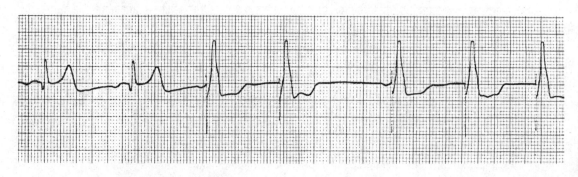

Figure 63. Example of failure to pace.

ACTION	RATIONALE

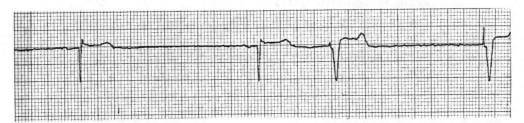

Figure 64. Example of failure to pace.

A. Check security of connections.

A. Poor connection of negative pole may cause intermittent or continuous loss of capture.

B. Increase ma.; evaluate threshold for stimulation.

B. Fibrosis and drug-induced changes in myocardium can alter threshold with time.

C. If lead is dislodged:
   (1) Notify physician of possible lead dislodgment. Repositioning of pacing electrode is usually indicated.
   (2) Occasionally lifting or repositioning patient's arm or turning patient to left side may serve as temporary method of forcing lead back into position.

D. Assess for pacing of diaphragm; this may be observed or palpated as muscle twitching in left lower chest with each paced beat.

D. With ventricular perforation, pacing may be unaffected, intermittent, or lost.

PRECAUTIONS

1. Provide defibrillator, emergency cart, and medications for immediate

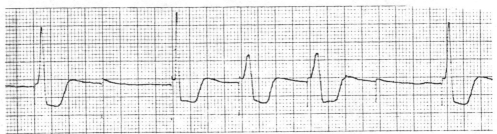

Figure 65. Example of failure to capture.

use. Pacemaker stimuli may inadvertently be delivered in vulnerable period, causing lethal dysrhythmias.
2. Wear rubber gloves when handling connector tips of pacing catheter electrode.
3. Follow electrical safety guidelines for patient with pacemakers.
4. Observe monitor carefully during threshold checking. Do not be distracted.

RELATED CARE

1. Monitor threshold profile daily. See the method for "Emergency Insertion of A Temporary Pacing Electrode (Assisting With)" for determining stimulation and sensitivity thresholds.
2. Perform site care daily; check external pacing electrode wire position and insulation; check security of catheter terminals within pacemaker connectors.
3. Assess pacemaker dressings for dryness. Change immediately if damp or wet.

COMPLICATIONS

Competitive dysrhythmias   Infection
Lethal dysrhythmias   Electromicroshock
Cardiac arrest   Equipment malfunction

REFERENCES

Hoechst Pharmaceuticals, Inc.: Cardiac Pacemaking: Directions in Cardiovascular Medicine. Somerville, N.J., Hoechst Pharmaceuticals, 1974, pp. 5–40.
Medtronic, Inc.: External Pacemaker. Minneapolis, Medtronic, 1976.
Peterson, C.R.: Temporary pacing: Indications, Techniques and Troubleshooting. Medtronic, Inc., no date.

PERMANENT PACEMAKER MANAGEMENT

Carolyn Chalkley, R.N., M.S.N.

OVERVIEW

An implanted cardiac pacing system is used in those instances which have potential risks for lethal dysrhythmias or altered electrodynamics and subsequent altered hemodynamics. (See the overview for "Temporary Pacemaker Management.")

Components of a permanent pacing system include a pulse generator and pacing catheter electrode. The pulse generator contains the energy source; this can be a lithium iodide battery, nuclear battery, or mercury-zinc oxide cells (Fig. 66). Some pulse generators have batteries that are rechargeable by means of a transcutaneous technique and the use of an external power source. The pacing electrode can be bipolar or unipolar. It may be positioned by using an endocardial implant through a transvenous approach, a myocardial implant using a thoracotomy approach, or an epicardial implant using a subcostal or subxyphoid approach.

This section will focus on select methods of permanent pacemaker management utilized within critical care. However, it is not intended to minimize nursing actions regarding patient responsibilities and follow-up pacemaker assessment. Such reinforcement teaching enhances patient retention and continuity of self-responsibilities. The transtelephonic transmission of a patient's ECG to the physician's office or manufacturer is an accurate method of determining pacemaker capture, sensing, dysrhythmia status, and rate, facilitating the need for planned or prompt hospitalization and/or medical intervention.

ASSESSING SELECT PARAMETERS OF A PERMANENT PACING SYSTEM

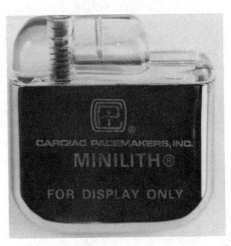

Figure 66. Permanent pacemaker. Courtesy of Cardiac Pacemakers, Inc.

OBJECTIVES

1. To determine proper functioning of the following parameters on a pulse generator: rate, current output, open circuit voltage, pulse duration, and sensitivity.
2. To determine the minimum intensity of a stimulus that causes depolarization of the heart via a permanently implanted pacing electrode.
3. To determine the adequacy of the intracavitary R wave signal to insure proper sensing by an implanted demand pulse generator.
4. To determine the integrity of the pacing electrode and its connection to a viable myocardium.

SPECIAL EQUIPMENT

Medtronic PSA Model 5300 (used for constant voltage fixed rate pacing)
Cordis PSA Model 290A
Pacemaker extension cable (used for constant current or constant voltage demand pacing)
ECG recorder
Defibrillator
Emergency cart and medications

METHOD

ACTION	RATIONALE
1. Establish ECG continuous recording.	
2. Determine proper functioning of the following parameters on a pulse generator: rate, current output, open circuit, voltage, pulse duration, and sensitivity.	
A. Using Medtronic PSA model 5300:	
(1) Connect test cable to PSA; do not remove pacing cable if continued pacing is desired.	
(a) Set PSA as follows if the patient requires pacing.	(a) When PSA is turned on it will pace patient on fixed rate throughout the testing method.
(1) Rate: 50	
(2) Current output: 6 ma.	

ACTION	RATIONALE

       (3)   Pulse duration: same as implanted pacemaker.

(2) Set function dial to the "pulse amplitude" position. Read and record the current in milliamperes indicated on the digital display.

    (a) The PSA will generally show a current reading higher than that indicated by the manufacturer of the pulse generator under test.

    (a) This variance occurs because the manufacturer measures the current at a point further into pulse than the 90-microsecond window of the PSA. Conversely, if the manufacturer measures the peak current of the generator at the leading edge of the pulse, the PSA will indicate a value up to 3% lower than the manufacturer's specifications.

(3) Check for proper sensing.

(3) When the R wave test switch is depressed, the PSA emits a train of 4.0-millivolt R waves at a rate of approximately 150 ppm. The simulated R waves should cause a ventricular-inhibited pulse generator to inhibit.

    (a) Switch function dial to "pulse amplitude" position.

       (1) Depress the R wave test switch.

       (2) Observe for a zero reading on the digital display in a ventricular-inhibited pulse generator.

       (2) This indicates proper sensing.

    (b) Set function selector to "pulse interval"

ACTION   **RATIONALE**

position to test a ven-
tricular-triggered or
atrial-triggered pulse
generator.

(1) Observe for
rhythmic display
of the normal in-
terval of the pulse
generator.

(2) Depress the R
wave button to
increase the rate
to the pacemaker
limit.

(3) Observe that dis-
play will change
from the normal
reading to ap-
proximately 500
milliseconds.

(4) Observe that R
reading will con-
tinue to flash off
and on rhyth-
mically.

(5) Observe for nor-
mal reading when
the button is re-
leased.

(4) Turn function dial to the
"pulse interval" position.
Read and record the interval in milliseconds indi-
cated on the digital
display.

(5) Turn function dial to
"pulse width" position.
Read and record pulse
width in milliseconds.

B. Using Cordis PSA Model
290A:

(1) Connect pacer test cable
to PSA and pacer to be
tested.

(2) Turn mode switch to
"pacer output or sensing."

ACTION   **RATIONALE**

    (a)   Program pacemaker to a high output prior to testing a Cordis Omni pacemaker.

(3)   Turn on PSA.

(4)   Push rate button; read digital display and record.

(5)   Push current output button; read digital display and record.

(6)   Push open circuit voltage button; read digital display and record.

(7)   Push pulse duration button; read digital display and record.

(8)   Push sensitivity button; increase the pacer sensitivity dial slowly while observing the digital display on screen of PSA.

    (a)   Determine pacer sensitivity; this is the last number seen before the screen reads 000.

3.   Perform stimulation threshold assessment.

     3.   This determines the minimum intensity of a stimulus that causes depolarization of the heart via a permanently implanted pacing electrode.

    A.   Using Medtronic PSA 5300 (Fig. 67).

      (1)   Set PSA as follows.

         (a)   Output: 5 V.

         (b)   Pulse width: at pulse width of implantable pulse generator.

         (c)   Rate: 10 beats per minute (bpm) above patient's rate.

         (d)   Function: off.

      (2)   Connect nonsterile end of pacemaker extension cable to PSA; sterile end of pacemaker extension cable will be connected to implanted lead.

ACTION	RATIONALE
(3) Turn PSA function dial to threshold.	
(a) Turn off external pulse generator, if used.	(a) This prevents competition between the two pulse generators.
(4) Decrease output gradually until capture is lost.	
(5) Increase output until capture is regained.	(5) Threshold is the minimum electrical stimulus required to cause depolarization.
(6) Record output (voltage threshold) and digital display (current threshold).	
B. Using Cordis PSA Model 290:	

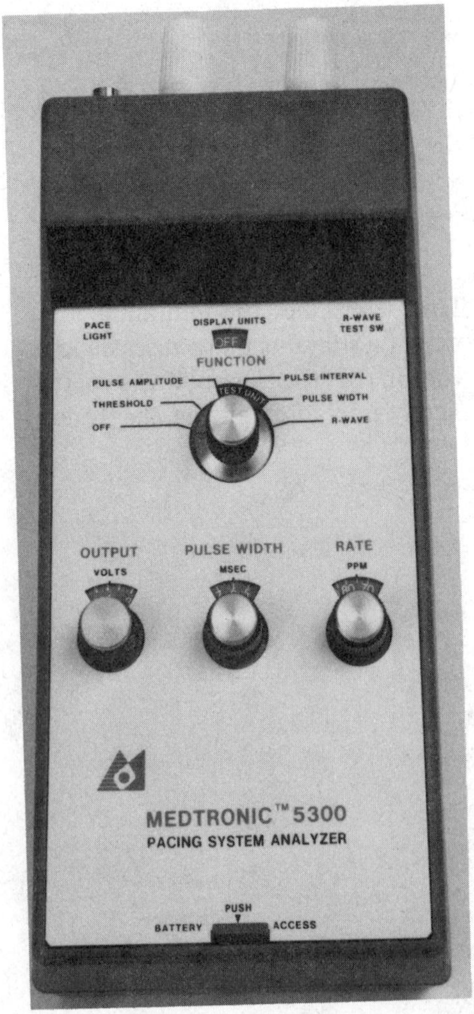

Figure 67. Pacing system analyzer. Courtesy of Medtronic, Inc., Minneapolis, Minn.

ACTION	RATIONALE
(1) Set up PSA as follows.	
(a) Rate: 70 or 10 bpm greater than patient's rate.	
(b) Pulse duration: same as pulse duration of implantable pacemaker.	
(c) Pacing threshold: 6 ma.	
(d) Mode: constant current or constant voltage, depending upon type of implantable unit.	
(2) Connect nonsterile end of cable to PSA; sterile end of cable will be connected to implanted lead.	
(3) Turn off external pulse generator, if used.	(3) This prevents competition between the two pulse generators.
(4) Turn PSA on. PSA will now pace on demand at the settings dialed in step 3-B-(1).	
(5) Determine voltage threshold by setting mode switch to "constant voltage;" depress voltage threshold button.	
(6) Determine current threshold by turning mode switch to "constant current"; depress current threshold button.	
(7) Observe ECG for capture continuously; turn down pacing threshold dial slowly until capture is lost.	
(8) Turn up pacing threshold dial until capture is regained.	(8) Threshold is the minimum electrical stimulus required to cause depolarization.
(9) Record reading on digital display.	
(a) Voltage threshold will	

ACTION

RATIONALE

read in millivolts
(mV.).
(b) Current threshold will
read in milliamps
(ma.).

4. Perform sensing threshold assessment.

    A. Using Medtronic PSA Model
5300:
    (1) Set up PSA as follows.
      (a) Output: 5 V.
      (b) Pulse width: at pulse
width of implantable
unit.
      (c) Rate: 10 bpm above
patient's rate.
      (d) Function: off.
    (2) Connect nonsterile end to
PSA; sterile end of extension cable will be connected to implanted lead.
    (3) Turn PSA function to
"R wave"; turn off external pulse generator, if
in use.
    (4) Depress R wave test switch
for 4 or 5 seconds.

    (5) Record digital reading;
this should be twice the
sensitivity of the pulse generator to be implanted.
    B. Using Cordis PSA Model
290A:
    (1) Set up PSA as follows.
      (a) Rate: 70.
      (b) Pulse duration: same

4. This determines the adequacy of the
intracavitary R wave signal to insure
proper sensing by an implanted pulse
generator.

    (3) This prevents competitive
rhythms and allows the
PSA to sense the patient's
natural beats.
    (4) Note that Medtronic PSA
operates at a fixed rate and
may cause competitive
rhythms. Further, a PSA
does not pace when the R
wave test switch is depressed. Monitor patient
closely for hemodynamic
deterioration when this
switch is depressed.

    (1) Patient may be demand-
paced immediately before
and after the sensing pro-

ACTION	RATIONALE
as pulse duration of implantable unit. (c) Pacing threshold: 6 ma. (d) Mode: constant current or constant voltage.	cedure at the parameters set by returning the PSA to pacing mode (constant voltage or constant current.
(2) Connect nonsterile end of cable to PSA; sterile end of cable will be connected to implanted lead.	
(3) Turn off external pulse generator, if used.	(3) This prevents competition between the two pulse generators and allows the PSA to sense the patient's natural beats.
(4) Turn PSA on. PSA will now pace on demand at settings dialed in 4-B-(1).	
(5) Turn mode dial to "sensing threshold."	(5) This automatically converts the pacing to 30 bpm, 10 ma., 1.0 msec pulse duration.
(6) Observe for hemodynamic deterioration if patient does not have intrinsic rate great enough to maintain cardiac output. If patient's rate is less than 30 beats per minute, the R wave cannot be sensed with this method.	
(7) Push sensing button.	
(8) Turn sensing threshold dial up until green sense light goes out and red output light comes on.	
(9) Record digital display; this value should be twice the sensitivity of the implantable unit.	
(10) Return mode dial to "constant current" or "constant voltage" to resume pacing at rate, ma., and pulse duration set in step 4-B-(1).	

ACTION	RATIONALE

5. Perform lead impedance (resistance) assessment.

    A. Using Medtronic PSA Model 5300:

      (1) Set lower three dials of PSA as follows.

        (a) Output dial: 5 volts.

        (b) Pulse width: at pulse width of implantable pulse generator.

        (c) Rate dial: at least 10 bpm above the patient's intrinsic rate.

        (d) PSA: off.

      (2) Turn function dial to "threshold" position and observe current reading on digital display. The reading should be between 7.1 ma. (700 ohms) and 16.7 ma. (300 ohms), except on small-tipped electrodes which exhibit a higher normal resistance value (example: 1000 ohms). Verify readings with manufacturer's specification for lead being tested. Convert ma. reading into ohms, using Table 1.

5. This determines the integrity of the pacing electrode and its connection to a viable myocardium.

      (1) With these settings, the voltage delivered to the implanted lead system is directly adjustable by the output dial. The current delivered into the lead system, which is a function of the lead system resistance and heart tissue, is displayed on the digital readout.

      (2) Current values less than 7.1 ma. may indicate poor electrical integrity (example: fractured lead). Erratic current readings may be due to fractured lead, loose connection between lead and PSA, or unstable electrode position. High resistance may indicate excessive fibrosis around lead.

TABLE 1.

Ohms	Milliamperes*
2000	2.5
1000	5
833	6
714	7
625	8
555	9
500	10
454	11

ACTION   RATIONALE

TABLE 1.   Continued.

Ohms	Milliamperes*
417	12
384	13
357	14
333	15
313	16
294	17
277	18
263	19
260	20
238	21
227	22
217	23
208	24
200	25

*As indicated on PSA digital display.

B. Using Cordis PSA Model 290A:

(1) Set PSA as follows.
  (a) Rate: 70.
  (b) Current output: 6 ma.
  (c) Pulse duration: same as implanted unit.

(1) Patient may be paced on demand at the settings before and after testing of lead impedance to maintain cardiac output.

(2) Connect nonsterile end of cable to the PSA; sterile end of extension cable will be connected to the implanted lead.

(3) Turn on PSA.

(4) Turn mode switch to "constant current."

(5) Press current threshold button.

(6) Turn pacing threshold dial to 1.0.

(6) The procedure must be performed quickly if patient is pacer-dependent and threshold is greater than 1.

(7) Press voltage threshold button.

ACTION	RATIONALE
(8) Record digital reading by moving decimal point three places to right as follows: (a) If reading is 0.5— resistance is 500 ohms. (b) If reading is 1.2— resistance is 1200 ohms.	
(9) Verify readings with manufacturer's specification for the lead being tested.	(9) Low resistance may indicate lead fracture. High resistance may indicate excessive fibrosis around electrode.

PRECAUTIONS

1. Provide defibrillator, emergency cart, and medications for immediate use.
2. Follow electrical safety guidelines for patients with pacemakers.

RELATED CARE

Monitor patient's ECG and hemodynamic responses during select assessment/reprogramming of permanent pacemaker.

COMPLICATIONS

Lethal dysrhythmias	Electromicroshock
Cardiac arrest	Equipment malfunction

SUPPLIERS

Cordis Corporation
Medtronic, Inc.

REFERENCES

Cordis Corporation: Technical Manual for Pacemaker Systems Analyzer Model 290A. Miami, Cordis, 1976.

Medtronic, Inc.: Technical Manual for Pacemaker Systems Analyzer Model 5300. Minneapolis, Medtronic, 1976.

Parsonnett, V., et al.: Implantable cardiac pacemakers: Status report and resource guideline. Circulation, 50:A–21, 1974.

INHIBITION OF PERMANENT PACEMAKER

OBJECTIVE

To assess the patient's underlying cardiac rhythm by inhibiting permanent pacing temporarily through the use of an external temporary pacemaker.

SPECIAL EQUIPMENT

Temporary external pacemaker
Pacemaker extension cable
  with alligator clips
Suction cup electrode

ECG recorder
Defibrillator
Emergency cart and medications

METHOD

ACTION	RATIONALE
1. Locate the pulse generator by inspection or gentle palpation.	
2. Obtain initial ECG recording.	2. This serves as baseline data.
3. Determine model of pulse generator. This information may be found on patient's I.D. card, earlier charts, or by x-ray identification of pulse generator.	3. The effectiveness of this method will depend upon the model of pulse generator and the distance between skin surface and pacing system; therefore, it cannot be used in all patients.
4. Apply suction cups to patient.	
A. If unipolar pacemaker is used, place one suction cup over pulse generator and another over tip of electrode.	
B. If bipolar pacemaker is used, place one suction cup over tip of electrode and other suction cup approximately 1 inch above and to the right (over the ring or proximal electrode).	
5. Connect suction cups to temporary external pacemaker, using extension cable (Fig. 68).	
A. Use positive clip connected to suction cup over pulse generator or proximal electrode.	

ACTION   RATIONALE

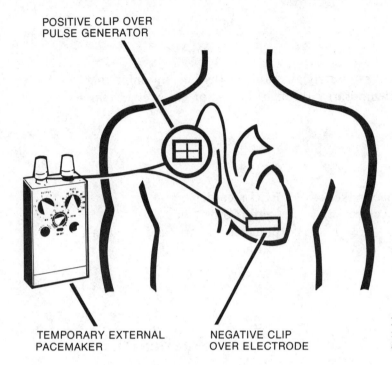

POSITIVE CLIP OVER
PULSE GENERATOR

TEMPORARY EXTERNAL   NEGATIVE CLIP
PACEMAKER   OVER ELECTRODE

Figure 68. Inhibition of permanent pacemaker using a temporary external pacemaker.

B. Use negative clip connected to suction cup over distal electrode.

6. Set sensitivity control of temporary external pacemaker on fixed rate.

7. Set rate of temporary external pacemaker at a value slightly higher than rate of the implanted unit; set amplitude at 4 ma. or higher, if necessary to inhibit permanent pacing.

8. Turn on temporary external pacemaker.

8. The external pulses will inhibit the implanted pacemaker completely or partially, depending upon the type of pacemaker.

9. Record and assess ECG in usual fashion.

9. Patient's own beats can be evaluated for change in the ECG which may not be evident during paced rhythm.

10. Disconnect the temporary external pacemaker.

11. Reprogramming to a lower rate may be done if patient's own heart rate is only slightly less than that of implanted pacemaker or if pacemaker cannot be inhibited by this method.

PRECAUTIONS

1. Follow electrical safety guidelines for patients with pacemakers.
2. Provide defibrillator, emergency cart, and medications for immediate use.

RELATED CARE

Monitor patient's hemodynamic responses.

COMPLICATIONS

Cardiac arrest   Altered Hemodynamics
Dysrhythmias   Equipment malfunction
Electromicroshock

SUPPLIERS

Cordis Corporation
Medtronic, Inc.

REFERENCES

Cordis Corporation: Technical Manual for Pacemaker Systems Analyzer Model 290A. Miami, Cordis, 1976.
Medtronic, Inc.: Technical Manual for Pacemaker Systems Analyzer Model 5300. Minneapolis, Medtronic, 1976.
Parsonnett, V., et al.: Implantable cardiac pacemakers: Status report and resource guideline. Circulation, *50*:A–21, 1974.

REPROGRAMMING A PERMANENT PACEMAKER _____

OBJECTIVE

To change the rate, current output, sensitivity, or pulse duration of a permanent pacemaker when there is a change in the patient's condition, using a pacemaker reprogrammer.

SPECIAL EQUIPMENT

Pacemaker programmer
(Fig. 69)
ECG recorder

Defibrillator
Emergency cart and medications

METHOD

ACTION	RATIONALE
1. Adjust programmer to desired settings (see manufacturer's specification manual).	1. Parameters which may be programmed vary among manufacturers.
2. Locate pulse generator by inspection or gentle palpation.	
3. Place programmer over reed switch	

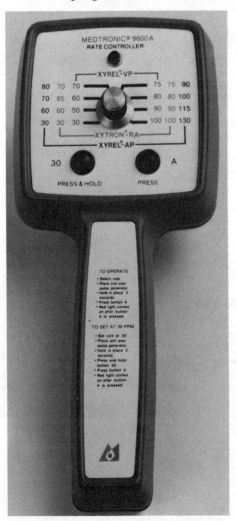

Figure 69. Programmer for a permanent pacemaker. Courtesy of Medtronic Inc., Minneapolis, Minn.

ACTION	RATIONALE

of pulse generator and activate programmer. Programmer must be
within 1 inch of the reed switch
of the pulse generator.
4. Verify change in rate by assessing
ECG.

PRECAUTIONS

1. Provide defibrillator, emergency cart, and medications for immediate
use.
2. Follow electrical safety guidelines for patients with pacemakers.

RELATED CARE

Monitor patient's ECG and hemodynamic responses during select
assessment/reprogramming of permanent pacemaker.

COMPLICATIONS

Lethal dysrhythmias	Electromicroshock
Cardiac arrest	Equipment malfunction

SUPPLIERS

Cordis Corporation
CPI
Medtronic, Inc.
Intermedics

REFERENCES

Cordis Corporation: Tehnical Manual for Pacemaker Systems Analyzer Model
290A. Miami, Cordis, 1976.
Medtronic, Inc.: Tehnical Manual for Pacemaker Systems Analyzer Model
5300. Minneapolis, Medtronic, 1976.
Parsonnett, V., et al.: Implantable cardiac pacemakers: Status report and resource
guideline. Circulation, *50*:A–21, 1974.

USE OF A MAGNET

OBJECTIVE

To temporarily convert a permanent demand pacemaker to fixed rate
through the use of a magnet for such purposes as determining pacing
rate, appropriate capture, or overriding dysrhythmias.

SPECIAL EQUIPMENT

Appropriate pacemaker magnet, supplied by same manufacturer as
pacemaker
ECG recorder
Defibrillator
Emergency cart and medications

METHOD

ACTION	RATIONALE
1. Initiate continuous ECG recording.	1. This provides baseline data.

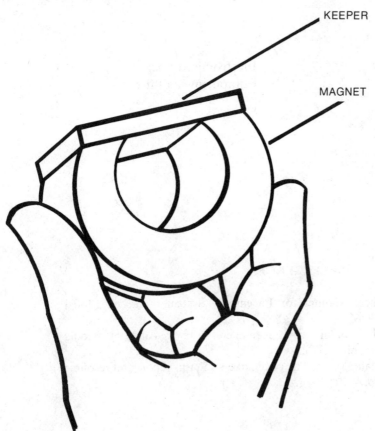

KEEPER

MAGNET

Figure 70. Keeper with magnet.

ACTION	RATIONALE
2. Remove keeper from magnet. (Fig. 70).	2. Keeper protects magnet until external application.
3. Apply magnet externally directly over the reed switch of the pulse generator (Fig. 71).	
A. Place the magnet within one inch of the pulse generator (Fig. 72).	A. This activates the reed switch.
B. Determine that the magnet is aligned parallel to the connectors of the pulse generator.	B. This activates the reed switch.
4. Maintain correct magnet position until pacemaker spikes are observed on the ECG recording.	
5. Examine ECG strip for pacemaker spike and appropriate capture.	5. Each pacemaker spike falling outside the retractory period should be followed immediately by a paced depolarization.
6. Remove magnet; apply keeper.	
7. Assess patient's ECG rhythm post-magnet application.	
8. Turn off ECG recorder.	

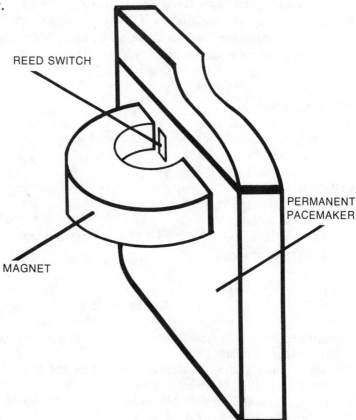

REED SWITCH

PERMANENT
PACEMAKER

MAGNET

Figure 71. Positioning magnet over reed switch. (Position of reed switch varies among manufacturers.)

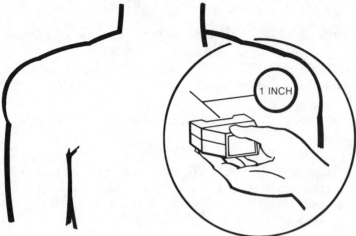

Figure 72. Placement of magnet within 1 inch of pulse generator.

PRECAUTIONS

1. Follow electrical safety guidelines for patients with pacemakers.
2. Provide defibrillator, emergency cart, and medications for immediate use.
3. Note that some pacemakers exhibit a 20% increase in rate when the magnet is applied.
4. Observe for competitive rhythms, ventricular tachycardia or ventricular fibrillation caused by fixed rate ventricular pacing.
5. Remove magnet immediately if competitive rhythms occur.
6. Protect against reed switch breakage by using only a magnet supplied by the pacemaker manufacturer.

RELATED CARE

Monitor patient's hemodynamic responses.

COMPLICATIONS

Cardiac arrest
Dysrhythmias
Electromicroshock

Altered hemodynamics
Equipment malfunction

REFERENCES

Cordis Corporation: Technical Manual for Pacemaker Systems Analyzer Model 290A. Miami, Cordis, 1976.

Medtronic, Inc.: Technical Manual for Pacemaker Systems Analyzer Model 5300. Minneapolis, Medtronic, 1976.

Parsonnett, V., et al.: Implantable cardiac pacemakers: Status report and resource guideline. Circulation, *50*:A–21, 1974.

NONINVASIVE PERIPHERAL VASCULAR
BLOOD FLOW MEASUREMENT

Karen Wheelock, R.N., M.A.

OVERVIEW

Monitoring changes in blood flow of the peripheral vascular system can often be accomplished through inspection, palpation, and auscultatory assessment. In persons with altered hemodynamics or acute onset of circulatory impairment due to thrombus, embolus, or spasms, the development of noninvasive peripheral vascular blood flow devices has enhanced the quality of obtaining data for rapid diagnosis of the patency and/or status of arteriovenous systems. An ultrasound blood flow detector consists of an ultrasound probe, stethoscope, and amplifier that assists in detecting pulses, blood pressure, and/or their alterations. A strain gauge Plethysmograph is an electronic measurement of blood volume flow in peripheral vessels and digital pulse volume in extremities. A pulse volume recorder (PVR) measures blood volume changes at select areas on extremities, using an inflatable cuff and an oscillometer. Data derived from these studies often provide meaningful contributions for more definitive therapy.

ULTRASOUND BLOOD FLOW DETECTOR

OBJECTIVES

1. To detect blood flow in arterial and venous systems of the periphery.
2. To obtain blood pressure readings when conventional auscultation is not reliable.
3. To aid in diagnosis and assessment of peripheral vascular problems.
4. To evaluate treatment of peripheral vascular problems.

SPECIAL EQUIPMENT

Ultrasound probe with stethoscope of automatic speaker amplifier (Fig. 73).
Ultrasound transmission gel

METHOD

ACTION	RATIONALE

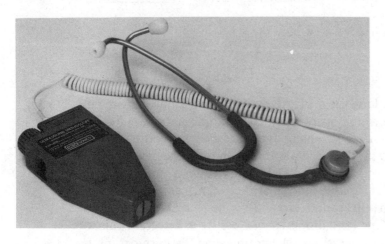

Figure 73. Ultrasound probe with stethoscope. Courtesy of Medsonics, Inc., Mountain View, Cal.

1. Apply ultrasound transmission gel to faceplate of probe.

2. Position probe on skin surface over the vessel; tilt probe slightly toward the axis of blood flow.

2. Tilting the probe produces a better signal.

3. Auscultate for arterial sound.
   A. Normal arterial sound is a loud, high pitched systolic sound with one or more softer, lower pitched diastolic sounds. These sounds are repeated with each cardiac cycle.

   A. The rapid forward blood flow in systole, a lesser reverse flow in early diastole, and slight forward flow late in diastole produces this auscultatory sound.

   B. Normal venous sound is cyclic with respirations, higher pitched on expiration, and resembles a windstorm.

4. Obtain blood pressure using an ultrasound blood flow detector, if desired.
   A. Use conventional method, substituting prelubricated ultrasound probe for regular stethoscope.
   B. Adjust volume as necessary.
   C. Inflate cuff until arterial sound disappears; release cuff pressure slowly while checking for systolic and diastolic pressures.

PRECAUTIONS

1. Avoid using probe in the vicinity of the eye due to risk of damaging delicate nerve tissue.
2. Diastolic pressure is difficult to detect in critically ill patients.
3. Clean ultrasound probe as directed by manufacturer to prevent face plate surface scratching; do not autoclave.
4. Avoid using alcohol as a transmission gel or to clean face plate of probe.

RELATED CARE

1. Integrate data with other information from circulation assessment.
2. Turn off instrument following each use to preserve battery life.
3. Check volume control and/or battery if no auscultatory signal is elicited. Replace battery a minimum of every 6 months.

COMPLICATIONS

Nerve tissue damage (with high intensity ultrasound)
Altered skin integrity
Equipment malfunction

SUPPLIERS

Corbin-Farnsworth
Medsonics Laboratories
Parks Electronics

REFERENCES

Dean, R.H., and Yas, J.S.: Hemodynamic measurements in peripheral vascular disease. Curr. Prob. Surg., *13*:1, 1976.

Felix, W.R., Jr., Sigel, B., and Popky, G.L.: Doppler ultrasound in diagnosis of peripheral vascular disease. Semin. Roentgenol., *10*:315, 1975.

Jarrett, F., and Detmer, D.E.: The use of noninvasive vascular studies in the diagnosis of peripheral vascular disease. Wis. Med. J. *76*:88, 1977.

Raines, J.K., Dir.: Criteria, Procedures, and Instrumentation for the Clinical Vascular Laboratory. Greenwich, CT, Life Sciences, Inc., Pamphlet developed by Vascular Laboratory, Dept. of Surgery, Massachusetts General Hospital, 1975.

Raines, J.K., Darling, R.C., Buth, J., Brewster, D., and Austen, W.G.: Vascular laboratory criteria for the management of peripheral vascular disease of the lower extremities. Surgery, *79*:21, 1976.

Soulen, R.L.: Doppler ultrasound in vascular disease. Int. Surg., *62*:298, 1977.

PULSE VOLUME RECORDER

OBJECTIVES

1. To detect blood volume change in the extremities.
2. To obtain systolic pressure readings in the extremities.
3. To aid in diagnosis and assessment of peripheral vascular problems, both arterial and venous.

SPECIAL EQUIPMENT

Pulse volume recorder (PVR), portable or cart model (Fig. 74)

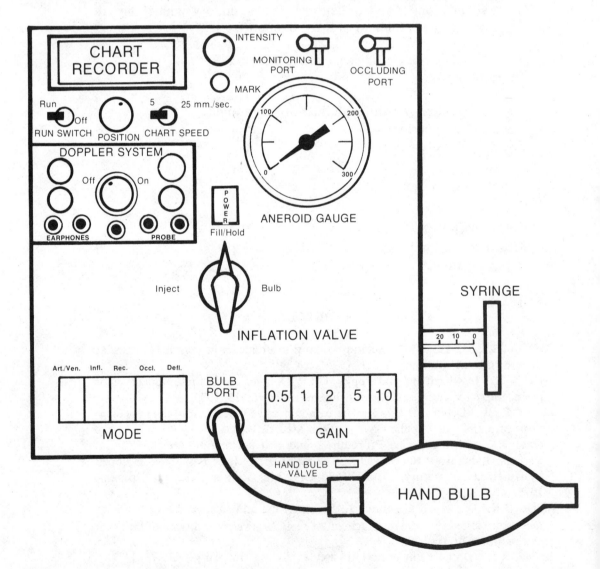

Figure 74. Pulse volume recorder.

Blood pressure cuffs:
    Thigh cuffs for above the knee
    Regular adult cuffs for upper arm, forearm, calf, and ankle
    Pediatric cuff for foot measurements

METHOD

ACTION	RATIONALE
1. Select appropriate cuff for site and place on extremity.	
2. Connect cuff to monitor port.	
3. Select inflation mode. Turn inflation valve to "bulb"; inflate cuff to arbitrary pressure.	3. Using an arbitrary pressure setting provides for constant cuff volume around the extremity from reading to reading.
A. Use valve to inflate large cuffs; usually about 65 mm. Hg. is required.	
B. Use syringe to inflate smaller cuffs.	
4. Check for the following.	4. If these criteria are not met, the cuff should be reapplied.
A. Approximately 400 ± 50 ml. of air is needed to inflate a thigh cuff to 65 mm. Hg.	
B. Approximately 75 ± 10 ml. of air is needed to inflate a calf cuff.	
5. Turn inflation valve to "fill/hold"; depress record button.	
6. Obtain chart recording.	
A. Turn run switch with the gain at 1.0 and the speed at 25 mm./second.	A. Machine is calibrated so that a 1.0 mm. Hg. change equals a 20 mm. deflection on the chart.
B. Record at least three consecutive and consistent cycles.	
7. Deflate cuff by pushing deflate button.	
8. Record systolic limb pressure (optional).	
A. Connect ultrasound blood flow probe to PVR; position over vessel.	
B. Inflate cuff to 20 mm. Hg. above brachial artery systolic pressure.	

ACTION	RATIONALE

    C.   Deflate cuff slowly, using valve on hand bulb.

    D.   Auscultate for systolic pressure, pressure at which ultrasound signal is first heard.

9.   Measure systolic and diastolic pressures with PVR (optional).

    A.   Place an occluding cuff proximal to the monitoring cuff.

    B.   Read lower limb systolic pressure at site of occlusive cuff when its pressure obliterates recordings from monitoring cuff.

    C.   Observe increase in amplitude of oscillation cuff. Pressure is slowly released from occlusion cuff.

    D.   Read diastolic pressure at the point at which maximum excursions occur.

PRECAUTIONS

1.   Monitor for cuff error.

    A.   At higher monitoring cuff pressures, distortion of recorded pulse wave form occurs.

    B.   Ideally, monitoring cuff pressure should be below limb diastolic pressure.

RELATED CARE

1.   Assess circulation of extremity prior to and after the diagnostic test.

2.   Integrate data with other information derived from circulation assessment.

COMPLICATIONS

Altered skin integrity
Equipment malfunction

SUPPLIERS

Life Sciences, Inc.

REFERENCES

Darling, R.C., Raines, J.K., Brenner, B.J., and Austen, W.G.: Quantitative segmental pulse volume recorder: A clinical tool. Surgery, 72:873, 1972.

Dean, R.H., and Yas, J.S.: Hemodynamic measurements in peripheral vascular disease. Curr. Probl. Surg., 13:1, 1976.

Jarrett, F., and Detmer, D.E.: The use of noninvasive vascular studies in the diagnosis of peripheral vascular disease. Wis. Med. J., 76:88, 1977.

Raines, J.K.: Criteria, Procedures, and Instrumentation for the Clinical Vascular Laboratory. Greenwich, CT, Life Sciences, Inc. Pamphlet developed by Vascular Laboratory, Dept. of Surgery, Massachusetts General Hospital, 1975.

Raines, J.K., Darling, R.C., Buth, J., Brewster, D., and Austen, W.G.: Vascular laboratory criteria for the management of peripheral vascular disease of the lower extremities. Surgery, 79:21, 1976.

STRAIN GAUGE PLETHYSMOGRAPHY

OBJECTIVES

1. To detect volume flow in the extremities.
2. To aid in diagnosis and assessment of peripheral vascular disease.

SPECIAL EQUIPMENT

Strain gauges
Special blood pressure cuff
Plethysmograph recorder

METHOD

ACTION	RATIONALE
1. Place select cuff at identified sites on larger extremity where a pressure reading will be taken; upper thigh, above knee, below knee, or ankle (Fig. 75).	
2. Place elastic strain gauge around digit.	
3. Turn on recorder; observe wave form.	3. This provides baseline data.
4. Inflate cuff until recorded pulses disappear. Gradually deflate cuff	4. At this point cuff pressure is equal to systolic pressure.

ACTION	RATIONALE

until small pulsations appear with each heartbeat.

5. Turn off recorder.

6. Complete systolic pressure measurements at four sites on each lower extremity: upper thigh, above knee, below the knee, and ankle, following steps 1 through 5.

7. Check for normal pressure gradients (see Fig. 75).

   A. High thigh: 170 mm. Hg.
   B. Above knee: 170 mm. Hg.
   C. Below knee: 170 mm. Hg.
   D. Ankle: 150 mm. Hg.

7. Pressure differences of 30 mm. Hg. or more indicate obstructive disease in the artery. Ankle pressure is normally within 15 mm. of brachial artery systolic pressure. Upper thigh pressure is normally 20 mm. or more above brachial artery systolic pressure.

PRECAUTIONS

Check for cuff errors; an extreme pressure gradient exists across an obstruction.

RELATED CARE

1. Determine the brachial artery and ankle pressures through a screening test.

2. Assess circulation of extremity prior to and after the diagnostic test.

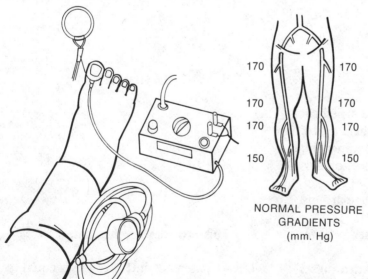

170   170
170   170
170   170
150   150

NORMAL PRESSURE
GRADIENTS
(mm. Hg)

Figure 75. Mercury strain gauge plethysmograph.

3. Integrate with other information derived from circulation assessment.

COMPLICATIONS

Altered skin integrity
Equipment malfunction

SUPPLIERS

Parks Electronics

REFERENCES

Dean, R.H., and Yas, J.S.: Hemodynamic measurements in peripheral vascular disease. Curr. Probl. Surg., *13*:1, 1976.

Felix, W.R., Jr., Sigel, B., and Popky, G.L.: Doppler ultrasound in diagnosis of peripheral vascular disease. Semin. Roentgenol. *10*:315, 1975.

Jarrett, F., and Detmer, D.E.: The use of non-invasive vascular studies in the diagnosis of peripheral vascular disease. Wis. Med. J., *76*:88, 1977.

Raines, J.K.: Criteria, Procedures, and Instrumentation for the Clinical Vascular Laboratory. Greenwich, Conn., Life Sciences, Inc., 1975. Pamphlet developed by Vascular Laboratory, Dept. of Surgery, Massachusetts General Hospital.

Raines, J.K., Darling, R.C., Buth, J., Brewster, D., and Austen, W.G.: Vascular laboratory criteria for the management of peripheral vascular disease of the lower extremities. Surgery, *79*:21, 1976.

ROTATING TOURNIQUETS

Karen Wheelock, R.N., M.A.

OVERVIEW

Rotating tourniquet therapy is one of many therapeutic interventions frequently prescribed in the medical emergency of pulmonary edema. By rotating tourniquets on extremities systematically, venous return to the heart is decreased. Automatic devices for sequential rotation are available, or the therapy may be performed manually. Application, monitoring, and assessment of clinical response during therapy, as well as the proper discontinuation of therapy and assessment of the effects of altered hemodynamics, are major components of the method.

OBJECTIVES

1. To decrease circulating volume in such instances as acute pulmonary edema or severe congestive heart failure.
2. To provide temporary support therapy until additional definitive treatment is initiated.

SPECIAL EQUIPMENT

Automatic rotating tourniquet equipment, *or*
Four wide, soft rubber tourniquets
Four soft pads

METHOD

ACTION	RATIONALE
1. Place patient in semi-Fowler's position.	
2. Obtain baseline blood pressure reading.	
3. Select mode for rotating tourniquet therapy.	
A. Automatic rotating tourniquets:	
(1) Place cuffs high on appropriate extremity.	
(2) Secure air tubes to valves located on portable auto-	

ACTION	RATIONALE

matic rotating tourniquet equipment.

(3)   Close all outlet valves.

(4)   Adjust cuff release timer to the prescribed cycle length; multiply time selected by 3 to determine total length of time each cuff is to be inflated.

(4)   Length of inflation is individualized and prescribed by physician.

(5)   Set pressure to be maintained in the cuffs just above patient's diastolic pressure, using pressure control knob.

(5)   This ensures impedance to venous return without interfering with arterial supply to the extremity.

(6)   Activate alarm system.

(6)   This permits an audible signal and a red alarm light to go on if machine fails to rotate cuffs or if there is an air leak.

(7)   Open valves, one at a time, observing effect on patient.

(7)   Machine will automatically inflate and deflate cuffs in rotation.

(8)   Monitor blood pressure frequently.
   (a)   Close valve to one of arm cuffs when deflated.
   (b)   Disconnect air tube from valve.
   (c)   Connect an aneroid sphygmometer to cuff.
   (d)   Obtain blood pressure.
   (e)   Reconnect to air tubing; open valve.

(8)   Use of rotating tourniquets may precipitate hypotension in some patients.

(9)   Facilitate safe transport and therapy, when necessary.
   (a)   Close all four valves.

   (b)   Leave cuffs connected and in place.
   (c)   Turn off power.

   (a)   This maintains pressure in three of the four cuffs.

   (c)   Never leave cuffs inflated longer than 45 minutes.

ACTION	RATIONALE
(d) Transfer patient to cart.	
(e) Turn on power; open valves.	
(f) Check and adjust pressure, as needed.	
(10) Discontinue therapy when prescribed. Close valve and disconnect air hose from cuff as each cuff deflates in a rotating fashion.	(10) This permits gradual return of trapped blood into systemic circulation.
B. Manual rotating tourniquets:	
(1) Place pads and tourniquets high on three extremities; position fourth pad and tourniquet next to, but not on, the fourth extremity.	
(2) Palpate arterial pulses in three extremities while tourniquets are in place.	(2) Tourniquets should not obliterate arterial pulses.
(3) Rotate tourniquets in a clockwise manner every 15 minutes (Fig. 76).	(3) Tourniquets should not be left in place on any extremity for longer than 45 minutes.
(a) Remove first tourniquet and apply tourniquet to fourth extremity.	
(b) Continue to rotate tourniquets in a clockwise manner every 15 minutes.	

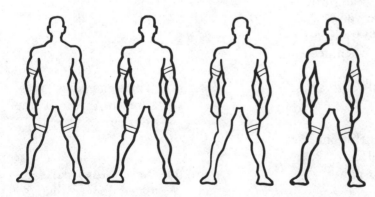

Figure 76. Pattern of 15-minute rotation of tourniquets.

BEGIN   FIRST ROTATION SECOND ROTATION   THIRD ROTATION

ACTION	RATIONALE
(4) Monitor blood pressure by placing cuff on arm that is tourniquet-free.	(4) Use of rotating tourniquets may precipitate hypotension in some patients.
(5) Discontinue therapy when prescribed; remove one at a time, at same time intervals, and in same clockwise rotation.	(5) This permits gradual return of trapped blood into systemic circulation.

4. Monitor patient status during and after therapy.

PRECAUTIONS

1. Assess extremities frequently for the presence of an arterial pulse and skin integrity. It is anticipated that discoloration and temperature change will occur in the extremity while treatment is in progress.
2. Closely monitor the total length of time venous flow is impeded. Never leave cuffs inflated or tourniquets in place on an extremity for longer than 45 minutes at any time.
3. Do not remove all tourniquets at once since this offers a high risk for circulatory overload and/or Pulmonary Edema.
4. Use of rotating tourniquets may precipitate hypotension in some patients.
5. Have emergency life support equipment available, if needed.

RELATED CARE

1. Assist in continuity of tourniquet rotation by keeping a diagram and times of rotation at bedside.
2. Facilitate pharmacologic therapy as prescribed by physician.

COMPLICATIONS

Hypotension   Peripheral ischemia
Cardiac/respiratory arrest   Altered skin integrity

SUPPLIERS

Kidde Rotating Tourniquets
R.P. Scherer Rotating Tourniquets

REFERENCES

Brunner, L.S., and Smith, D.S.: Textbook of Medical-Surgical Nursing, 3rd ed. Philadelphia, J.B. Lippincott, 1975, pp. 397–398.

Luckmann, J., and Sorensen, K.C.: Medical-Surgical Nursing: A Psychophysiologic Approach, 2nd ed. Philadelphia, W.B. Saunders, 1980.

Mercy Methods of Care. Procedure Manual. Cedar Rapids, Iowa, Mercy Hospital, 1976.

THERAPEUTIC PHLEBOTOMY

Janice Casper, R.N., B.S.N.

OVERVIEW

The altered hemodynamic status of a critically ill patient can be purposefully improved by multidimensional and aggressive medical therapy. A therapeutic phlebotomy may be indicated: (1) when it is necessary to remove blood from a patient to decrease the number of red blood cells in polycythemia; (2) to decrease intravascular volume in acute pulmonary edema; or (3) for potential autotransfusion. A phlebotomy is performed electively or as an emergency intervention within the critical care setting.

OBJECTIVES

1. To safely remove 250 to 500 ml. of blood in order to decrease central blood volume or red cell mass.
2. To insure proper collection of blood for potential autotransfusion.

SPECIAL EQUIPMENT

500-ml. sterile vacuum bottle containing anticoagulant solution
Blood collection tubing with 16-gauge, 18-gauge, or 19-gauge needle
Tourniquet
Sterile gauze pads
Povidone-iodine prep swabs
Tape
Povidone-iodine ointment

METHOD

ACTION	RATIONALE
1. Prepare vacuum collection bottle, ascertaining that vacuum is intact.	
A. Shake bottle; listen for splashing sound.	A. A splashing sound indicates loss of vacuum; bottle should be discarded.
B. Close tubing clamp; insert needle-to-bottle into inlet port, using sterile technique; invert bottle and observe for bubbles.	B. Bubbles indicate an air leak; bottle should be discarded.
2. Apply tourniquet and, using sterile	

ACTION	RATIONALE

technique, perform venipuncture.

A. Select large vein and the largest needle possible.

    A. A large needle lumen prevents clotting and decreases red cell lysis if autotransfusion is desired.

B. Observe for flashback of blood; open tubing clamp.

C. Prepare venipuncture site.

    (1) Secure needle to skin with tape.

    (2) Apply povidone-iodine ointment; cover with sterile gauze dressing.

    (2) Povidone-iodine ointment provides a seal around needle at entry site and controls for infection.

3. Position inverted vacuum collection bottle approximately 6 to 12 inches below level of venipuncture.

3. Blood flows through anticoagulant solution; positioning the bottle at this level decreases the risk of air emboli.

4. Rotate the vacuum collection bottle gently and at frequent intervals.

4. Rotation facilitates mixing of blood with the anticoagulant solution.

5. Assess patient continuously; closely monitor cardiopulmonary status during therapy.

5. Patients are high risk for altered hemodynamics.

6. Close tubing clamp when the prescribed amount of blood has been collected; remove needle from patient preserving sterility of system.

7. Apply a sterile gauze pressure dressing to venipuncture site.

8. Rotate gently and invert collection bottle post therapy.

8. Rotation facilitates mixing of blood with anticoagulant solution.

9. Send collection bottle to blood bank immediately, when autotransfusion is anticipated.

9. Refrigeration and storage must be initiated promptly.

PRECAUTIONS

1. Establish one intravenous route for potential emergency intervention prior to therapy.
2. Monitor patient's hemoglobin and hematocrit before and after therapy.
3. Do not remove more than 500 ml. blood at one time.
4. Bleed patient at a slower rate and provide a longer rest time after therapy when phlebotomy is prescribed electively.

RELATED CARE

1. Monitor patient's vital signs, cardiac rhythm, and clinical symptomatology prior to and during therapy, and every 15 minutes until stable following therapy.
2. Assess venipuncture site frequently for delayed hematoma formation.

COMPLICATIONS

Hypovolemia	Nausea, vomiting
Syncope	Hematoma
Convulsions	Vascular trauma
Cardiac or respiratory arrest	Infection

SUPPLIERS

Travenol, Inc. (vacuum bottles)

REFERENCES

American Association of Blood Banks: Technical Methods and Procedures of the American Association of Blood Banks, 5th ed. Chicago: American Association of Blood Banks, 1971.

Metzer, Lawrence E. (ed.): Concepts and Practice of Intensive Care for Nurse Specialists. Bowie, Md., The Charles Press Publishers, 1976, p.132.

CARDIOCENTESIS (ASSISTING WITH)

Karen Wheelock, R.N., M.A.

OVERVIEW

A cardiocentesis is surgical aspiration into the pericardial space to relieve pressure on the heart and/or remove fluid for diagnostic testing. Fluid can be caused by pericardial effusion, myocardial perforation or rupture, and effusion from a tumor or chest trauma. In the life-threatening situation of cardiac tamponade, a cardiocentesis is performed as an emergency therapeutic intervention. Early assessment of altered hemodynamic parameters, facilitation of the emergency intervention, and follow-through monitoring of the patient for complications are vital contributions.

OBJECTIVES

1. To facilitate safe removal of fluid from the pericardial space by needle aspiration in such instances as pericarditis with effusion, post-trauma, acute rheumatic fever, other infections, tumors, or in the emergency intervention for cardiac tamponade.
2. To assess the patient's hemodynamic response to therapy.

SPECIAL EQUIPMENT

16- to 18-gauge short bevel needle
50-ml. syringe with three-way stopcock
Povidone-iodine prep solution
Local anesthetic
Sterile gloves

Ground wire
Clip or clamp for attachment of ECG lead to needle
ECG recorder
Defibrillator and resuscitation equipment

METHOD

ACTION	RATIONALE
1. Place patient in semirecumbent position, with head elevated approximately 60°.	1. This position facilitates needle insertion.
2. Obtain baseline blood pressure.	
3. Attach limb leads of grounded ECG.	

186

ACTION	RATIONALE
4. Prepare resuscitation equipment and medications as appropriate.	4. Serious dysrhythmias can occur during the therapy.
5. Attach lead V of ECG to aspiration needle.	5. This enhances safe position, since a sharp increase in QRS complex can be observed during needle penetration of the pericardial sac.
6. Prep skin site with povidone-iodone solution. The most common insertion site is subxyphoid, with the needle being inserted in the angle between the xyphoid and costal margin, directed towards the right shoulder.	
7. Monitor effect of therapy on patient during needle insertion and aspiration of fluid.	7. Aspiration fluid may be clear, cloudy, or bloody, but should not clot.
8. Facilitate care and transport of specimen for appropriate laboratory analysis.	

PRECAUTIONS

1. Observe presence of marked ST elevation, elevation of PR segment, or dysrhythmias, which indicate contact with epicardium or poor grounding.
2. Monitor blood pressure, pulse, and heart rhythm during entire procedure, and for 24 hours posttherapy.
3. Assess for signs and symptoms of cardiac tamponade.

RELATED CARE

1. Facilitate obtaining written consent unless performed as an emergency intervention.
2. Assess skin integrity at site; provide site care posttherapy.

COMPLICATIONS

Cardiac tamponade
Perforation of ventricle
Cardiac arrest
Dysrhythmias
Hydropneumothorax

Laceration of coronary artery
Aspiration of blood from cardiac chambers
Air embolism
Infection

REFERENCES

Beeson, P.B., McDermott, W., and Wyngaarden, J.B. (eds.): Textbook of Medicine, 15th ed. Philadelphia, W.B. Saunders, 1979.

Pories, W.J., and Gaudiani, V.A.: Cardiac tamponade. Surg. Clin. North Am. 55:573, 1975.

Wintrobe, M., et al. (eds.): Harrison's Principles of Internal Medicine, 6th ed. New York, McGraw-Hill, 1970, p. 1217.

THE
PULMONARY
SYSTEM

AIRWAY MANAGEMENT

Jeannette McCann McHugh, R.N., M.S.N.

OVERVIEW

Situations can arise in which patients are unable to maintain a patent airway and/or adequate ventilation independently. In an acute situation, temporary measures may be taken until definitive airway management is possible. In certain cases airway obstruction may be due to a flaccid tongue falling against the posterior pharyngeal wall. This may be relieved by hyperextension of the neck or forward displacement of the mandible, or by the use of nasopharyngeal or oropharyngeal airways. Also used for rescue purposes is the esophageal obturator airway which, when placed properly, blocks air flow into the stomach and allows ventilation through apertures located at the pharyngeal level.

When these measures are inadequate, or when a respiratory crisis is not resolved quickly, the patient will most likely require endotracheal intubation. Endotracheal intubation may be performed on critically ill patients in order to facilitate bronchial hygiene, prevent aspiration, and provide mechanical ventilation and/or high concentrations of oxygen. Although intubation may be necessary for adequate respiratory care, the artificial airway interrupts the upper airway functions of humidification, filtration, and warming of inspired gases, and also interferes with the cough and gag reflexes. Intubation also entails the potential hazard of tracheal injury. Once a patient is intubated, measures must be taken to compensate for the interrupted upper airway functions. Inspired gases must be humidified to prevent dryness of the respiratory mucous membrane, filtered to prevent deposition of foreign material in the lungs, and warmed to prevent loss of body heat.

Scrupulous attention to these details is essential, since the upper airway is the respiratory system's first line of defense against pathogenic organisms and sensitizing foreign particles. A breakdown in the respiratory mucous membrane, for example, may provide direct entry for pathogens into the cardiovascular network, and thereby to the whole body. In addition, the intubated patient's inability to generate an effective cough necessitates the use of aseptic endotracheal suctioning to facilitate secretion removal. Additional techniques such as postural drainage, percussion, and vibration may be needed to move secretions from peripheral airways to a level within the tracheobronchial tree that is accessible to a suction catheter. (We cannot suggest that these techniques mitigate against evacuation of air from lung segments; so many factors promote suction-induced atelectasis.)

For the patient unable to maintain effective ventilation and oxygenation, a mechanical ventilator may be provided to assist or control respiratory rates, inspiratory/expiratory ratios, inspiratory volumes, and varying flow patterns. Pressures of different levels and types above atmospheric pressure can be supplied to improve oxygen transport across the respiratory membrane.

For prolonged respiratory support, a tracheostomy is performed to improve access to the tracheobroncheal tree and prevent upper airway trauma resulting from endotracheal tube pressure on the mouth, uvula and larynx, as well as to alleviate patient discomfort and increased salivation. Indications for an emergency tracheostomy include severe facial and/or neck trauma and upper airway obstructions (e.g., tumors). When the respiratory crisis approaches resolution, consideration is given to termination of ventilatory support as well as eventual extubation. This weaning process may occur quickly or may be prolonged, and requires additional innovative measures and devices that allow the patient to increase respiratory strength and decrease dependence on supportive measures. The prospect of a ventilator-dependent patient rightfully encourages the implementation of this process as early as possible.

INSTRUMENTATION

An emergency artificial airway is usually provided first by insertion of a plastic oropharyngeal device that generally conforms to the mouth from the lips to the base of the tongue. It is designed to hold the tongue of an unconscious patient forward, preventing obstruction of the posterior pharynx.

The esophageal obturator airway (EOA) is a transparent device similar in appearance to an endotracheal tube. However, as a temporary airway it is quite different in several ways; the major differences are that the tube is inserted into the esophagus, instead of the trachea, and its distal end is blocked. When inserted, an esophageal cuff is inflated, a mask is applied firmly to seal the nose and mouth, and air is forced into the trachea through tube perforations in the pharyngeal area. It is inserted blindly and can be accomplished quickly and easily. Those patients requiring further airway management will have an endotracheal tube inserted prior to removal of the EOA.

Both endotracheal and tracheostomy tubes are composed of polyvinyl chloride (PVC), silicone, and/or nylon, and are disposable, although some silicone and nylon tubes can be steam- or gas-sterilized for reuse. These products are lightweight, soft, nontoxic, and have a longer shelf life than rubber. Standard size fittings (15 mm. male) provide easy connection to respiratory equipment. In addition, cuffs are bonded to the tube, resulting in less opportunity for cuffs to slip and herniate over the tip. Tubes should be selected with large volume (Fig. 77), low pressure cuffs that create a seal

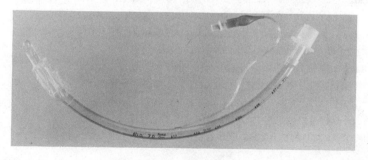

Figure 77. Endotracheal tube with large volume, low pressure cuff.

with less than 25 cm. H_2O (approximately 20 mm. Hg) pressure measured during expiration. Continuous in-line pressure gauges are available to assist in monitoring cuff pressures. Self-inflating foam cuffs are also available; these do not require monitoring but it has been reported that they sometimes lose their elasticity within 48 hours.

The endotracheal tube is generally the airway of choice in an emergency. The tube may be inserted via the oral or nasal route in about 1 to 5 minutes, while a tracheostomy takes approximately 15 minutes. Endotracheal tubes are radiopaque or have radiopaque markings to permit verification of tip position by x-ray. Although endotracheal tubes with large volume, low pressure cuffed tubes are preferred, red rubber low volume, high pressure cuffed tubes are commonly used for short-term airway management during surgical procedures. Methods are described in the literature for softening and stretching rigid cuffs so as to make them into high volume, low pressure cuffs.

When an artificial airway must remain in place for prolonged airway management, a tracheotomy is performed and a tracheostomy tube inserted. Tracheostomy tubes are available in four styles: single-cannula, double-cannula, fenestrated, and "speaking" (Fig. 78). Double-cannula tubes are frequently used in the critical care unit for the patient requiring mechanical ventilation. The inner cannula is removable and allows cleaning of built-up secretions in the cannula. Fenestrated tubes, a type of double-cannula tube, have an opening above the cuff that permits air to flow through to the larynx. If mechanical ventilation is required, an inner cannula in some models occludes the fenestration. However, with the occluding inner cannula removed, the fenestration permits the patient to speak and, additionally, with the proximal end occluded, it is possible to evaluate the patient's ability to breathe spontaneously. "Speaking" tubes permit delivery of humidified air or oxygen through an accessory line to an outlet just above the cuff. The gas flows upward through the larynx, enabling the patient to speak.

Swivel connectors are available for lightweight, flexible connections to the ventilating system, providing improved patient comfort and positioning flexibility. They may be an integral part of the tracheostomy tube, or they may be added to either the tracheostomy or endotracheal tube. Two highly desirable features to look for in swivel adapters are (1) a suction port, to permit suctioning without disconnecting the mechanical ventilator; and (2) an

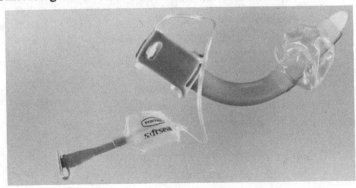

Figure 78.   Single cannula tracheostomy tube.

effective antidisconnect method of securing the adapter to the ventilator tubing and add-on swivel adapter to the tracheostomy or endotracheal tubes.

Respiratory instrumentation continues to proliferate and become increasingly sophisticated. Careful, critical evaluation of these devices' positive and negative features regarding usefulness, efficiency, and safety must be undertaken; the devices will either hinder or improve airway management, depending upon how they are used.

ESOPHAGEAL OBTURATOR AIRWAY INSERTION

OBJECTIVES

1. To provide a route for direct ventilation of the lungs rapidly.
2. To prevent insufflation of air into the patient's stomach, with consequent risk of vomiting and aspiration.

SPECIAL EQUIPMENT

Esophageal obturator airway (EOA) and attached mask
50-ml. syringe
Self-inflating bag/mask

METHOD

ACTION	RATIONALE
1. Assess patient's respiratory and reflexic state.	1. The esophageal obturator airway is recommended for resuscitation of unconscious, areflexic, apneic, or near apneic adults.
2. Administer mouth-to-mouth ventilations, or ventilate with bag/mask and supplemental oxygen. Ventilation is established while the esophageal obturator airway is obtained and prepared for use (mask attached, balloon fully deflated).	2. Mouth-to-mouth ventilation allows the rescuer to assess the patency of the upper airway.
3. Open the patient's mouth using crossed finger technique with patient's head in a neutral position (Fig. 79).	
4. Grasp patient's tongue and mandible, and pull forward.	

ACTION   **RATIONALE**

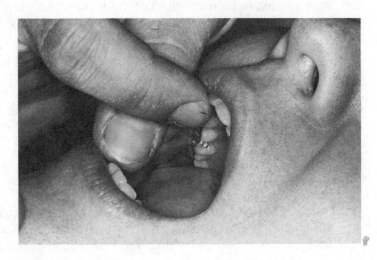

Figure 79. Crossed finger technique.

5. Use other hand to hold esophageal obturator airway (connected to the mask); insert into patient's mouth with tip pointing upward toward the hard palate.

6. Advance tube into posterior pharynx, rotating it 180° and insert into esophagus.

7. Apply steady, gentle pressure to advance tube until mask is securely seated on patient's face.

8. Blow into tube or ventilate with bag/mask, checking tube position during ventilations.
   A. Observe chest excursion.
   B. Auscultate breath sounds.

9. Inflate balloon with 30 ml. of air.

10. Ventilate the patient with positive pressure.

6. This prevents pushing the tongue against the posterior pharynx obstructing insertion.

7. The balloon must be seated below the level of the tracheal bifurcation; positive pressure ventilation is not possible if the mask is not seated firmly upon the patient's face.

8. If tracheal obturation has occurred the chest will not rise and breath sounds will be absent during ventilations.

9. This seals off esophagus and directs inspiratory tidal volumes from pharynx into trachea and lungs.

PRECAUTIONS

1. Minimize risk of esophageal rupture by utilizing the esophageal obturator airway in patients who are of adult proportion (over 60 inches in height) and age (over 16 years). Avoid forcing the airway during insertion. If difficulties arise, discontinue the intubation and administer mouth-to-mouth ventilation.

2. Minimize esophageal trauma by avoiding the use of esophageal obtur-
    ator airways in patients with known or suspected esophageal pathology.
    This includes patients with esophageal varices or strictures and patients
    who have swallowed caustic substances.
3. Always deflate esophageal balloon before removing tube.
4. Reduce the risk of aspiration of vomitus during esophageal extubation
    by ensuring a protected trachea. This is usually achieved by tracheal in-
    tubation and cuff inflation prior to the removal of the esophageal obtur-
    ator airway.

RELATED CARE

1. Assess adequacy of ventilation frequently by auscultating both lung
    fields and observing for symmetric lung excursion continuously.
2. Insert nasogastric tube through aperture in esophageal airway and aspir-
    ate stomach contents prior to removal of airway.
3. Place the patient on his side, deflate the esophageal balloon, and remove
    the airway quickly when consciousness returns rapidly and gagging or
    retching begins.

COMPLICATIONS

Esophageal rupture/perforation
Tracheal intubation
Vomiting with aspiration during extubation

REFERENCES

Don Michael, T.A., et al.: Mouth-to-lung airway for cardiac resusciation. Lancet,
    2:1329, 1968.
Gordon, A.S.: Technique of cardiopulmonary resuscitation (CPR) and pitfalls in
    performance. (In Meltzer, L.E., et al. (eds.): Textbook of Coronary Care.
    Amsterdam, Excerpta Medica, 1973, pp. 421–422.
Greenbaum, D.M., et al.: Esophageal obstruction during oxygen administration:
    A new method for use in resuscitation. Chest, 65:188, 1974.
Schofferman, J., et al.: The esophageal obturator airway. A clinical evaluation.
    Chest, 69:167, 1976.

ENDOTRACHEAL INTUBATION

OVERVIEW

There are three routes by which an endotracheal tube may be placed.

Tracheotomy. An endotracheal tube may be inserted through a tracheostomy when the upper airway is obstructed (e.g., tumor, severe facial trauma) or when the physical characteristics of the neck make nasal or oral placement impossible.

Nasotracheal Intubation. A nasotracheal tube is often more comfortable for conscious patients than an oral tracheal tube. However, a nasotracheal tube is generally more time-consuming to insert and its diameter is limited by upper airway anatomy.

Oral Tracheal Intubation. Oral tracheal intubation is generally preferred as the quickest and least traumatic means of emergency airway placement. This method will present the technique for oral endotracheal intubation.

OBJECTIVE

To establish a patent airway by correct placement of an oral endotracheal tube.

SPECIAL EQUIPMENT

Anesthesia bag and oxygen source
Topical anesthesia: 4% lidocaine or 4% cocaine
Suction source
Sterile suction catheter
Sterile glove
Sterile normal saline solution
Laryngoscope with curved and straight blades
Low pressure cuffed endotracheal tube (usually 36 Fr. for adult males and 32 to 34 Fr. for adult females; however, a range of sizes should be available).
Water-soluble anesthetic lubricating jelly
Malleable plastic or metal stylet
Magill forceps
Bite block or oral pharyngeal airway
Adhesive tape, alcohol swabs, tincture of benzoin
Swivel adapter

METHOD

ACTION	RATIONALE
1. Check tube cuff, laryngoscope batteries, and bulbs.	1. This insures properly functioning equipment.

ACTION	RATIONALE

2. Insert stylet into selected tube.
   A. Shape to desired curve for insertion.
   B. Lubricate tip of tube and stylet.

   B. This decreases mucosal trauma and makes insertion of tube easier.

3. Remove headboard from bed.

   3. This provides access to head of patient.

4. Prepare patient.
   A. Place patient's head on 2 to 4 inches of firm padding.

   A. This aligns the axes of oral cavity, pharynx, and trachea.

   B. Remove patient's dentures and/or partial plates and suction airway, if needed.

   B. This prevents damage to dental prostheses and maintains a patent, visible insertion pathway.

   C. Hyperventilate the patient with 100% oxygen.

   C. This decreases the lowering of PaO_2 during the insertion process.

5. Open patient's jaw widely, using cross finger technique with right hand (see Fig. 79); spray pharynx with topical anesthetic.

   5. This decreases gagging and discomfort.

6. Hold laryngoscope in non-dominant hand and introduce blade along right side of mouth. Advance blade and move centrally to displace tongue to left.
   A. Epiglottis is seen at base of tongue.
   B. Insert a straight blade beyond the epiglottis; a curved blade is positioned with its tip anterior to epiglottis.

   B. Inserting the blade too deeply causes entire larynx to be elevated, exposing the esophagus.

7. Hold wrist rigid; lift laryngoscope forward and upward at a 45° angle. At no time is leverage against the teeth used to effect exposure.

   7. This elevates the mandible and exposes the larynx. Leverage on teeth may cause tooth loss or damage and possible airway obstruction.

8. Insert endotracheal tube, with cuff deflated and concavity oriented laterally, into larynx until cuff disappears beyond vocal cords. Magill forceps may be used to assist placement when nasal route is used.

9. Remove stylet, inflate cuff, and, if necessary, suction tube, using sterile technique; then insert pharyngeal airway or bite block.

ACTION	RATIONALE
10. Ventilate the patient with 100% oxygen and auscultate chest to check tube placement.	
11. Obtain a chest x-ray to ascertain exact tube position; endotracheal tube tip should be at least 3 cm. above carina.	11. An x-ray provides visual observation of tube placement so that, if the tube has been inserted into the right main stem bronchus, it can be pulled back to proper position.
12. Cleanse patient's cheeks with alcohol, apply benzoin, and tape tube securely. (see also the method for "Securing Airways").	
13. Mark tube at level of mouth.	13. This mark is checked at intervals to make sure that the tube has not been inadvertently pulled out or inserted deeper into the trachea.
14. Connect patient to humidified oxygen source or mechanical ventilator using swivel adapter.	14. The swivel adapter reduces motion of the tube in the patient's mouth and trachea.
15. Recheck cuff volume to ascertain that minimum amount of air necessary to protect airway and permit ventilation is used.	15. Minimal occlusive volume for cuff inflation or intracuff pressure less than 25 cm. of water is an essential measure for preventing tracheal necrosis (see also the method for "Prevention of Tracheal Injuries").

PRECAUTIONS

1. Avoid traumatizing mouth, pharynx, larynx, and esophagus; bruises, lacerations, and abrasions may occur during an emergency intubation. Trauma to lips may be avoided by spreading them away from laryngoscope blade and teeth; damage to teeth that are in poor repair may be unavoidable.
2. When the patient cannot be intubated within a reasonable period of time, prevent hypoxia by discontinuing the procedure and ventilating with 100% oxygen.
3. Observe for indications of esophageal intubation; these include abdominal distention and eructations with manual ventilation and absent breath sounds across the lung fields. In such cases the tube must be removed and the patient reintubated.
4. Obtain information regarding possible cervical neck injury; extreme care must be taken in this case to prevent transection of the spinal cord.

RELATED CARE

1. Insert a nasogastric tube to avoid gastric distention and aspiration. It may be connected to intermittent gastric suction, in the event of a paralytic ileus, or it may be used for feedings and/or antacid administration.
2. Monitor patients undergoing intubation whenever possible. A wide variety of ectopy and conduction disturbances have been observed during intubation and have been ascribed to hypoxia and vago-vagal reflexes. Careful preoxygenation and quick atraumatic intubation will minimize cardiovascular sequelae.

COMPLICATIONS

Bruises, lacerations, and abrasions
Tooth loss or damage
Hypoxemia
Cardiac dysrhythmias
Esophageal intubation

Vomiting with aspiration
Laryngeal trauma
Intubation of right main stem bronchus
Tracheal rupture
Tracheoesophageal fistula

REFERENCES

Dripps, R.D., Eckenhoff, J.E., and Vandam, L.D.: Introduction to Anesthesia, 5th ed. Philadelphia, W.B. Saunders, 1977, pp. 220–227.

Eagan, D.F.: Fundamentals of Respiratory Therapy, 3rd ed. St. Louis, C.V. Mosby, 1977, pp. 390–406.

Knowlson, G.T.G., and Bassett, H.F.M.: The pressures exerted on the trachea by endotracheal inflatable cuffs. Br. J. Anesthesiol., 42:834, 1970.

Schofferman, J., Dill, P., and Lewis, A.J.: The esophageal obturator airway, a clinical evaluation. Chest, 69:67, 1976.

Snow, J.C.: Manual of Anesthesia, 1st ed. Boston, Little, Brown and Company, 1977.

ENDOTRACHEAL SUCTIONING

OVERVIEW

Endotracheal intubation is often necessary to maintain airway patency. Ironically, however, introduction of an endotracheal tube makes effective coughing difficult and reduces the patient's ability to raise tracheobronchial secretions. Under these circumstances removal of accumulated secretions must be accomplished by endotracheal suctioning.

In addition, some disease states, pain, and surgical procedures will make effective coughing difficult and reduce the ability to raise tracheobronchial secretions. Endotracheal intubation may not be desirable, or the patient may have been recently extubated. In such cases, removal of accumulated secretions may be accomplished by blind endotracheal suctioning.

OBJECTIVES

1. To remove tracheobronchial secretions, using sterile technique.
2. To mobilize tenacious secretions for removal, using sterile suctioning technique.

SPECIAL EQUIPMENT

Sterile glove
Sterile catheter with intermittent suction control port
Sterile normal saline solution
Suction source
Anesthesia bag connected to 100% oxygen

METHOD

ACTION	RATIONALE
1. Assess patient's need for endotracheal suctioning; indications include: A. Coarse adventitious sounds. B. Coughing. C. Increasing inspiratory pressures for patients receiving mechanical ventilation.	1. Since endotracheal suctioning can be hazardous and cause discomfort, it is not recommended in the absence of apparent need.
2. Pour sterile saline solution into sterile cup.	
3. Open catheter packaging, maintaining catheter sterility. A 14 Fr. catheter is commonly used in adult patients; however, catheter should not exceed one-third the inner diameter of the airway.	3. Catheters exceeding one-third the airway diameter increase the possibility of suction-induced hypoxia and atelectasis.
4. Preoxygenate patients with 100% oxygen. A. Use anesthesia bag, or B. Change oxygen setting on me-	4. Preoxygenation may help minimize suction-induced hypoxia.

ACTION	RATIONALE
chanical ventilator to 100%. Remember that ventilators cycle for variable lengths of time before oxygen delivery reaches 100%.	
5. Glove and maintain sterility of dominant hand.	5. This decreases the incidence of contamination and infection of the clinician, and the possible transmission to other patients.
6. Using nondominant hand, remove ventilator or open suctioning port on swivel adapter. Ventilator tubing end may be: A. Placed on a sterile drape. B. Slipped inside a nonpowdered sterile glove. C. Held by a colleague. If contamination occurs, attachments should be replaced with sterile ones.	6. This prevents contamination of the ventilator tubing.
7. Using sterile gloved dominant hand, pick up catheter and connect to suction source; thumb of opposite "clean" gloved hand controls suction port.	
8. Dampen catheter in sterile saline solution to lubricate.	8. Surgical lubricant is usually unnecessary and may accumulate on inner surface of the endotracheal tube.
9. Using sterile gloved hand, insert catheter fully into endotracheal tube. Do not force if an obstruction is encountered.	
10. Apply intermittent suction by quickly opening and closing suction port; withdraw catheter, using a rotating motion. Entire suctioning pass should not exceed 10 seconds in duration.	10. Intermittent suction minimizes tissue damage from invagination of tracheal mucosa into the catheter tip; the rotating motion sweeps the catheter tip against all sides of the airway wall as the catheter is withdrawn.
11. Hyperinflate patient's lungs with 100% oxygen.	11. This re-expands sections of the lungs which may have been evacuated of air and collapsed, and minimizes hypoxemia due to suction-induced atelectasis.
12. Reconnect patient to ventilator or close the suction port of the swivel adapter.	

ACTION	RATIONALE
13. Assess effectiveness of suctioning pass. If adventitious sounds, ventilatory difficulty, or patient discomfort persist, repeat steps 7 through 12.	
14. If secretions are tenacious, introduce 5 to 10 ml. of sterile saline solution into airway, and follow with several ventilatory cycles.	14. Introduction of saline may help mobilize secretions and aid in their removal.

PRECAUTIONS

1. Immediately prior to suctioning, preoxygenate patients with 100% oxygen to minimize suction-induced hypoxia by raising PaO_2.
2. Minimize suction-induced atelectasis and hypoxemia.
   A. Avoid the use of catheters larger than one-third the diameter of the airway.
   B. Administer one or more postsuctioning hyperinflations, using either an anesthesia bag or the manual "sigh" of a mechanical ventilator.
3. Maintain rigorous sterile technique when suctioning the intubated patient. Impaired pulmonary defense systems and invasive instrumentation of the pulmonary tract predisposes these patients to colonization and infection. Never use the same catheter to suction the nose or mouth and then the trachea.
4. Limit the frequency of suctioning and avoid, as much as possible, catheter impaction in the bronchial tree when the patient is anticoagulated or when hemorrhage from suction-induced trauma is evident.
5. Minimize the frequency and duration of suctioning when the patient is on PEEP or CPAP. Small suctioning-induced changes may have profound effects on these marginally oxygenated patients.
6. Maintain awareness of the limitations of endotracheal suctioning. Maneuvers and catheter designs have been proposed to increase the likelihood of catheter passage into the left bronchus; however, these have been shown to be of limited success. Because the left main stem bronchus emerges from the trachea at a 45-degree angle from the vertical, suction catheters are almost inevitably passed into the right bronchus.

RELATED CARE

1. Include strategies to move secretions through peripheral airways. These measures are appropriate hydration, adequate humidification of inspired gases, coughing and deep breathing, frequent position changes,

chest physiotherapy, and bronchodilating agents.

2. Monitor the patient carefully during endotracheal suctioning for ectopic dysrhythmias aggravated by suction-induced hypoxemia and other dysrhythmias, particularly conduction disturbances, related to catheter irritation of vagal receptors within the respiratory tract.

COMPLICATIONS

Hypoxemia

Atelectasis

Dysrhythmias

Nosocomial pulmonary tract infection

Mucosal trauma with increased secretions

REFERENCES

Adlkofer, R., and Powaser, M.: The effect of endotracheal suctioning on arterial blood gases after cardiac surgery. Heart Lung, 7:1011–1014, 1978.

Bryant, L.R., Trinkle, K., Kazi, M.U., Baker, J., and Griffin, W.O.: Bacterial colonization profile with tracheal intubation and mechanical ventilation. Arch. Surg. 104:647, 1972.

Bushnell, S.S.: Respiratory Intensive Care Nursing. Boston, Little, Brown and Company, 1973, pp. 197–199.

Jaquette, G.: To reduce the hazards of endotracheal suction. Am. J. Nurs., 71:2362, 1971.

Johnson, W.G., Pierce, A.K., Sanford, J.P., and Thomas, G.D.: Nosocomial respiratory infections with gram negative bacilli. The significance of colonization of the respiratory tract. Ann. Intern. Med., 77:701, 1972.

Kirimili, B., King, J.E., and Pfaeffle, H.H.: Evaluation of tracheobronchial suction techniques. J. Thorac. Cardiovasc. Surg., 59:340, 1970.

Massachusetts General Hospital, Department of Nursing: Massachusetts General Hospital Manual of Nursing Procedures. Boston, Little, Brown and Company, 1975, pp. 269–271.

Naigow, D., and Powaser, M.: The effect of different endotracheal suction procedures on arterial blood gases in a controlled experimental model. Heart Lung, 6:808–816, 1977.

Stevens, R.M., Teres, D., Skillman, J.J., and Feingold, D.S.: Pneumonia in an intensive care unit. A 30 months experience. Arch. Intern. Med., 134:106, 1974.

Zwillic, C.W., Pierson, D.J., Creagh, C.E., Sutton, F.D., Schatz, E., and Petty, T.L.: Complications of assisted ventilation—a prospective study of 354 consecutive episodes. Am. J. Med., 57:161, 1974.

BLIND ENDOTRACHEAL SUCTIONING

OBJECTIVES

1. To remove accumulated tracheobronchial secretions, using sterile technique.
2. To mobilize pulmonary secretions by stimulation of cough reflexes.

SPECIAL EQUIPMENT

Sterile glove
Sterile catheter (14 to 16 Fr. for adult patients), with intermittent suction control port
Sterile normal saline solution
Suction source
Oxygen source and mask capable of delivering high concentrations of oxygen
Sterile water-soluble lubricant
Sterile gauze pad
Soft rubber nasopharyngeal airway
Tissues

METHOD

ACTION	RATIONALE
1. Assess patient's need for blind endotracheal suctioning.	1. The patient does not need suctioning: A. If evidence of accumulating secretions is not present. B. And/or, if the patient can be educated and encouraged to cough and deep breathe effectively.
2. Prepare patient. A. Raise head of patient's bed to high or semi-Fowler's position, as tolerated. B. Insert lubricated soft rubber nasopharyngeal airway, if appropriate or requested by the patient. C. Preoxygenate patient with high concentration of oxygen for 5 minutes or more.	C. Arterial oxygen tensions are increased in anticipation of suction-induced decreases in PAO_2 and PaO_2.
3. Turn on suction source.	

ACTION	RATIONALE
4. Open sterile saline.	
5. Squeeze adequate quantity of lubricant onto sterile gauze pad.	
6. Don sterile glove on dominant hand.	
7. Using gloved hand, pick up catheter and roll tip generously in lubricant.	
8. Insert catheter into patient's nasal passage and advance into pharynx, approximately 8 to 10 cm.	
9. Ask patient to breathe slowly and deeply as catheter is advanced.	
A. Listen for airway sounds transmitted through catheter.	
B. If absent, withdraw catheter into pharynx and repeat.	B. The absence of airway sounds transmitted through the catheter suggests entry into the esophagus.
10. Continue to advance catheter as fully as possible into trachea, withdrawing 1 to 2 cm. if obstruction is met at level of carina.	
11. Attach catheter to suction source; apply intermittent suction with ungloved hand while rotating and withdrawing catheter.	
12. Hyperoxygenate patient as described in step 2-C, and encourage maximal deep breaths.	12. These measures are employed to reverse suction-induced hypoxia and atelectasis.
13. Clear tubing by aspirating sterile saline solution through catheter.	
14. Assess effectiveness of suctioning, repeating steps 8 through 11, if necessary.	
15. Discard glove and catheter and turn off suction.	
16. Return patient to comfortable position.	

PRECAUTIONS

1. Preoxygenate for 5 minutes or more prior to suctioning in anticipation of suctioning-induced reductions in alveolar and arterial oxygen tensions.
2. Maintain scrupulous sterility during the suction process in order to minimize the risk of respiratory tract infection. Recognize that patients

with excessive, poorly mobilized secretions frequently have compromised pulmonary and systemic defenses against infection.

3. Recognize that oral and nasotracheal suctioning, even when performed with rigorous sterile technique, risks inoculation of lower airways with nose and mouth flora. Minimize spread of bacteria within the airways by limiting the frequency of blind endotracheal suctioning as much as possible.

4. Limit or avoid the use of blind endotracheal suctioning when there is a predisposition to or evidence of hemorrhage from suction-induced trauma. Conditions that predispose to hemorrhage include any bleeding disorder, esophageal varices, and treatment with anticoagulants.

5. Limit suctioning and catheter-induced trauma by using the nasopharyngeal airway, when appropriate, and avoiding the use of large suction catheters or high suction pressures.

6. Minimize suction-induced asystole or ectopy by scrupulous preoxygenation. Avoid the use of blind endotracheal suctioning in patients with increased vagal sensitivity, unstable conduction disturbances, and/or acute myocardial ischemia. Patients at any risk of suction-induced dysrhythmias should be monitored during suctioning.

7. Minimize the risk of catheter-induced gagging and consequent aspiration of vomitus by sitting the patient upright prior to suctioning. Avoid suctioning patients within an hour of feeding and never suction patients who complain of nausea.

8. Avoid hyperoxygenation of patients with lung disorders characterized by chronic hypercapnea. Strategies other than nasotracheal suctioning may need to be used in aiding these patients to mobilize secretions.

RELATED CARE

1. Encourage postsuctioning deep breathing to reverse suctioning-induced atelectasis. If the patient cannot deep breathe voluntarily, administer several hyperinflations with an anesthesia bag and mask.

2. Pursue measures aimed at mobilizing peripheral airway secretions in any program of pulmonary hygiene. These measures include adequate hydration, humidification of inspired gases, chest physiotherapy, bronchodilators, frequent position changes and, if possible, ambulation.

COMPLICATIONS

Hypoxemia
Atelectasis
Vomiting and aspiration
Dysrhythmias

Mucosal trauma with increased secretions
Nosocomial pulmonary tract infections
Hemorrhage

REFERENCES

Massachusetts General Hospital, Department of Nursing: Massachusetts General Hospital Manual of Nursing Procedures. Boston, Little, Brown, and Company, 1975, pp. 281–283.

TRACHEOSTOMY CARE

OVERVIEW

Tracheostomy care is performed at least every 8 hours, or more frequently if needed, in order to keep the airway patent and free of sources of infection, as well as to make the tracheostomy more esthetically acceptable to the patient and visitors.

OBJECTIVES

1. To provide aseptic wound care and dressing of the tracheostomy and to keep the double-walled tracheostomy tube aseptically clean.
2. To maintain ventilation of the patient.

SPECIAL EQUIPMENT

Two sterile bowls
Sterile gauze pads
Cotton swabs
Forceps
Sterile water and sterile hydrogen peroxide
Tracheostomy care adapter for outer cannula
Tracheostomy brush or sterile pipe cleaners
Sterile gloves
Tracheostomy ties
Tracheostomy dressing
Equipment for endotracheal suctioning

METHOD

ACTION	RATIONALE
1. Assist patient to position of comfort that exposes tracheostomy and surrounding skin.	
2. Remove soiled dressing, using forceps.	

ACTION	RATIONALE

3. Pour hydrogen peroxide and water into separate sterile bowls.

4. Dampen sterile applicators in hydrogen peroxide and swab secretions from area around tracheostomy.

    4. This decreases odor and medium for bacterial growth.

5. Dampen sterile gauze pads with saline, maintaining sterility, and place on skin for several minutes if secretions are encrusted. Repeat step 4.

    5. This moistens and softens dry secretions.

6. Perform the following steps if patient has a double-walled tracheostomy tube:

    A. Remove inner cannula and immerse in hydrogen peroxide.

    B. Suction outer cannula, if necessary (see the method for "Endotracheal Suctioning").

    C. Using tracheostomy care adapter, reconnect ventilation or oxygen source to outer cannula.

    D. Don sterile gloves and, using tracheostomy brush or bent pipe cleaners, clean secretions from inside inner cannula.

    E. Rinse inner cannula in bowl of sterile water.

    F. Reinsert inner cannula into tracheostomy, making certain that locking mechanism is engaged, and reconnect ventilator or oxygen source.

7. Change tracheostomy ties, if soiled; apply and secure clean ties *before* removing old ones. Ties should fit snugly against the skin, but should be loose enough to allow two fingers to be slipped beneath them.

    7. A tracheostomy tube that is untied, no matter how briefly, is in danger of being coughed or pulled out. Ties that are too tight will cause patient discomfort; ties that are too loose allow the cannula to slide too freely within the trachea and may cause mucosal damage.

8. Apply new tracheostomy dressing.

PRECAUTIONS

1. Observe for tracheal obstruction caused by accumulated secretions or cuff malfunction.
   A. In such a case, a catheter is passed into the tracheostomy to ascertain the nature of the obstruction, and the cuff is deflated.
   B. If the obstruction is not relieved, the tracheostomy tube is removed, the stoma covered and the patient ventilated with a bag/mask and supplemental oxygen until a new tracheostomy tube is inserted.
2. Prevent accidental decannulation by tying the tube securely in place and providing adequate slack in ventilator or oxygen connections. Restrain or sedate disoriented and agitated patients who are at risk of removing airways.
3. See also the method for "Prevention of Tracheal Injuries."
4. Suction the oropharynx before deflating a cuff to prevent accumulated oral secretions from draining into the tracheobronchial tree.
5. Prevent obstruction secondary to accumulated secretions by providing adequate humidification of inspired gases, appropriate patient hydration, proper endotracheal suctioning, and chest physiotherapy.

RELATED CARE

1. Obtain cultures of the wound site and sputum daily.
2. Change the tracheostomy tube every 24 to 48 hours, depending upon the amount of secretions or crusting. The change should be made rapidly, no more than 10 to 15 seconds, with all necessary instruments available.
3. Change nebulizers and tubing connected to the tracheostomy tube daily, since they are potential sources of infection.
4. Use a large volume, low pressure cuff when using cuffed tracheostomy tubes to reduce tracheal complications.

COMPLICATIONS

Tracheal obstruction
Accidental decannulation
Tracheal mucosal damage
Wound infection

Tracheobronchial tree infection
Stomal stenosis
Tracheal stricture
Tracheoesophageal fistula

REFERENCES

Bushnell, S.S.: Respiratory Intensive Care Nursing. Boston, Little, Brown and Company, 1973, pp. 203–207.
Eagan, D.F.: Fundamentals of Respiratory Therapy, 3rd ed. St. Louis, C.V. Mosby, 1977, pp. 395–406.
Massachusetts General Hospital, Department of Nursing: Massachusetts General

Hospital Manual of Nursing Procedures. Boston, Little, Brown and Company, 1975, pp. 272–273.

PREVENTION OF TRACHEAL INJURIES _____

OVERVIEW

Endotracheal intubation is often a necessary support for critically ill patients. However, cannulation of the trachea has been observed to cause a range of injuries, including tracheomalacia, tracheoesophageal fistula, tracheoinnominate artery fistula, and ulceration and scarring of the vocal cords.

Tissue changes, including necrosis of the posterior portions of the larynx, are common among patients treated with nasal and oral tracheal tubes. Although damage to larynx and vocal cords may be avoided by tracheostomy, the most common site of injury for all intubated patients is at the site of the endotracheal or tracheostomy tube cuff. Various nursing measures may be undertaken to minimize these tracheal injuries.

OBJECTIVES

1. To minimize traction or torsion on the patient's endotracheal tube.
2. To inflate a tube cuff, permitting tracheal wall capillary perfusion.

SPECIAL EQUIPMENT

10-ml. syringe
Swivel adapter

Intracuff pressure measuring gauge

METHOD

ACTION	RATIONALE
1. Suspend ventilator tubing above level of patient by adjustable support arms attached to ventilator. Tubing should be long enough to permit patient to turn from side to side.	1. Tubing that is too short or draped on bed or side rail will put traction on the patient's endotracheal/tracheostomy tube.
2. Connect relatively rigid ventilator tubing to patient's endotra-	2. This allows freer movement of the patient's head, neck, and torso and pre-

ACTION	RATIONALE

cheal/tracheostomy tube with a fully flexible adapter (one type is the Morsh swivel adapter).

vents undue torsion on the endotracheal/tracheostomy tube.

3. Keep patient comfortable and at ease. Sedate or restrain confused or agitated patients, as appropriate, when a safe airway cannot otherwise be assured.

3. An agitated patient may dislodge or pull out a tracheal tube; thrashing and struggling may cause permanent vocal cord injury in patients with oral or nasal tracheal tubes.

4. Select technique for cuff inflation.
   A. Inflate tube cuffs with minimal occlusive volume of air.
      (1) Determine minimal occlusive volume while patient receives positive pressure ventilation. An anesthesia bag may be used for patients who do not require mechanical ventilation.
      (2) Auscultate neck for inspiratory air leaks while air is injected slowly into inflation port of cuff.
      (3) Continue to fill cuff with air until inspiratory air leak is obliterated.
      (4) Withdraw a small amount of air until a slight leak is noted at peak inspiratory pressures.

A. Tracheal injury at the cuff site is due to distortion of tracheal anatomy and occlusion of tracheal capillaries. Necrosis is especially common with the use of low volume, high pressure cuffs. High volume, low pressure cuff designs conform more closely to tracheal contours and can achieve an airway seal at pressures which do not occlude mucosal blood flow. Overinflation of any cuff, however, can cause tracheal ischemia, distortion, and consequent injury.

   B. Inflate a high volume, low pressure tube cuff with a minimal pressure of between 15 and 25 cm. H_2O.
      (1) Determine minimal occlusive volume as in step 4-A.
      (2) Attach cuff pressure measuring gauge to cuff inflation tube.
      (3) Fill 10-ml. syringe with air and attach to self-sealing inflation port attached to gauge.
      (4) Auscultate neck for inspiratory air leaks while air is injected slowly into inflation port.

B. Pressure less than 15 cm. H_2O increases risk of aspiration around the cuff. Pressure greater than 25 cm. of water increases risk of complications associated with diminished blood flow to tracheal wall capillaries. 27 cm. H_2O pressure is the approximate tracheal mucosal capillary blood pressure. When cuff pressure is maintained below this, capillary perfusion occurs.

ACTION	RATIONALE
(5) Continue to fill cuff with air slowly until inspiratory air leak is obliterated.	
(6) Leave cuff pressure measuring gauge connected to cuff. Pressure should be less than 25 cm. H_2O.	(6) This permits continuous in-line pressure monitoring.

PRECAUTIONS

1. Suspect tracheomalacia at the cuff site when increasing amounts of injected air are required to achieve the minimal occlusive volume or maintain a given pressure.
2. Observe for stridor or respiratory distress following extubation; have emergency reintubation supplies immediately available.
3. To prevent aspiration and possible infection, suction accumulated upper airway secretions from above the cuff before deflating and reinflating the cuff.

RELATED CARE

Deflate and inflate large volume, low pressure cuffs only when required to maintain the minimal occlusive volume or maintain the given low pressure. Routine periodic cuff deflations have been demonstrated to be of little or no value in preventing tracheal ischemia.

COMPLICATIONS

Tracheomalacia   Tracheoesophageal fistula
Laryngeal edema   Infection

REFERENCES

Bushnell, S.S.: Respiratory Intensive Care Nursing. Boston, Little, Brown and Company, 1973, pp. 203–207.

Grillo, H.C., Cooper, J.D., Geffin, B., and Pontoppidan, H.: A low pressure cuff for tracheostomy tubes to minimize tracheal injury. A comparative clinical trial. J. Thorac. Cardiovasc. Surg., 62:898, 1971.

Hedden, M., Ersoz, C.J., Donnelly, W.H., and Safar, P.: Laryngotracheal damage after prolonged use of orotracheal tubes in adults. J.A.M.A., 207:703, 1969.

Hedley-White, J., et al.: Applied Physiology of Respiratory Care. Boston, Little, Brown and Company, 1976, pp. 3–11.

Knowlson, G.T.G., and Bassett, H.F.M.: The pressures exerted on the trachea by endotracheal inflatable çuffs. Br. J. Anesthesiol., *42*:834, 1970.

Massachusetts General Hospital, Department of Nursing: Massachusetts General Hospital Manual of Nursing Procedures. Boston, Little, Brown and Company, 1975, p. 274.

Powaser, M.M., Brown, M.C., Chezem, J., Woodburne, C.R., Rogenes, P., and Hanson, B.: The effectiveness of hourly cuff deflation in minimizing tracheal damage. Heart Lung, *5*:734, 1976.

SECURING AIRWAYS

OBJECTIVES

1. To prevent inadvertent removal of the airway.
2. To minimize tracheal erosion by limiting sliding movements of the airway.

SPECIAL EQUIPMENT

Tracheostomy tube
Twill tape, single strand, 30 to 34 inches in length
Scissors
Hemostats or tweezers
Endotracheal tube
Twill tape, 30 to 34 inches
½-inch width adhesive tape, 4 to 6 inches

METHOD

ACTION	RATIONALE
Tracheostomy Tube	
1. Obtain single length of twill tape prior to beginning tracheostomy care.	1. Mucous-encrusted tracheostomy ties should be changed as a part of routine tracheostomy care. Prepackaged kits may not include adequate lengths of twill tape.
2. Complete tracheostomy care regimen without removing old ties.	2. Untied tracheostomy cannulas are always at risk of being removed by sudden patient movements, even when handheld by a second person.
3. Slip end of the clean twill tape	

ACTION	RATIONALE

under tracheostomy flange, and use hemostats or tweezers to pull tape through the tie slot.

4. Thread this end of tape behind and around patient's neck.

5. Slip this same end of twill tape under second flange and, using hemostat or tweezers, through tie slots.

6. Bring opposite end of clean twill tape behind and around patient's neck, but do not bring through tie slot.

7. Pull gently on two ends of twill tape until tie fits snugly around neck and tracheostomy flanges are flat against skin.

8. Tie a firm knot at side of patient's neck.

8. The knot is less likely to become mucous-encrusted when tied some distance from the tracheostomy. The knot should not be over a cervical prominence where it can cause discomfort.

9. Carefully distinguish between old and new ties; snip and remove old ties.

10. Recheck tracheostomy ties for snugness.

10. Loose-fitting ties may initially be obscured by close-fitting, soiled ties.

Endotracheal Tube

1. With old ties removed, hold endotracheal tube and find mark which indicates proper point of tube emergence from mouth or nares (see also the method for "Endotracheal Intubation").

1. This mark indicates proper position of tube end below the level of the cords and above the tracheal bifurcation; if not marked, recheck tube position and mark point of emergence.

2. Tie a length of twill tape tightly around tube, immediately below mark of emergence, and knot tape firmly.

2. Obscuring mark with tape will make future assessment of tube position difficult.

3. Wrap a 4 to 6 inch length of adhesive tape around tube and over twill tape.

4. Bring ends of twill tape around and behind patient's neck; pull tape gently until snug against skin.

ACTION	RATIONALE

5. Tie in secure knot at side of patient's neck.

PRECAUTIONS

1. Do not remove old ties on the tracheostomy tube prior to replacing with clean ones.
2. Use care not to extubate the patient inadvertently when replacing endotracheal tube ties.

RELATED CARE

1. Ensure snug fit of airway ties. Ties should be close-fitting and allow minimal in and out movements of endotracheal or tracheostomy tubes. They should be loose enough to allow two fingers to be slipped between the ties and the patient's neck.
2. Limit the movement of the tracheostomy and endotracheal tubes during tie changes. This minimizes stimulation of tracheolaryngeal reflexes and consequent patient discomfort.

COMPLICATIONS

Extubation

EXTUBATION _____

OBJECTIVES

1. To remove oral or nasotracheal tubes safely and atraumatically.
2. To observe for and minimize the hazards of laryngeal tissue reaction following extubation.

SPECIAL EQUIPMENT

Materials for endotracheal suctioning (see p. 201)
Anesthesia bag with universal adapter
Syringe
T tube

Face mask
Humidifier (usually heated)
Supplemental oxygen source
Materials for endotracheal intubation (see p. 197)

METHOD

ACTION	RATIONALE

1. Assess patient's readiness for extubation. The patient should:
   A. Be completely weaned from mechanical ventilation.
   B. Be conscious and/or possess competent pharyngeal reflexes.
   C. Be capable of generating an effective cough.
   D. Have regained muscular control (e.g., is able to lift head and has adequate hand grasp).
   E. Have acceptable respiratory parameters.
      (1) Minute volume (90 ml./kg.).
      (2) Inspiratory force (20 to 25 cm. H_2O).
      (3) Forced vital capacity (15 ml./kg.).
   F. Have no serious cardiac dysrhythmias.
   G. Have a stable pulse and blood pressure.

2. Preoxygenate patient with 100% oxygen.

3. Lower head of patient's bed into a dependent position, when possible and if tolerated.

   3. This minimizes the risk of draining pooled oral secretions into the lungs when the cuff is deflated.

4. Attach anesthesia bag to endotracheal tube and administer a maximal inflation with anesthesia bag as cuff is deflated.

   4. This forces accumulated secretions away from lower airways as the cuff is deflated.

5. Attach patient to T tube and allow several breaths with cuff deflated.

   5. The patient may need time to cough and stabilize respiratory pattern before proceeding.

6. Suction endotracheal tube, if necessary.

7. Remove suction catheter from endotracheal tube and reoxygenate patient with 100% oxygen via T tube.

   7. Catheter contact with vocal cords during extubation may precipitate trauma, spasm, or hemorrhage.

8. Ask patient to inspire maximally or inflate lungs maximally with

   8. This allows easier and less traumatic tube removal with expiration.

ACTION	RATIONALE
anesthesia bag, and remove endo-tracheal tube at point of maximal inspiration.	
9. Suction pharynx, as necessary, and elevate head of bed if blood pressure is stable.	
10. Administer prescribed mixture of humidified oxygen via face mask.	10. Humidified inspired gases will aid in minimizing laryngeal edema.
11. Observe closely for increasing hoarseness or respiratory stridor.	11. Laryngeal edema or spasm may necessitate reintubation.

PRECAUTIONS

1. Anticipate the presence of pooled oral secretions above the endotracheal tube cuff. Although suctioning above the cuff prior to extubation may be of some value, the removal of all secretions cannot be assured. Promote drainage of pooled secretions away from lower airways by placing patient in head down position prior to cuff deflation and administering a positive pressure breath with the anesthesia bag simultaneously with deflation.

2. Observe for signs of respiratory stridor, gasping for air, increasing hoarseness, or increased swallowing that may indicate development of laryngospasm or edema. Minimize laryngeal tissue reaction by providing warm humidification via face mask following extubation. Keep an endotracheal intubation tray at bedside in the event that laryngeal tissues begin to compromise airway patency.

RELATED CARE

1. Provide constant calm reassurance and support to extubated patients. They may experience air hunger, thus heightening their anxiety level.

2. Encourage slow, deep breaths and, unless contraindicated, encourage patients with accumulating secretions to cough.

3. Provide heated humidified oxygen for most extubated patients to assist secretion mobilization. However, the patient who has had traumatic intubations or who otherwise exhibits signs of laryngeal edema may benefit from cold humidified oxygen.

4. Allow no oral intake for approximately 6 hours after extubation because the larynx is not usually competent for several hours. After this, only clear liquids should be permitted until the patient swallows with ease.

5. Assess arterial blood gas levels postextubation to determine minimal safe inspired oxygen level. Additional blood gas determinations should be performed as indicated.

6. Administer chest physiotherapy as necessary, usually four times a day.

COMPLICATIONS

Aspiration of pooled oral secretions into lower airways
Laryngospasm and/or laryngeal edema

REFERENCES

Bushnell, S.S.: Respiratory Intensive Nursing Care. Boston, Little, Brown and
    Company, 1973, p. 57.
McConnell, E.A.: After surgery. Nurs. '77, 7:32–39, 1977.

VENTILATORY MANAGEMENT

Jeanette McCann McHugh, R.N., M.S.N.

OVERVIEW

Critical care nurses should be thoroughly acquainted with ventilator control settings, displays, and alarms. These features not only provide valuable data about the patient's pulmonary status but have a major impact upon it. Table 2 has been provided to help identify the controls of several types of ventilators in common use. Information for ventilators not listed may be obtained from the manufacturer's operating manuals, respiratory therapists, and several texts.

Pressure-preset ventilators are characterized by inspiratory cycles which terminate at preset peak pressures. Under these conditions, delivered tidal volumes may be decreased by increased airway resistance, or by decreased lung-chest compliance. For this reason these ventilators are not preferred for prolonged mechanical ventilation.

Volume preset ventilators are characterized by inspiratory cycles which terminate after a preset tidal volume has been delivered. Because of their greater precision and the availability of special features, these ventilators are preferred for complex respiratory care.

INSTITUTING MECHANICAL VENTILATION

OBJECTIVES

1. To institute respiratory support.
2. To determine appropriate ventilator settings.

SPECIAL EQUIPMENT

Ventilator
Pressure-preset ventilator (Bird and Bennett Series)
Volume-preset ventilator

METHOD

ACTION	RATIONALE
1. Institute mechanical ventilation, using following criteria:	1. A total clinical picture must be considered before instituting mechnical

ACTION	RATIONALE
A. Vital capacity less than 10 ml./kg.	ventilation. Laboratory findings and shunt calculations aid the decision-making process.
B. $AaDO_2$ of 300 to 350 mm. Hg or more on 100% oxygen.	
C. Acute alveolar hypoventilation, causing pH of 7.25 or less.	
2. Intubate the patient (see the method for "Endotracheal Intubation").	
3. Calculate or derive appropriate ventilator settings from normograms.	3. These settings provide a minute volume approximately twice normal. This is appropriate for most patients in respiratory failure since their pathology is commonly associated with an increased physiologic dead space. When respiratory failure is secondary to nonpulmonary pathology (barbiturate overdose, neuromuscular disease), minute volumes may be diminished by reducing the respiratory rate.
A. Tidal volume = 10 ml./kg. body weight.	
B. Rate = normal adult rate; approximately 15 breaths/min.	
C. $FIO_2 = \dfrac{AaDO_2 + 100 \text{ mm. Hg}}{\text{barometric pressure}}$	
D. Determine appropriate airflow patterns.	
4. Be familiar with ventilator:	
A. Displays and data provided about the patient.	
B. Alarms, and their meanings.	
C. Current settings.	
5. Repeat arterial blood gas determinations 30 minutes after the patient has stabilized on the ventilator (see the method for "Arterial Puncture").	5. Blood gas results are used to verify that the ventilator settings are providing adequate ventilation and oxygenation.

PRECAUTIONS

1. Observe carefully for signs and symptoms of reduced cardiac output, especially in those patients with hypovolemia or limited autonomic responses. Venous return and cardiac output may be reduced, particularly during prolonged inspiratory:expiratory ratio or during positive end expiratory pressure (PEEP).
2. Prevent atelectasis with larger tidal volumes, thorough tracheobronchial hygiene, and regular position changes.
3. Detect a positive fluid balance and predict patient's fluid needs by maintaining accurate intake and output records and obtaining daily weights. A positive fluid balance may be due to complex physiologic changes induced by mechanical ventilation. In addition, properly humidified

Table 2.   CONTROLS, DISPLAYS, ALARMS, AND SPECIAL FEATURES OF SEVERAL MECHANICAL VENTILATORS

	Servo	Bennett MA-1	Bennett MA-2
Flow Pattern	May be altered in several ways: (1) flow wave switch allows operator to select sine or square wave; (2) altering spring tension will increase or decrease driving pressure; (3) altering minute volume, inspiratory time %, or rate controls will alter flow.	May be altered with peak flow control setting.	Same as MA-1.
Inspiratory Volume Control	Minute volume and rate are set by operator; tidal volume is determined by the ventilator. Imprudent unilateral changes in either minute volume or rate may therefore cause profound change in the tidal volume. On assist mode patient tidal volume remains constant. Patient may increase minute volume by increasing rate.	Tidal volume and rate determined by operator. Patient may increase minute volume by increasing rate.	Same as MA-1.
Inspiratory to Expiratory Ratio	A function of several settings: (1) rate; (2) minute volume; (3) inspiratory time %; (4) inspiratory hold %.	Expiratory time determined by inspiratory plateau and expiratory retard settings. Inspiratory time determined by volume and flow settings. Alarm sounds if inspiratory to expiratory ratio exceeds 1:1.	Same as MA-1.
Display/Monitoring Capabilities	Expiratory minute volume/inspiratory:expiratory ratio/tidal volume, and airway pressure/lung mechanics calculator/CO_2 analyzer calculates: end volume CO_2, effective/ineffective tidal volume, CO_2 production.	Tidal volume spirometer/temperature inspiratory gases/inspiratory pressure gauge/assist light; indicates patient-initiated breath/sigh light/oxygen light; indicates oxygen enrichment.	Tidal volume spirometer/digital display of temperature of inspiratory gases/inspiratory pressure gauge/digital display of rate/digital display of FIO_2/oxygen light/assist light/sigh light.
Alarms/Alerts	Alarm sounds if changes in controls effect a minute volume that is too high or too low. Upper limit pressure alarm/electric power failure.	Pressure limit alarm/oxygen failure alarm/adverse inspiratory:expiratory time ratio alarm/failure of spirometer to receive set volume within a set time initiates an alarm. Excessive inspiratory gas temperature alarm.	Pressure limit alarm/oxygen failure alarm/adverse inspiratory:expiratory time ratio alarm/failure of spirometer to receive set volume within a set time initiates an alarm. Excessive inspiratory gas temperature alarm/low pressure alarm/failure to cycle alarm.
Special Features	PEEP/CPAP/IMV/inspiratory hold.	PEEP (optional attachments)/negative expiratory pressure (optional attachments)/inspiratory hold/expiratory retard.	IMV/CPAP/PEEP/inspiratory hold.

Table 2. **CONTROLS, DISPLAYS, ALARMS, AND SPECIAL FEATURES OF SEVERAL MECHANICAL VENTILATORS**

	Bourns Bear-1	Ohio CCV-2	Emerson 3-PV(Post op)
Flow Pattern	Wave form alteration control allows operator to select sine or square wave.	Adjustable inspiratory flow control.	Provides inspiratory gases in a sine wave flow pattern.
Inspiratory Volume Control	Tidal volume and rate determined by operator. Patient may increase minute volume by increasing rate.	Tidal volume set by operator. Expiratory time control is titrated until desired rate is achieved.	Stroke volume adjustment knob is located in front of machine at approximately shin level. Rate is set by titrating inhalation and exhalation time controls (see below).
Inspiratory to Expiratory Ratio	Inspiratory to expiratory time will not exceed 1:1 when I:E switch is in "on" position.	A function of inspiratory volume flow and hold settings and expiratory time setting.	Inspiratory and expiratory times are set with two independent controls. When both controls are set similarly (both at 12 o'clock, for example) inspiratory and expiratory times are equal. Turning either control clockwise shortens the inspiratory or expiratory phase. Counterclockwise turns lengthen either phase. Turning *both* controls equal distance in similar directions will increase or decrease respiratory rate.
Display/Monitoring Capabilities	Airway pressure/digital display of expiratory volume/minute volume accumulate/inspiratory: expiratory ratio.	Tidal volume displayed by bellows spirometer. Digital display of rate/system pressure and patient pressure gauge/patient manifold thermometer.	A revolving needle spirometer is an available accessory. Zeroed during the inspiratory phase, the needle moves during expiration to a setting that will approximate tidal volume.
Alarms/Alerts	Low oxygen pressure alarm/low air pressure alarm/high inspiratory pressure alarm/adverse inspiratory:expiratory time ratio alarm/low CPAP alarm/low PEEP alarm apnea alarm/ventilator failure alarm.	Oxygen failure alarm/power failure alarm/high inspiratory pressure alarm/failure to cycle alarm.	An alarm will sound to indicate power failure, massive leak or disconnection of the patient. This alarm is an accessory and may not be present on all Emerson 3-PV ventilators.
Special Features	IMV/CPAP/PEEP/ inspiratory hold.	PEEP/IMV/inspiratory hold.	PEEP is an available accessory. However, patient assist sensitivity cannot be adjusted to accommodate positive airway pressure. Patients must generate negative pressure to initiate an assisted cycle.

gases block insensible water loss from the respiratory tract in mechanically ventilated patients.

4. Employ every practical means of improving ventilation/perfusion relationships to make the need for high oxygen concentrations as temporary as possible. Alveolar damage occurs when high concentrations of inspired oxygen are delivered for prolonged periods of time.

5. Auscultate the chest carefully and frequently to detect early development of subcutaneous emphysema and pneumothorax. They are especially likely to occur following damage to airways or visceral pleura which allows air leaks during positive pressure inspiration. They are also more likely to occur among patients ventilated with PEEP and/or high inspiratory pressures. Chest tubes may be necessary to prevent total lung collapse.

6. Be prepared to relieve the building intrathoracic pressure of a tension pneumothorax rapidly. This may appear as sudden patient distress and/or ventilator malfunction, with the patient rapidly losing consciousness and the face appearing plethoric and cyanotic. The neck veins are distended and the trachea may be deviated away from the tension pneumothorax. A quick inspection of the chest shows one hemithorax becoming distended and tympanic to percussion. Insert one or more large bore needles between the intercostal spaces and ventilate the patient manually until help is summoned and chest tubes are placed.

RELATED CARE

1. Maintain strict asepsis in airway and bronchial hygiene measures and in the care of respiratory equipment. Respiratory disease and/or its treatment may impair nearly all host defenses.
   A. Change all tubing every 24 hours.
   B. Drain liquid condensed in the tubing in the same direction as the air flow. Never drain condensed liquid back into the humidifier.
   C. Wash hands thoroughly between patients as well as between "dirty" nursing tasks (such as Foley care) and "clean" tasks (such as endotracheal suctioning).

2. Use positive end expiratory pressure (PEEP) to maintain above atmospheric pressure in patient airways throughout and between respiratory cycles. This increases functional residual capacity and balances the distribution of inspired tidal volumes throughout the lungs, thereby reducing shunt hypoxemia. PEEP frequently results in improved oxygenation at lower inspired oxygen concentrations and improved ventilation at lower peak inspiratory pressures. However, PEEP increases the risk of barotrauma and may be associated with decreased cardiac output.

3. Return arterial pCO_2 to normal in tachypneic patients who are overriding the ventilator respiratory rate settings and developing hypocapnia. When pharmacologic suppression of the patient's respiratory drive is not appropriate, add additional tubing between the patient's airway and

the inspiratory arm of the ventilating circuit. This increased mechanical dead space causes the patient to rebreathe a portion of the CO_2 expired and reverses respiratory alkalosis.

4. Suppress the respiratory drive of patients who are tachypneic and grossly overdriving a mechanical ventilator to prevent fatigue, decrease oxygen consumption, and improve blood gas levels. Patients who also, because of fear, cerebral hypoxia, or dyspnea asynchronously "fight" the ventilator will require respiratory drive suppression. Respiratory drive may be suppressed by:

    A. Manual hyperinflation, with an oxygen concentration that satiates oxygen and carbon dioxide chemoreceptors.

    B. Narcotics, such as morphine sulfate, given IV. These suppress central respiratory control centers and sedate the anxious patient.

    C. Neuromuscular blocking agents. These paralyze the respiratory muscles. These agents do not alleviate the patient's confusion, fear, or dyspnea, but only block muscular responses to them. The nurse must be acutely aware of the patient's needs for constant reassurance and explanation regarding his temporary paralysis. The nurse should be aware of the pharmacology of drugs employed to suppress respiration, since they may be associated with reduced cardiac output, bronchospasm, or other remote effects.

5. Monitor stool and/or nasogastric aspirate daily, guaiac, as patients receiving prolonged mechanical ventilation are at increased risk of gastrointestinal bleeding. In addition, prophylactic antacid therapy to maintain gastric pH above 5 may be instituted. This is accomplished with hourly testing of gastric pH and titration with antacids, as needed.

COMPLICATIONS

Equipment malfunction
Nosocomial infection
Instrumentation error
Microshock
Positive fluid balance
Oxygen toxicity
Hypocapnia/hypercapnia
Hypoxia/anoxia

Gastrointestinal bleeding
Subcutaneous emphysema
Tension pneumothorax
Atelectasis
Reduced cardiac output/venous
   return
Hyperthermia
Cardiopulmonary arrest

SUPPLIERS

Bourns, Inc. (Bourns Bear-1)
J. H. Emerson, Inc. (Emerson 3-PV (Post op))
Ohio Medical Products (Ohio CCV-2)
Puritan-Bennett Corporation (MA1, MA2)
Siemens-Elema (Servo)

REFERENCES

Eagan, D.F.: Fundamentals of Respiratory Therapy, 3rd ed. St. Louis, C. V. Mosby, 1977, pp. 322–387.

Falke, K.J., Pontoppidan, H., Kumar, A., Leith, D.E., Geffin, B., and Mayer, M.B.: Ventilation with end expiratory pressure in acute lung disease. J. Clin. Invest., *51*:2315, 1972.

Hedley-White, J., et al.: Applied Physiology of Respiratory Care. Boston, Little, Brown and Company, 1976, pp. 18–23.

Hunsinger, D.L., et al.: Respiratory Technology: A Procedure Manual, 2nd ed. Reston, Va., Reston Publishing, 1976, pp. 169–197.

McPherson, S.P.: Respiratory Therapy Equipment. St. Louis, C. V. Mosby, 1977, pp. 168–190.

Rogers, R.M., Weiler, C., and Ruppenthal, B.: The impact of the respiratory intensive care unit on survival of patients with acute respiratory failure. Heart Lung, *1*:475, 1972.

Skillman, J.J., et al.: Intensive Care. Boston, Little, Brown and Company, 1975.

WEANING FROM MECHANICALLY ASSISTED VENTILATION

OBJECTIVES

1. To assess the readiness of the patient before weaning is attempted.
2. To wean a patient effectively.
3. To monitor qualitative (behavioral) and quantitative (ventilatory functions, vital signs) indications of blood gas derangements that may occur during weaning.

SPECIAL EQUIPMENT

Source of heated humdified oxygen of prescribed concentration
T piece adapter

METHOD

ACTION	RATIONALE
1. Assess patient's readiness for weaning. 　A. AaDO$_2$ should be 350 mm. Hg or less on 100% oxygen. 　B. Dead space to tidal volume	

ACTION	RATIONALE
ratio (VD/VT) should not exceed 0.60.	
C. Patient should be able to generate -25 cm. H_2O pressure and/or have a vital capacity of 10 ml./kg. body weight.	
2. Suction patient, as necessary, and give sufficient time to recover from suction-induced dyspnea and hypoxia.	
3. Elevate head of patient's bed, if possible.	3. Proper positioning will reduce intra-abdominal resistance to diaphragmatic excursion.
4. Remove patient from ventilator and connect to source of humidified oxygen, keeping ventilator connections sterile during weaning intervals. Oxygen concentrations are prescribed by the physician and are generally higher than those supplied while on the ventilator.	
5. Measure vital capacity, tidal volume, arterial blood gas concentrations, and vital signs before and after weaning periods. They may be measured during weaning periods as needed.	5. Weaning attempts are terminated if any symptoms of hypoxia or alveolar hypoventilation develop (see precautions, below).
6. At prescribed termination of weaning period: A. Remove T piece. B. Place the patient back on mechanical ventilation. C. Assist patient into a comfortable position.	
7. Reduce length of intervals between weaning periods gradually as weaning periods are lengthened.	

PRECAUTIONS

Observe for signs of blood gas derangements during weaning, including rapid, shallow respirations with or without dyspnea. In addition, hypotension, cyanosis, ectopy and/or conduction disturbances, behavior changes, or decreased level of consciousness may also occur. In particular, agitation, fear, and/or air hunger during weaning should not be dismissed as functional complaints but should be investigated in terms of alterations in vital signs, ventilatory parameters, and blood gas levels. Weaning should be terminated at any point if hypoxia or alveolar hypoventilation is suspected.

RELATED CARE

1. Prepare patients for weaning from the beginning of mechanical ventilation. They should be reassured that the use of a ventilator is "temporary." Patients are also told of any signs of improvement in their condition, and are encouraged to look forward to trial periods off the ventilator.
2. Remain with the patient during weaning. Since he is unattached from ventilator alarms and unable to summon help, a patient's deterioration may go unnoticed. In addition, patients are entitled to close support and encouragement during a procedure that they may perceive as threatening and frightening.
3. Weaning should not be attempted at night until prolonged daytime periods of spontaneous ventilation are well established. Lack of staff for close supervision and patient fatigue at night results in suboptimal weaning.
4. Intermittent mandatory ventilation (IMV) is a more physiologic approach to weaning patients during mechanical ventilation. It permits the patient to remain attached to the ventilator while spontaneously breathing a humidified oxygen mixture. The ventilator is set to deliver a mandatory breath at specific intervals. These intervals are gradually lengthened until the patient breathes entirely independently of the ventilator.

COMPLICATIONS

Hypoxia	Hypotension
Dysrhythmias	Respiratory arrest

REFERENCES

Eagan, D.F.: Fundamentals of Respiratory Therapy, 3rd ed. St. Louis, C. V. Mosby, 1977, 456–460.

Falke, K.J., Pontoppidan, H., Kumar, A., Leith, D.E., Geffin, B., and Mayer, M.B.: Ventilation with end expiratory pressure in acute lung disease. J. Clin. Invest., 51:2315, 1972.

Fitzgerald, L.M., and Huber, G.L.: Weaning the patient from mechanical ventilation. Heart Lung, 5:228, 1976.

Hedley-White, J., et al.: Applied Physiology of Respiratory Care. Boston, Little, Brown and Company, 1976, 133–144.

Hunsinger, D.L., et al.: Respiratory Technology: A Procedure Manual, 2nd ed. Reston, VA, Reston Publishing, 1976, 197–198.

McPherson, S.P.: Respiratory Therapy Equipment. St. Louis, C. V. Mosby, 1977, p. 189.

Rogers, R.M., Weiler, C., and Ruppenthal, B.: The impact of the respiratory intensive care unit on survival of patients with acute respiratory failure. Heart Lung, *1*:475, 1972.

Sahn, S.A., and Lakshminarayan, S.: Bedside criteria for discontinuation of mechanical ventilation. Chest, *63*:1002, 1973.

Sahn, S.A., Lakshminarayan, S., and Petty, T.L.: Weaning from mechanical ventilation. J.A.M.A., *235*:2208, 1976.

Skillman, J.J., et al.: Intensive Care. Boston, Little, Brown and Company, 1975.

AMBUING WITH POSITIVE END AIRWAY PRESSURE (PEEP)

OBJECTIVES

1. To maintain increased functional residual capacity (FRC) and minimize shunting in patients removed from mechanical ventilation with PEEP.
2. To provide optimal oxygenation and alveolar ventilation for patients who must be removed from mechanical ventilation with PEEP for transport, bronchial hygiene, or other purposes.

SPECIAL EQUIPMENT

Anesthesia bag with universal adapter
Oxygen source
Source of expiratory resistance (water column, PEEP valve, etc.)

METHOD

ACTION	RATIONALE
1. Begin flow of oxygen into anesthesia bag.	
2. Attach source of expiratory resistance (Fig. 80).	
3. Remove ventilator hose from airway at end inspiration.	
4. Attach anesthesia bag to airway during passive expiratory phase.	
5. Observe patient's abdomen and	5. Tidal volumes, and therefore alveolar

ACTION   **RATIONALE**

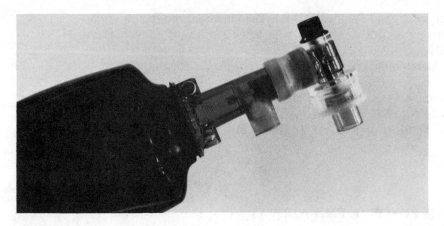

Figure 80.   Anesthesia bag with PEEP valve.

chest for inspiratory efforts and supply breaths "on demand."

ventilation, will be diminished if breaths are delivered against resistance or asynchronously with patient efforts.

6. Encourage patient to breathe slowly and deeply.
7. Administer slow, full breaths at a rate of 10 to 12 per minute to apneic or paralyzed patients.
8. Release inflation hold at end inspiration and allow patient to exhale against expiratory resistance.
9. Repeat respiratory cycles as described in steps 5 through 8 until patient can be returned to mechanical ventilation with PEEP.

PRECAUTIONS

1. Minimize the risk of nosocomial pulmonary infections by employing aseptic technique in the management of all ventilatory equipment. Provide each patient with a sterilized anesthesia bag at least every 24 hours. Avoid using the same bag for more than one patient, thus reducing sources of cross-infection. Replace any anesthesia bag that becomes contaminated.
2. Observe for sudden deterioration in ventilatory status that may indicate formation of a pneumothorax. Patients with poor compliance who are ventilated with PEEP are at risk of pulmonary tissue rupture with consequent leakage of air into the pleural space (see the precautions for "Instituting Mechanical Ventilation").

RELATED CARE

Maintain desired levels of PEEP when ventilating with Boehringer valves by holding the valve upright at all times. Expiratory resistance is provided by the Boehringer valve by means of weighted balls in a cylinder. If the cylinder becomes tilted the balls roll within the cylinder, opening the aperture and allowing free exhalation. Also, inverting the cylinders will occlude the exhalation port entirely.

COMPLICATIONS

Infection   Pneumothorax
Inadequate or excessive alveolar
   ventilation

REFERENCES

Manufacturer's Literature
Massachusetts General Hospital, Unpublished procedure.

CONTINUOUS POSITIVE AIRWAY PRESSURE (CPAP)   _____

OBJECTIVES

1. To increase functional residual capacity (FRC) and decrease the degree of pulmonary shunting.
2. To obviate the need for intubation and mechanical ventilation in acute, potentially reversible pulmonary pathology.

SPECIAL EQUIPMENT

Oxygen source
Oxygen/air mixer
Reservoir bag
Source of warm humidification
Clear face mask of rigid material with soft, pliable seal
Straps for face mask
Inspiratory and expiratory tubing with one-way valves
CPAP device with safety pop-off feature
   PEEP valve
   Water column
   Spring-loaded membrane
   PEEP system of mechanical ventilator

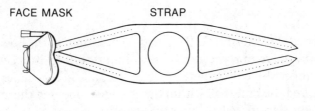

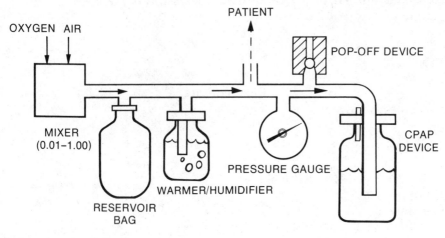

Figure 81. CPAP system.

Pressure gauge (cm. H_2O pressure)
Skin lotion

METHOD

ACTION	RATIONALE
1. Obtain baseline blood gas levels, vital signs and, if possible, central venous and pulmonary vascular pressures.	1. CPAP has profound respiratory and circulatory effects. The clinician must be able to detect early adverse as well as desirable reactions.
2. Explain procedure to patient and his significant others, including purpose and potential discomforts of CPAP.	2. Mask CPAP is a stressful experience that may last an indefinite amount of time. Patient cooperation is essential for success. The patient in turn needs maximal emotional support of staff and significant others.
3. Begin flow of warm humidified oxygen mixture through system.	
4. Apply face mask to patient and strap in place without in-line expiratory resistance.	4. Allows the patient a few moments to adjust to the tight-fitting mask.
5. Connect CPAP device to expiratory tubing.	

ACTION	RATIONALE
6. Explain to patient that he/she may begin to sense a change in the work of breathing.	6. Dyspneic patients may panic if they suddenly sense interference in their already labored respirations.
7. Slowly adjust expiratory resistance until desired level of positive airway pressure is achieved.	
8. Remain with patient and encourage regular, relaxed respiratory pattern.	
9. Assess vital signs and central venous and pulmonary vascular pressures as soon as patient is stabilized. Determine blood gas levels as appropriate or prescribed.	9. These data provide a baseline from which the response to CPAP can be assessed.
10. Check the system frequently for air leaks, with particular attention to the face mask seal.	10. Air leaks will reduce the positive airway pressure.
11. Assess respiratory and circulatory parameters hourly, and more frequently as indicated.	11. CPAP imposes an increased workload on critically ill patients who are therefore at risk of slipping into respiratory failure.
12. Continue to provide close physical presence and emotional support.	
13. Discontinue CPAP for 10 minutes every 2 hours and provide warmed humidified oxygen via face tent.	13. The patient will need periods of rest from increased ventilatory workload as well as opportunity for verbalization, oral hygiene, and nourishment.
14. Assess skin around bony prominences of face and under any tubes (nasogastric tubes, etc.) that may protrude from under mask.	
15. Massage reddened areas with lotion.	
16. Reassess non-CPAP respiratory and circulatory parameters as appropriate.	
17. Reinstitute CPAP as described in steps 3 through 10.	
18. Continue intermittent mask CPAP until pulmonary pathology resolves, or until more definitive respiratory support measures become necessary.	

PRECAUTIONS

1. Provide an expiratory tubing system that has an integral pop-off valve between the patient and the CPAP device. The valve should release to

allow free exhalation if the system pressure exceeds desired levels of positive pressure; this could occur if the CPAP device malfunctions.

2. Ensure consistent levels of CPAP by checking the pressure gauge and observing the system for air leaks frequently. Air leaks around the face mask are particularly common.

3. Perform careful, periodic chest assessment in order to detect signs of pneumothorax. CPAP in patients with diseased, poorly compliant lungs may precipitate rupture, with the escape of air into the pleural space. The clinician should be particularly alert to this possibility if high levels of CPAP are being attempted or if a sudden deterioration in ventilatory status occurs.

4. Observe respiratory efforts and chest excursion, as well as respiratory rate and depth frequently. Patients treated with CPAP are subjected to an increased respiratory workload on top of diseased, poorly compliant lungs. Fatigue and resultant hypercapnea may occur. An anesthesia bag with face mask, and in some cases an intubation tray, should be kept at the bedside.

5. Minimize the risk of infection by applying aseptic management of all CPAP equipment. Patients with pulmonary disease have compromised defense systems and are susceptible to infection. CPAP systems provide a warm, moist environment for bacterial growth and should be changed at least every 48 hours.

6. Avoid the use of opaque face masks, since they obscure patient vomiting and promote aspiration. Further minimize the risk of aspiration by checking the abdomen for distention frequently. Immediately attend to patient complaints of nausea by replacing the CPAP mask with the face tent and humidified oxygen.

RELATED CARE

Provide the patient with an alternative means of communication while the CPAP mask is in place. If the patient must be left alone momentarily, provide a bell, buzzer, or other device for summoning help.

COMPLICATIONS

Ventilatory fatigue and failure   Excoriation of face
Pneumothorax   Infection
Diminished cardiac output

SUPPLIERS

Boehringer Laboratories (Boehringer valve)
Puritan-Bennett Corporation (Spring-loaded membrane obtained from
  MA-1 ventilator)

REFERENCES

University of Wisconsin Hospitals Manual of Respiratory Therapy Procedures.
  Unpublished.

Jeannette McCann McHugh, R.N., M.S.N.

OVERVIEW

The visceral and parietal pleura form a potential intrathoracic space that is filled with only 4 ml. of lubricating pleural fluid. Between these two membranes, which line the chest wall and cover the lungs, there is a fluctuating but always negative intrapleural pressure. Disease, chest trauma, or surgery may cause disruption of the lung, thorax, or pleura and enable air or fluid to flow into the pleural space. This interrupts full inspiratory excursion and may lead to complete lung collapse. Some injuries can result in a tension pneumothorax in which the lung collapses, mediastinal structures are displaced, and the heart and great vessels are compressed, leading to sudden death.

Patients requiring intensive respiratory care are subject to pleural space disruptions secondary to thoracic surgery and ventilatory barotrauma, as well as their own pulmonary pathology. For this reason the critical care nurse must know how to manage chest drainage systems safely as well as assist with chest tube placement.

After chest tubes have been inserted into the pleural space to remove air or fluid, they are connected to a chest drainage system. A chest drainage system may be composed of one, two, or three parts, each of which provides a specific function. These functions can be described in terms of the classic three-bottle chest drainage system, and provided by a bottle chest drainage system or a disposable chest drainage unit.

CHEST TUBE PLACEMENT (ASSISTING WITH)

OBJECTIVES

1. To identify the signs of intrapleural air and fluid.
2. To assist the physician by anticipating needs during chest tube placement.
3. To attach the chest tubes to a drainage system and maintain chest tube patency.

SPECIAL EQUIPMENT

Antiseptic skin prep and swabs
Sterile drape(s)
Sterile gloves
Anesthetic with 2-ml. syringe and 5/8" 28-gauge and 21-gauge
   1¼" needles

Scalpel blade and handle

Chest tubes with obturators in varying sizes

Suture material (000) needle and needle holder

Kelly clamps (two)

Hemostat

Forceps

Dressing materials:

    Sterile gauze pads/Scissors/Occlusive dressing (petroleum jelly gauze)/Occlusive tape

Connecting tube and straight and Y connectors

Drainage/water seal/suction source

METHOD

ACTION	RATIONALE

1. Auscultate/percuss chest.
  A. Pleural space disruptions may be manifested by decreased compliance and increased peak inspiratory pressures. Decreased PaO_2, and increased $AaDO_2$.
  B. Intrapleural air may be manifested by distant to absent breath sounds, hyperresonance, or tympany to percussion.
  C. Intrapleural fluid may be manifested by distant to absent breath sounds, dullness, or flatness to percussion.
	1. This identifies area of pleural space disruptions.

2. Prepare drainage system (see the method for "Three-Bottle Closed Chest Drainage System"). In an emergency, water seal may be provided by placing distal end of chest tube into bottle of sterile saline or water at a depth of about 2 cm.	2. If the tube is immersed under too much H_2O, accumulating pressure within the chest cannot escape.
3. Assist physician with chest tube insertion. Chest tubes are usually placed in the second intercostal space anteriorly to remove intrapleural air and in the eighth or ninth intercostal space posteriorly to remove fluid. If the pleural space contains both air and fluid,	

ACTION	RATIONALE
chest tubes may be placed at both sites.	

4. Connect tubing to drainage system.
  A. Wire and tape connections securely.
  B. If two tubes are placed, a Y connector may be used to connect them to a single drainage system.	

5. Apply occlusive dressing to tube insertion site.	
6. Turn on suction source, as appropriate.	
7. Place vertical strip of tape along collection bottle(s). Mark level of drainage and monitor every hour, or as circumstances indicate.	
8. Coil tubing and secure to bottom sheet in loose loop. Connecting tubing should be long enough for patient to turn 120° and sit upright.	8. Fluid accumulating in lengths of dependent tubing interferes with flow of drainage into collecting system.
9. "Strip" accumulated clots, fibrin, and drainage out of tubing each hour. Pinch tubing with both hands, sliding fingers of one hand distally along tube. The entire length of each tube should be stripped hourly, or as indicated.	

10. Make the following observations hourly.
  A. Water seal is maintained at 2 cm.
  B. Prescribed amount of suction is maintained.
  C. Continuous gentle bubbling is present in suction control bottle.
  D. Color and quantity of drainage is noted.	

PRECAUTIONS

Keep Kelly clamps readily available at the bedside. If a disconnection occurs, a leak develops, or bottle No. 1 or No. 2 breaks, the tube should be clamped and a physician notified. Since there is a risk of tension pneumothorax under these circumstances, the patient should not be left unattended and should be observed for any signs of respiratory difficulty. If a developing tension pneumothorax is suspected, the clamps are released and accumulated pleural air is allowed to escape.

RELATED CARE

1. Auscultate and percuss the chest to determine if a nonfluctuating water seal column is due to an obstructed chest tube or re-expansion of the lung. A patient breathing spontaneously should cause fluid in the water seal column to rise slightly with inspiration.
2. Observe for bubbling in the water seal bottle; this indicates an air leak into the pleural space from the lung or bronchus. Continuous slow bubbling should always be present in the suction control bottle, however. Lack of bubbling may indicate failure of the suction source or an "upstream" leak within the system or around the chest tube.

COMPLICATIONS

Infection   Hemothorax
Hemorrhage   Equipment malfunction
Tension pneumothorax

REFERENCES

Bushnell, S.S.: Respiratory Intensive Care Nursing. Boston, Little, Brown and Company, 1973, p. 249.
Clinical Aspects of Chest Drainage. St. Louis, Sherwood Medical.
Van Meter, M.: Chest tubes—basic techniques for better care. Nurs. '74, *4*:48, 1974.

THREE-BOTTLE CLOSED CHEST DRAINAGE SYSTEM _____

OBJECTIVES

1. To re-expand the involved lung in a pneumothorax.
2. To observe and measure drainage via the chest tubes.

SPECIAL EQUIPMENT

Three sterile wide-mouthed gallon bottles

Three sterile caps or stoppers (two caps with two vents, third cap with
   three vents)
Two sterile glass pipets (longer than the depth of the bottles) and five
   small glass vents
Four lengths of sterile tubing
50-ml. irrigation syringe
Sterile water
1″ adhesive tape and wire
Centimeter ruler
Sterile gloves
Needle holder
Kelly clamps (two)

METHOD

| ACTION | RATIONALE |

1. Open sterile packages of bottles and
   related equipment.
2. Don sterile gloves.
3. Prepare water seal bottle (Fig. 82).

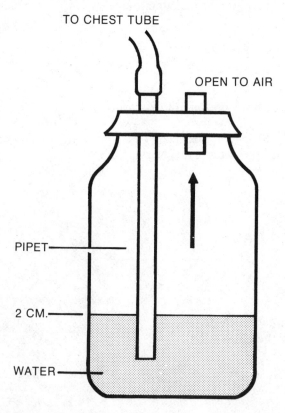

Figure 82.   Water seal bottle.

ACTION	RATIONALE
A. Cap one bottle with a two-vented cap.	
B. Insert long glass pipet through one hole and a small glass vent in second hole.	
C. Attach long tubing to long glass pipet.	
4. Prepare the suction control bottle (Fig. 83).	
A. Cap the bottle with three-vented cap.	
B. Insert a long glass pipet through middle vent and small glass vents into other holes.	B. This is used to control the amount of suction applied by the system.
C. Attach small glass vent of water seal bottle to a small glass vent of suction control bottle with a piece of tubing.	
D. Attach a long piece of tubing to remaining glass vent on suction control bottle.	D. This is connected to the suction source.

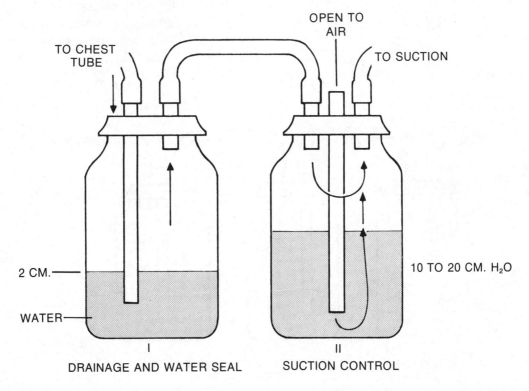

Figure 83. Two-bottle chest drainage system.

ACTION	RATIONALE

5. Prepare collection bottle (Fig. 84).
    A. Cap bottle with remaining two-vented cap.
    B. Insert two small glass vents into holes.
    C. Attach long tubing from long glass pipet of the underwater seal bottle to small glass vent of collection bottle.
    D. Attach a long tubing to remaining glass vent. Keep the end of this tube sterile.

    D. This connects the chest tubes to the collection bottle.

    E. Remove gloves.
    F. Add sterile water to underwater seal bottle; position glass pipet tip 2 cm. under water level.

    F. As the patient inspires, generating negative intrathoracic pressure, water rises in the pipet but air is blocked from entering the pleural space.

    G. Add prescribed amount of sterile water to suction control bottle.

    G. The amount of suction delivered to the chest tube is determined by the length (cm.) of pipet beneath the water surface. Chest drainage systems are usually set to deliver 10 to 20 cm. H_2O negative pressure to the chest tube.

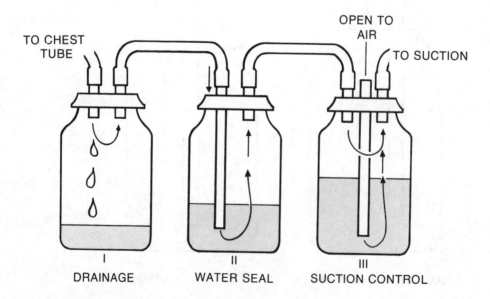

Figure 84.   Three-bottle chest drainage system.

ACTION	RATIONALE
H. Wrap tubing connections twice with wire. Using needle holder, grasp wire ends and twist them several times.	H. This secures the connection and prevents separation.
I. Wrap 1'' adhesive tape around wire, overlapping it to cover both connectors and wired tubing.	I. The tape prevents cuts to the fingers and hands when the tubing is handled, and provides additional protection from separation.
J. Tape bottles to floor.	J. This prevents accidental separation of tube connections or bottle caps in case the bottles are jarred or hit.

PRECAUTIONS

Place the underwater seal pipet only 2 cm. under the water level. If an intrathoracic air leak is present, accumulating interpleural air may safely escape through the chest tube and pipet, causing bubbling at the point of the water seal. Placing the pipet below more than 2 cm. of water may cause a hazard by increasing the amount of intrathoracic pressure which must develop before accumulated pleural air can be blown off. Placing the pipet below less than 2 cm. of water risks loss of water seal from evaporation, and a subsequent pneumothorax.

RELATED CARE

1. Precalibrate a collection bottle for measuring the drainage.
2. Observe the fluid level in the underwater seal column; it should rise and fall during the respiratory cycle. A single underwater seal bottle should be used only for a pneumothorax, since draining interpleural fluids will cause a rising fluid level and create a progressive resistance to drainage. If underwater seal alone is used, the air vent is left open to air.
3. Provide suction when air enters the pleural cavity faster than it is forced out through the underwater seal.

COMPLICATIONS

Pleural erosion and hemorrhage

Hematomas of lungs and chest wall

Failure of lung to re-expand

Tension pneumothorax

Infection

REFERENCES

Bushnell, S.S.: Respiratory Intensive Care Nursing. Boston, Little, Brown and Company, 1973, pp. 225–261.

Clinical Aspects of Chest Drainage. St. Louis, Sherwood Medical.

Van Meter, M.: Chest tubes—basic techniques for better care. Nurs. '74, 4:48, 1974.

DISPOSABLE CHEST DRAINAGE UNIT _____

OBJECTIVES

1. To re-expand the involved lung in a pneumothorax.
2. To observe and measure drainage via the chest tubes.

SPECIAL EQUIPMENT

Chest drainage unit   1'' adhesive tape and wire
50-ml. irrigation syringe   Needle holder
Sterile water   Two Kelly clamps

METHOD

ACTION	RATIONALE
1. Arrange tubings so they will not fall on floor. Make sure protective caps are securely attached to connectors.	1. This prevents contamination while equipment is being readied.
2. Attach sterile 50-ml. irrigation syringe, without barrel, to rubber tubing of water seal chamber.	
3. Fill water seal chamber up to 2-cm. line. If the patient will be on straight drainage, connector will be left off; otherwise, reapply.	
4. Remove cap from suction control chamber and, using same method as in step 3, fill to level necessary for desired amount of suction. Replace cap.	4. This will keep bubbling at minimum.
5. Fill the third chamber, found on some units, to a specified level in a similar manner.	

ACTION	RATIONALE
6. Hang unit from the bed or place in support device.	
7. Wire and tape the chest tube connection to the long tubing (see the method for "Three-Bottle Closed Chest Drainage System").	7. This prevents accidental disconnection and resulting pneumothorax.

PRECAUTIONS

See precautions for the "Three-Bottle Closed Chest Drainage System."

RELATED CARE

See related care for the "Three-Bottle Closed Chest Drainage System."

COMPLICATIONS

See complications for the "Three-Bottle Closed Chest Drainage System."

SUPPLIERS

Argyle "Double Seal" chest drainage unit
Deknatel, division of Howmedica, Inc. (Pleur-evac)

REFERENCES

Bushnell, S.S.: Respiratory Intensive Care Nursing. Boston, Little, Brown and Company, 1973, pp. 255–261.

Clinical Aspects of Chest Drainage. St. Louis, Sherwood Medical.

Van Meter, M.: Chest tubes—basic techniques for better care. Nurs. '74, *4*:48, 1974.

CHEST PHYSIOTHERAPY

Jeannette McCann McHugh, R.N., M.S.N.

OVERVIEW

Airway obstruction is a common contributing factor in respiratory failure which causes ventilation/perfusion defects and frustrates the usefulness of ventilatory and oxygen therapy. Therefore, measures are taken to alleviate bronchospasm and move secretions from peripheral to central airways from which they are more easily removed. In addition to the use of bronchodilating drugs, these measures include adequate hydration, deep breathing, and coughing exercises, postural drainage, and chest physiotherapy.

Postural drainage employs specific body positions to facilitate drainage of secretions from affected lung segments into the major airways. When several segments are involved, upper lobes are drained first, then middle, and finally lower lobes (Figs. 85 through 93 illustrate the position employed for each segment of lung.) Each position is maintained for 20 to 30 minutes if possible. Percussion and vibration are used in conjunction with postural drainage to loosen tenacious secretions and enhance drainage.

OBJECTIVES

1. To determine and place the patient in the appropriate drainage positions.
2. To percuss and vibrate the chest effectively, loosening secretions and enhancing drainage.

SPECIAL EQUIPMENT

Towels   Several pillows

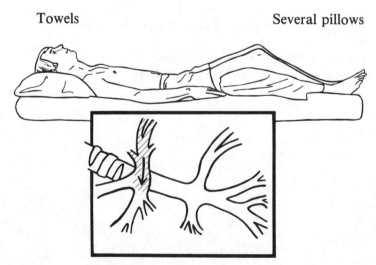

Figure 85. Upper lobes, anterior segments. (Adapted from Bushnell, S.S.: Respiratory Intensive Care Nursing, 1st ed. Boston, Little, Brown, and Company, 1973, Fig. 37, p. 79. Reproduced by permission.)

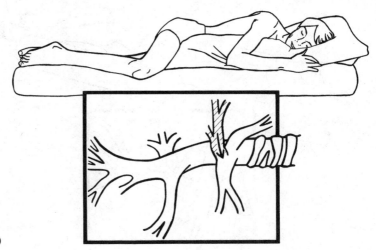

Figure 86. Upper lobe, posterior segment, right posterior bronchus. (Adapted from Bushnell, Fig. 38, p. 80. Reproduced by permission.)

METHOD

ACTION	RATIONALE
1. Conduct an assessment using chest x-rays and auscultation to locate involved areas and estimate severity of obstruction.	1. The most severely obstructed airways permit less air movement and have *fewer* adventitious sounds. Diminished, absent, or bronchial breath sounds may indicate more severe pathology than loud rales and rhonchae.
2. Position patient appropriately and ensure that he is comfortably supported and relaxed.	

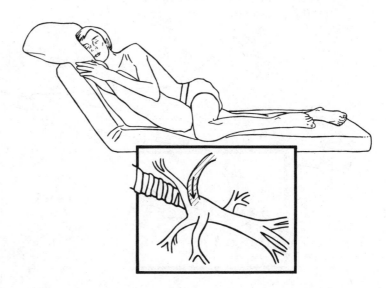

Figure 87. Upper lobe, posterior segment, left posterior bronchus. (Adapted from Bushnell, Fig. 39, p. 80. Reproduced by permission.)

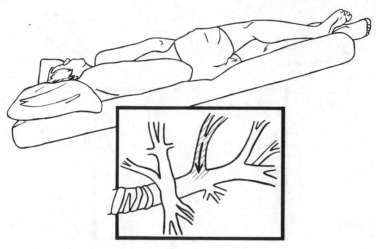

Figure 88.   Right middle lobe. (Adapted from Bushnell, Fig. 35, p. 78. Reproduced by permission.)

ACTION	RATIONALE
3. Provide tissues and receptacle for nonintubated patients or patients with deflated endotracheal tube cuffs.	
4. Drape chest with towel.	
5. Position yourself opposite site requiring therapy. Rhythmically clap chest wall. Hands should be held in cupped position; thumbs and fingers held together. Snap is applied only from the wrists. Elbows and shoulders are held loose and relaxed.	5. Air is caught under the cupped hand as it meets chest wall, causing an abrupt but cushioned blow. Percussion in the absence of chest trauma should not be strong enough to produce pain.
6. Stop periodically to encourage deep breathing and coughing.	

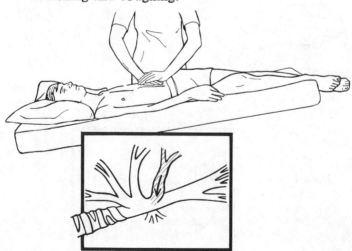

Figure 89.   Left lingula. (Adapted from Bushnell, Fig. 36, p. 78. Reproduced by permission.)

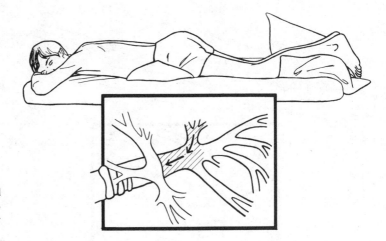

Figure 90. Lower lobes, apical segment. (Adapted from Bushnell, Fig. 31, p. 76. Reproduced by permission.)

ACTION	RATIONALE

7. Vibrate chest wall.
  A. Place one hand over affected segment and second hand on top of first.
  B. Ask patient to inspire deeply and then exhale.
  C. Holding moderate pressure against chest wall, vibrate hands during expiration.
  D. If patient is being mechanically ventilated, synchronize vibration with passive expiratory phase.
	7. This assists the movement of secretions up and out of the tracheobronchial tree.

8. Allow a few respiratory cycles for rest and/or coughing.	8. This avoids fatiguing and hyperventilation.

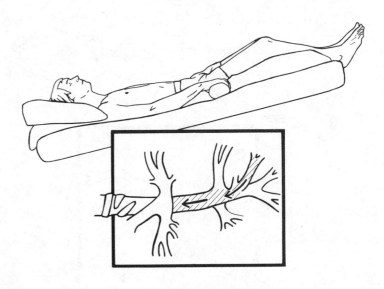

Figure 91. Lower lobes, anterior basal segment. (Adapted from Bushnell, Fig. 32, p. 76. Reproduced by permission.)

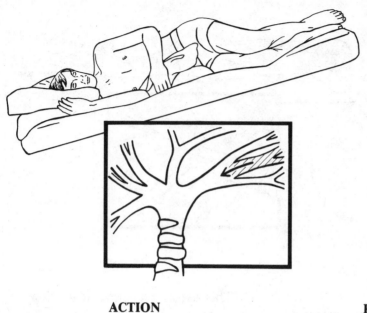

Figure 92. Lower lobe, lateral basal segment. (Adapted from Bushnell, Fig. 33, p. 77. Reproduced by permission.)

ACTION	RATIONALE

9. Repeat. The amount of physiotherapy given to each segment is a clinical judgment based upon:
    A. Number of segments involved.
    B. Character and amount of secretions.
    C. Patient's ability to tolerate the total procedure.
10. Allow several minutes for drainage.
11. Advance to next involved segment, and repeat physiotherapy as indicated.

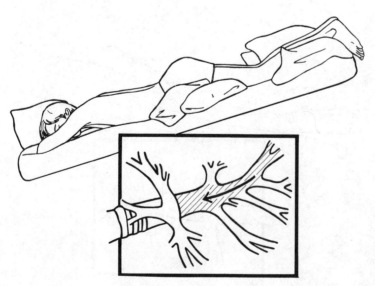

Figure 93. Lower lobes, posterior basal bronchus. (Adapted from Bushnell, Fig. 34, p. 77. Reproduced by permission.)

PRECAUTIONS

1. Avoid head-down and supine postural drainage after eating, since these positions may cause vomiting and aspiration. Head-down positioning may also be avoided in the presence of increased intracranial pressure.
2. Avoid postural drainage and physiotherapy during weaning intervals. Fatigue and/or abdominal pressure against the diaphragm may cause hyperventilation.
3. Do not percuss and vibrate in the presence of intrathoracic or intracranial bleeding, serious cardiac arrhythmias, or localized pulmonary infections which may be disseminated to unaffected lung tissue.

RELATED CARE

Make every effort to see that pain medication, aerosolized bronchodilator therapy, and chest physiotherapy are given in a coordinated fashion and integrated into the patient's overall care plan.

COMPLICATIONS

Dysrhythmias
Altered hemodynamics
Hypoventilation/hyperventilation
Fatigue

Disseminated pulmonary infections
Trauma
Rib fractures

REFERENCES

Bushnell, S.S.: Respiratory Intensive Care Nursing. Boston, Little, Brown and Company, 1973, pp. 71–80.
Waterson, M.: Teaching your patients postural drainage. Nurs. '78, 8:51, 1978.

THORACENTESIS (ASSISTING WITH)

Janice Casper, R.N., B.S.N.

OVERVIEW

Thoracentesis is performed to remove fluid and/or air from the pleural space or to instill sclerosing and/or antineoplastic agents between the two pleurae. This is accomplished by inserting a needle or trocar cannula instrument into the thoracic cavity at a select site, predetermined by x-ray findings and physical examination.

Thoracentesis using an anterior approach is usually performed as an emergency intervention for air removal and requires precise instrumentation and an understanding of thoracic anatomy. Thoracentesis using a posterior approach, however, is usually performed as a therapeutic intervention for fluid drainage or for obtaining a specimen for laboratory analysis. The critical care nurse shares responsibility in patient assessment before, during, and after this therapeutic intervention, and must be cognizant of its potential effects.

OBJECTIVES

1. To remove fluid or air from the pleural space for the prompt relief of lung compressions or respiratory distress.
2. To obtain a fluid specimen for laboratory analysis.
3. To instill therapeutic agents into the pleural space.

SPECIAL EQUIPMENT

Thoracentesis tray
Sterile gloves
Sterile drapes
Local anesthetic
25-gauge, 20-gauge, and
    18-gauge needles
Thoracentesis needles:
    15-gauge, 17-gauge, 3-inch,
    short bevels
Two 10-ml. syringes
Two 50-ml. syringes

Three-way stopcock with 10 to
    20 inches of tubing
Hemostat
Kelly clamp
Sterile fluid collection container
Scalpel blade (No. 11)
Laboratory specimen tubes
Sterile gauze pads
Povidone-iodine swabs
Povidone-iodine ointment
Tape

METHOD

ACTION	**RATIONALE**
1. Assess patient; obtain vital signs prior to therapy.	1. This information provides baseline data.
2. Position patient.	
A. Anterior thoracentesis approach:	A. An anterior-superior approach is used for air removal.
(1) Use supine position, with arm positioned under head.	
B. Posterior thoracentesis approach (options):	B. A posterior-inferior approach is used for fluid removal.
(1) Dangle patient at bedside with arms resting over a padded overbed table and feet resting on footstool.	
(2) Use chair-straddle technique with arms resting on high back of chair or padded overbed table.	
2. Don sterile gloves; mask and gown all persons in immediate area.	
3. Prepare skin site with povidone-iodine solution; drape area.	
4. Assess patient continuously while the thoracentesis is being performed.	
A. Support patient's position while skin zones are anesthetized; various gauges and lengths of needles are used for infiltration until parietal fluid is reached.	A. The patient may experience momentary pain on initial skin penetration and needle contact with the highly sensitive pleura prior to anesthesia infiltration.
B. Observe for pleural fluid return as needle is slowly advanced; as needle is withdrawn, note depth of penetration.	B. The depth of needle penetration to reach the pleural fluid is approximated and used as a guide during the advancement of the thoracentesis needle.
C. Instruct patient to breathe shallowly and to refrain from coughing as thoracentesis needle is advanced to pre-estimated depth and with constant aspiration; the thoracentesis needle is equipped with a preconnected 50-ml. syringe, three-way stopcock, and drainage tubing.	C. Shallow controlled breathing while the needle is in position minimizes risk of lung trauma. Also, the lung is re-expanding as fluid is removed; this brings the lung closer to the needle tip.

ACTION	RATIONALE
D. Support patient's position during immobilization period as thoracentesis needle is secured with Kelly clamp at skin puncture site and fluid is aspirated from pleural space (Fig. 94).	D. Securing the needle prevents inadvertent advancement during accidental movement.
E. Apply firm pressure to puncture site following removal of needle.	
F. Assess puncture site; apply povidone-iodine ointment and secure sterile dressing.	
5. Instruct patient to rest in bed postthoracentesis; monitor patient's vital signs and assess for pallor, cyanosis, dyspnea, tachycardia, hypotension, and bilateral breath sounds.	
6. Note amount and appearance of fluid removed; facilitate prompt transport of specimen for prescribed laboratory analysis.	
7. Assess postthoracentesis chest films.	7. A chest x-ray provides data regarding the presence or absence of a pneumothorax or residual pleural effusions.

PRECAUTIONS

1. Assess health history for information regarding:
   A. Bleeding disorders and/or current medications, such as heparin or Coumadin, which could increase the risk of complications.

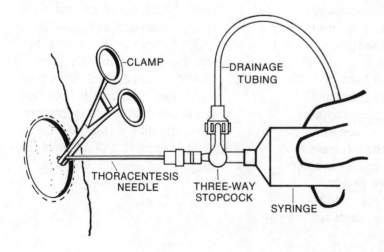

Figure 94. Thoracentesis.

    B.   Length of time of pleural effusion. Complete removal of a large pleural effusion present for longer than 3 months increases the risk of complications. Approximately 500 to 1000 ml. should be removed at one time in such cases.

2. Monitor the patient closely for perforation of the diaphragm or abdominal viscera if the puncture site is quite low in a posterior-inferior approach.

3. Recommend equipment testing prior to thoracentesis needle insertion to determine proper connections and ensure familiarity with directional stopcock positions. Air can enter pleural space owing to faulty instrumentation and cause a pneumothorax.

4. Control coughing, singultus, and patient movement; these will increase the risks of lung, nerve, and vessel trauma while needle is in position.

RELATED CARE

1. Adapt method from needle to cannula insertion for therapeutic agents or to facilitate abundant drainage over a 24-hour, but less than a 48-hour, period.

2. Consider using vacuum collection bottles rather than a syringe-aspiration method for large volumes of pleural fluid evacuation. The vacuum method offers potential for lung tissue aspiration.

3. Assess puncture site for pain, erythema, edema and warmth after 24 hours.

COMPLICATIONS

Pneumothorax	Hypovolemic shock
Respiratory arrest	Pleural shock
Hemothorax; hemorrhage	Infection
Diaphragmatic injury	Protein depletion
Penetration of abdominal viscera	Electrolyte imbalance

SUPPLIERS

Kendall-Curity
Monoject
Pharmaseal
Tomac

REFERENCE

Dryer, B.V. (ed.): Thoracentesis, Nutley, N.J., ROCOM, 1973.

THE
RENAL
SYSTEM

ACUTE HEMODIALYSIS

Anna J. Lavelle, R.N., B.S.N., and
Cheryl Tomich Wyman, R.N., B.S.N.

OVERVIEW

Hemodialysis can be defined as a modality whereby desirable elements are retained on the blood side of a membrane, unwanted particles are passed through to a bath, and dangerous agents such as bacteria and viruses are prevented from entering the blood. The removal of these elements from the blood occurs by virtue of the differences in their diffusion rates through a semipermeable membrane.

There are a variety of clinical situations in which hemodialysis is therapeutically prescribed. Acute hemodialysis is used in cases of acute renal failure, congestive heart failure, and drug overdose or intoxication. Chronic hemodialysis is used in cases of chronic renal failure. All of these clinical situations lead to some degree of renal impairment, resulting in fluid and electrolyte imbalances. The interpretation of blood chemistries, a diagnostic tool, is utilized to assess renal function, and this information can indicate the need for hemodialysis. It should be noted that some chronic hemodialysis patients do tolerate higher serum levels of electrolytes without manifesting clinical symptoms. To understand the basic principles of hemodialysis fully, the physiology of the processes of osmosis, diffusion, and ultrafiltration must be understood.

A patient's complete physiologic status must always be assessed before therapy is initiated. Such parameters may include:

1. Coagulation status or presence of fresh wounds since heparinization is required to permit free flow of blood through the artificial kidney. Many patients in the critical care unit have undergone surgery, trauma, and/or have bleeding problems. It is therefore important to administer heparin judiciously to avoid precipitating and/or increasing bleeding.
2. Cardiovascular status. Critically ill patients often cannot tolerate the sudden decrease in volume that is needed to fill the extracorporeal circuit when dialysis is initiated.
3. Pharmacologic profile. Special attention must be given to antihypertensives, vasopressors, or antibiotics a patient may be receiving. Some medications are dialyzed from the blood, and extra doses may need to be given postdialysis. Blood levels of medications may need to be determined pre- and postdialysis.

INSTRUMENTATION

When hemodialysis therapy has been prescribed, a means of vascular access must be created. There are various ways to accomplish this.

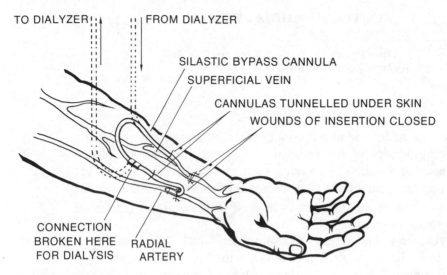

Figure 95.   A-V cannula.

Shunt/Cannula.   These are artificial external shunts which create a connection between an artery and a vein (Fig. 95). Cannulas are commonly made of Silastic because of its flexibility, resistance to clot formation, and ability to withstand external mechanical trauma. The cannula can be inserted immediately during a crisis and can be left in place indefinitely, unless complications arise. Common insertion sites are the distal portion of the arm or leg. The methods presented will be directed to cannula access technique.

Fistula.   This is an alternative method of obtaining vascular access by which an internal connection between an artery and a vein is created (Fig. 96). This type of access is not used in the critical care setting unless the patient presents with an already mature fistula. Access to the bloodstream is accomplished through venipuncture, using large bore needles which are then connected to the blood tubing on the dialysis machine.

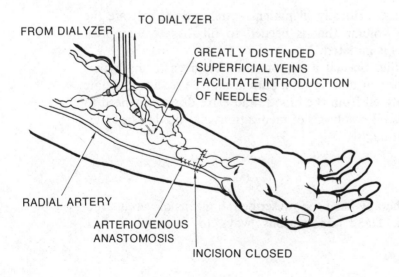

Figure 96.   A-V fistula.

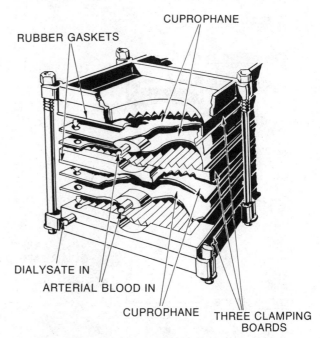

RUBBER GASKETS

CUPROPHANE

DIALYSATE IN

ARTERIAL BLOOD IN

CUPROPHANE   THREE CLAMPING
BOARDS

Figure 97. Cutaway view of parallel plate dialyzer.

Femoral Vein Dialysis. This is sometimes used in the critical care setting when *immediate* access to the bloodstream is required. A catheter is inserted into the femoral vein and connected to the blood tubing on the machine using a Y connector, thus creating a venous and arterial access. A special accessory pump is used to facilitate blood flow through the dialyzer, thereby avoiding admixing of blood. Opinion varies as to how long this catheter should be left in place; however, as a rule, 72 hours is generally acceptable. The catheter must be kept patent between dialysis treatments by infusing a constant heparinized saline solution and kept secure by sterile, protective dressings. The cannulated leg should be assessed frequently for circulatory compromise, hematoma formation, and catheter position.

Artificial Dialyzers

There are three major types of artificial dialyzers presently in use.

Parallel Plate. Sheets of cellophane membrane are placed in double layers like sandwiches and then placed between supporting plates. The plates are constructed so that the bath fluid can flow over the outside of the membrane, with the blood flowing between the cellophane layers. The parallel plate dialyzer operates on the principle of countercurrent flow—blood flows in one direction and dialysate flows in the opposite direction (Fig. 97).

Hollow Fiber. This utilizes between 10,000 and 20,000 tiny, hollow cellulose tubes through which the blood flows, with the dialysate fluid surrounding the fibers. This type of dialyzer also utilizes countercurrent flow (Fig. 98).

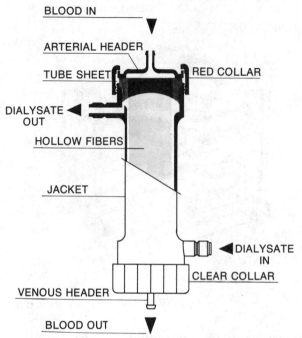

BLOOD IN

ARTERIAL HEADER

TUBE SHEET   RED COLLAR

DIALYSATE OUT

HOLLOW FIBERS

JACKET

DIALYSATE IN

CLEAR COLLAR

VENOUS HEADER

BLOOD OUT

Figure 98.   Hollow fiber dialyzer.

Coil.   This is composed of a long, flat envelope of cellulose tubing which is concentrically wound with a mesh supporting screen around a central core; bath fluid is pumped at a high flow rate through the support screen in a direction 90 degrees to that of the blood flow (Fig. 99).

Essentially, all hemodialysis machines have similar basic components (Fig. 100). Each hemodialysis machine contains several monitoring systems.
1.   The extracorporeal circuit contains:
    A.   Blood leak detector, which monitors outflowing dialysate for the presence of blood.

BLOOD INFLOW TUBES

BLOOD OUTFLOW TUBES

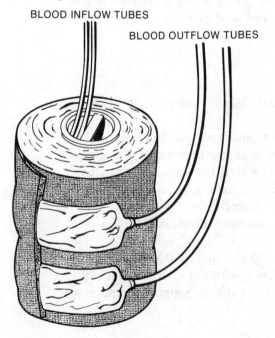

Figure 99.   Coil dialyzer

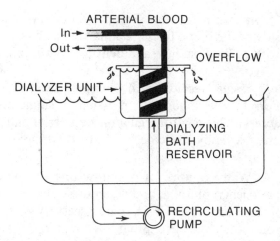

ARTERIAL BLOOD

In→

Out←

OVERFLOW

DIALYZER UNIT→

DIALYZING
BATH
RESERVOIR

RECIRCULATING
PUMP

Figure 100. Hemodialysis set-up

    B.   Blood line pressure monitors, which measure the pressure in the extracorporeal circuit.

    C.   Air leak detector, which monitors the presence of air in the extracorporeal circuit.

2.   The dialysate circuit contains:

    A.   Power "off," which monitors the failure of power to reach the machine.

    B.   Bath temperature, which monitors the temperature of the dialysate. The temperature of the bath should be that of normal body temperature; temperatures over 41°(105°*F)* may cause hemolysis and could be fatal.

    C.   Bath conductivity, which monitors the ion concentration in the dialysate. Dialysis against hypotonic or hypertonic solutions produces hemolysis and cerebral and cardiac symptoms. Prolonged contact may result in death.

       It should be noted that if either the temperature or conductivity violates preset limits, the machine will go into "bypass." This mode diverts the dialysate down the drain instead of having it flow through the dialyzer, thus preventing contact between blood and dangerous dialysate. This is indicated by the float being in the "down" position in the dialysate flow meter.

Related Equipment

    Related equipment includes various types of mechanical equipment used for the hemodialysis treatment, such as:

    Blood Pump.   The blood must be circulated through the dialyzer at a given rate; without adequate blood flow, effective dialysis is not accomplished. Acceptable blood flow rates for adults average 200 to 250 ml./minute. The blood pump is usually placed on the arterial blood line side and is regulated by a variable speed control knob.

Heparin Infusion Pump.   This device delivers heparin to the arterial side of the blood line at a constant fixed rate. Most of these pumps operate with a 30 ml. syringe and deliver heparin in ml.'s (or fractions of) per hour.

Single-Needle Timed Clamping Device.   This device is used in addition to the blood pump when a single-needle device is used for the access. This control regulates the arterial pull and venous return through the one needle by cyclic occlusion of the blood tubing.

Water Source.   Concentrations of sodium, calcium and magnesium vary geographically, and when these elements are present in high concentrations, water softeners may be necessary. State health departments conduct routine surveillance programs, and their analyses can be the basis for deciding what means are needed to treat the water to make it safe for dialysis. Some of these means are softening, filtration, distillation, deionization, and reverse osmosis.

Electrical Power.   Familiarity with the manufacturer's recommendations regarding the power source for the machine is of high priority. Correct voltage must be used to prevent overload to the circuitry, as well as damage to the equipment. Also, it is necessary to ground the machine, especially when accessory equipment draws its power from the machine itself. When initiating hemodialysis, determine the closest emergency power outlet in case it becomes necessary to switch to emergency circuitry.

INITIATING HEMODIALYSIS

OBJECTIVES

1. To obtain entrance to the patient's blood stream by the established blood access.
2. To ensure safe, aseptic hemodialysis initiation.

SPECIAL EQUIPMENT

Figure 101 illustrates the special equipment needed for initiating and terminating hemodialysis; only that needed for initiating hemodialysis is listed here.

Sterile bowl
Masks
Hemastix
Normal saline solution,
    500-ml. bag

Cup with alcohol to soak
    blood tubing caps
Alcohol prep pads
Monitor lines
Cannula connector-Teflon
    connector

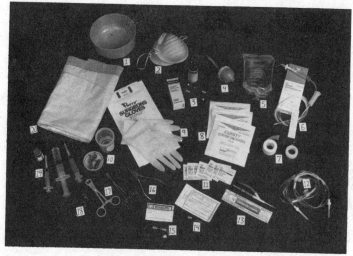

Figure 101. Equipment for initiating and terminating hemodialysis; 1, sterile bowl; 2, masks; 3, hemastix; 4, air pump; 5, normal saline, 500-ml. bag; 6, macrodrip tubing and 18-gauge needle; 7, 1-inch paper tape and ½-inch plastic tape; 8, sterile gauze pads; 9, sterile gloves; 10, cup with alcohol to soak blood tubing caps; 11, alcohol sponges; 12, monitor lines; 13, single needle; 14, cannula connector-Teflon connector; 15, cannula infusion T; 16, cannula separators; 17, hemostats; 18, "bulldogs," cannula clamps; 19, syringes and heparin; 20, linen saver.

Macrodrip tubing and 18-gauge
   needle
1" paper tape and ½" plastic
   tape
Sterile gauze pads
Sterile gloves

Cannula separators
Hemostats
"Bulldogs" or cannula clamps
Syringes and heparin
Linen saver

METHOD

ACTION	RATIONALE
1. Obtain and record patient's temperature, pulse, blood pressure, and weight.	1. This provides baseline information on the patient's condition.
2. Position patient comfortably in bed and make sure that blood lines are at same level as the bed.	2. This facilitates blood flow through machine and dialyzer, thereby not flowing against gravity.
3. Don mask and wash hands thoroughly.	3. This prevents infection of patient's cannula and prevents cross contamination between patients.
4. Don sterile gloves.	4. This protects self from blood contamination.
5. Place sterile gauze pads under cannula connection point and surrounding area of extremity.	5. This provides a sterile field when cannulas are disconnected.
6. Cleanse cannula connection with alcohol prep pad.	6. This decreases the possibility of contamination.

7. Clamp cannulas.
  A. Clamp arterial cannula with cannula clamp.
  B. Then clamp venous cannula with cannula clamp.
	7. This prevents accidental separation due to arterial pressure, stops cannula blood flow, and prevents any blood loss.

ACTION	RATIONALE
8. Separate cannulas with cannula separator.	
9. Draw predialysis blood for analysis, as prescribed.	
10. Insert sterile Teflon connector into both arterial and venous cannula ends.	10. This accommodates the blood lines of the machine.
11. Cleanse end of arterial cannula with alcohol prep pad and connect to arterial blood line of machine.	
12. Place end of venous line into sterile basin.	12. This allows the saline solution in the dialyzer and lines to flow out of the venous line into the basin.

13. Remove all clamps.
  A. Begin with clamp at venous blood line.
  B. Then proceed to clamp on arterial line.
  C. Finally, remove clamp on arterial cannula.
	13. This allows free flow of blood through the extracorporeal blood circuit.

14. Instill heparin prime, as prescribed, as blood enters the arterial drip chamber.	14. This anticoagulates the blood before it reaches the dialyzer.
15. Clamp venous blood line at basin when saline in venous drip bulb is light pink.	15. This prevents blood loss from the cannula and dialyzer.
16. Cleanse end of venous cannula with alcohol prep pad; attach end of venous blood line to venous cannula.	16. This completes the extracorporeal circuit.

17. Remove clamps:
  A. From venous blood line.
  B. From venous cannula.
	17. This allows free flow of blood through the circuit.

18. Tape cannula connections securely and tape blood tubing to patient's extremity.	18. This prevents accidental separation of connections during dialysis.
19. Record initiation time of hemodialysis.	
20. Monitor patient's vital signs; assess effect of initial therapy on patient.	

PRECAUTIONS

1. Ascertain patient's hepatitis status before dialysis is initiated and monthly thereafter while on maintenance dialysis. If a positive HAA patient

is placed on the machine unknowingly, the virus may be transmitted to the internal workings of the machine and may then be passed on to another patient. In some institutions, the machine is then considered to be contaminated and should only be used for the dialysis of HAA-positive patients.

Minimize the possible spread of hepatitis by proper hand washing between patients, restricting eating or drinking within the unit, and by careful disposal of all needles and equipment.

2. Avoid inadvertent contamination when dialyzing a patient who is critically ill or immunosuppressed by utilizing sterile technique.
3. Observe for initial untoward effects that may be due to:
   A. Initial hypovolemia resulting from filling dialyzer (the amount of blood required to fill the dialyzer varies; it averages between 90 and 300 ml., depending upon the type of dialyzer used).
   B. Removal of metabolic waste products.
   C. Electrolyte shifts.

RELATED CARE

1. Anticoagulate the blood as it enters and passes through the artificial kidney. The critically ill patient should have a baseline clotting time drawn prior to heparinization in order to assess individual needs. Methods include:
   A. Constant: Most patients receive a "prime" or loading dose based on body weight and clotting status at the initiation of dialysis, and may then receive from 500 to 2000 units per hour by infusion to keep the patient's clotting times below 1 hour.
   B. Low Dose: Usually 500 to 1000 units or less per hour is used to keep the patient's clotting times less than 15 minutes, which is important in the patient with bleeding difficulties.
   C. Regional: Protamine, the antidote for heparin, may be prescribed for infusion into the venous side of the blood tubing in order to decrease the patient's clotting time in the presence of a bleeding problem. Protamine is infused simultaneously with heparin while adjustments are made to keep the patient's clotting time between 5 and 15 minutes. The artificial kidney clotting time should be greater than 30 to 40 minutes.
2. Facilitate the removal of waste products, add select substances, and prevent the removal of desired substances with the proper dialysate bath.
   A. Two types of dialysate delivery systems are widely used.
      (1) Proportioning system: This requires the use of a liquid concentrate which can be purchased commercially or mixed by personnel. Through the use of a proportioning pump operated by various devices, tap water and concentrate are constantly mixed at a specified dilution rate.
      (2) Batch system: A given volume of dialyzing fluid is premixed at a certain concentration and stored in tanks from 100 to 300 liters or more in size.

B.   A standard dialysate bath composition may be:

Substance	Concentration (mEq./liter)
Total sodium	135
Sodium chloride	97
Sodium acetate	38
Calcium Chloride	3.0
Magnesium chloride	1.0
Potassium chloride	Adjusted according to patient's own serum potassium level.

Additions such as urea, dextrose and sodium bicarbonate can be used, if the patient's status warrants. All these substances can be adjusted to the individual patient.

3.   Establish the blood flow rate to determine an adequate dialysis process (usually 4 to 6 hours). An ideal blood flow rate is 200 to 250 ml./minute. Blood flow rate can be determined by measuring the "bubble time." This measurement is made by timing the progress of an air bubble through a 50-cm. length of tubing specifically marked on the blood line. An ideal bubble time is 2.0 to 3.0 seconds. Factors affecting blood flow include condition of cannula, blood pressure, and cardiac output. Blood flows are measured at each dialysis, after initiating treatment or anytime during dialysis when flows appear to be altered. Also, consult manufacturer's information, since flow rates are dependent upon the lumen size of the blood tubing.

COMPLICATIONS

Altered integrity of vascular
  access
Emboli
Hepatitis

Infection
Disequilibrium syndrome
Mechanical complications

MONITORING HEMODIALYSIS

OBJECTIVES

1.   To assess patient status during prescribed hemodialysis therapy to determine tolerance of procedure.
2.   To ascertain equipment performance and take corrective action, as needed.

SPECIAL EQUIPMENT

Figure 102 illustrates equipment for monitoring hemodyalisis.

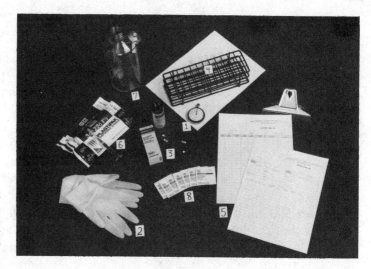

Figure 102. Monitoring equipment for hemodialysis: 1, stopwatch; 2, gloves; 3, hemastix; 4, clotting rack and glass tubes; 5, log-sheets; 6, syringe with needles; 7, needle discard receptacle; 8, alcohol sponges.

Stopwatch
Gloves
Hemastix
Clotting rack and glass tubes
Normal saline solution

Macrodrip tubing and 18-gauge
 needle
Logs
Syringes with needles
Needle discard receptacle
Alcohol prep pads

METHOD

ACTION	RATIONALE
1. Infuse heparin, as prescribed.	1. This maintains adequate blood flow through the dialyzer and prevents clotting.
2. Instill air into each drip chamber to displace blood approximately ½'' below top of chamber.	2. This allows visualization of blood flow rate into drip chambers, maintains patency of monitor lines, and provides accurate pressure reading.
3. Connect monitor lines on both arterial and venous drip bulbs, as specified by manufacturer.	3. This establishes mechanism for reading pressures.
4. Set alarm parameters.	4. This detects pressure changes.
5. Assemble photocell mechanism on venous drip chamber.	5. This provides a means to detect air in the system and prevent air embolus to the patient.
6. Hemastix the dialysate outflow.	6. This ensures operation of blood leak detector and detects blood leaks within the dialyzer.
7. Perform initial machine check and document on log sheet (includes checking of monitoring system).	7. This establishes baseline of machine functioning and assesses functioning of alarm system.

ACTION	RATIONALE
8. Assess patient; document on log sheet (blood pressure and pulse).	8. This establishes baseline tolerance level of patient to the initial volume depletion.
9. Obtain clotting times and record on clotting log.	
10. Gradually begin to increase negative pressure, if prescribed.	10. Prevents rupture in membrane of artificial kidney, achieves ultrafiltration and prevents sudden hypotension.
11. Place 500 ml. of normal saline with macrodrip tubing and 18-gauge needle attached on an IV pole within easy reach.	11. This will treat hypotension immediately and may be used to discontinue dialysis quickly, if necessary.

PRECAUTIONS

1. Keep cannula clamps (smooth-surfaced and without teeth) on cannula dressing at all times. In case of accidental separation, these must be used on the Silastic cannulas as opposed to hemostats to avoid puncturing cannulas.
2. Keep two hemostats available at all times. In an emergency (e.g., air embolus, clots in blood line returning to patient, or failure of bypass mechanism) these must be used on the blood line tubing.

RELATED CARE

1. Check machine and patient (including clotting times) at least every hour (or more frequently, if warranted).
2. Monitor the patient for signs and symptoms of intolerance to the hemodialysis therapy. The following are possible causes of hemodialysis intolerance:
    A.   Rapid blood flow rate in a patient with known cardiac disease.
    B.   Myocardial oxygen deprivation.
    C.   Rapid shift in serum potassium.
    D.   Altered electrodynamics.
    E.   Initial hypovolemia.
    F.   Air entrapment during fluid administration.
    G.   Blood line separation or dialyzer leak or rupture.
    H.   Excess ultrafiltration.
    I.   Too rapid return of dialyzer contents at termination of dialysis.
    J.   Pyrogenic/transfusion reaction.
    K.   Disequilibrium syndrome.
    L.   Fluid or sodium depletion.
    M.   Improper heparinization.

3. Support blood pressure, as prescribed by physician. The following may be used to treat hypotension and/or support the blood pressure:
    A. Normal saline.
    B. Plasmanate/albumin.
    C. Blood.
    D. Vasopressors.
4. Administer medications, as prescribed, via the venous blood line through a designated blood port.
5. Identify equipment malfunction. When a monitoring system is violated, prompt intervention is necessary to insure patient safety.
6. Monitor the patient's response to heparin. There are special blood ports or rubber sleeves on the arterial and venous blood lines; these are used to draw blood from the machine. For regional dialysis blood drawn from arterial sleeve is the *patient's* clotting time, while blood drawn from the venous sleeve (before protamine infusion) is considered the *machine's* clotting time.

COMPLICATIONS

Angina	Headache
Dysrhythmia	Convulsion
Air embolus	Muscle cramps
Exsanguination	Nausea, vomiting
Hypotension	Pruritus
Shortness of breath	Clotting in dialyzer
Hemolysis	Power failure
Fever/chills	

TERMINATING HEMODIALYSIS

OBJECTIVES

1. To conclude hemodialysis safely, and to reinfuse the blood within the extracorporeal system.
2. To re-establish blood flow through cannulas.
3. To assess patient's status post hemodialysis therapy.

SPECIAL EQUIPMENT

Masks	Alcohol prep pads
Air pump	Cannula connector-Teflon
Normal saline solution, 500-ml.	connector and/or
bag	cannula infusion T

Macrodrip tubing and 18-gauge
   needle
1'' paper tape and ½'' plastic
   tape
Sterile gauze pads
Sterile gloves

Cannula separators
Hemostats
"Bulldogs" or cannula clamps
Linen saver

METHOD

ACTION	RATIONALE
1. Reduce negative pressure to zero.	1. This minimizes blood volume in dialyzer.
2. Cancel venous/arterial pressure alarms and air leak alarm.	2. This prevents alarms during procedure.
3. Drape venous blood line on bed.	3. This allows visualization of all tubing as rinse progresses.
4. Don mask.	
5. Remove dressings and tape; expose cannula connection sites; preserve integrity of blood tubing system.	
6. Don gloves.	
7. Place sterile gauze pads under connection points of tubing.	7. This provides a sterile field for separated cannulas.
8. Cleanse arterial connection with alcohol prep pad.	
9. Clamp arterial cannula and arterial blood line tubing.	9. This prevents blood loss when cannulas are separated.
10. Use separating forceps to separate arterial tubing from cannula.	
11. Connect IV of normal saline solution to arterial tubing; then open clamps until approximately 100 to 150 ml. of saline is infused.	11. This initiates saline rinse of blood tubing.
12. Clamp saline and arterial lines.	
13. Return blood to patient, using either saline or air pump.	13. This facilitates maximum return of patient's RBC's.
14. Cleanse venous connection with alcohol prep pad; separate tubing.	
15. Insert Teflon connector or infusion T halfway into venous cannula; attach arterial cannula over exposed area of connector and remove clamps from venous and then arterial cannulas.	
16. Tape connection securely.	

ACTION	RATIONALE
17. Perform cannula site care.	
18. Remove all needles, syringes, and traces of blood from machine and work area; dispose in safe manner, as required by institution.	18. This prevents possible spread of hepatitis.
19. Obtain postdialysis weight, pulse, temperature, and blood pressure.	19. This determines the efficiency of dialysis in regard to weight loss and patient's tolerance of procedure.

PRECAUTIONS

Avoid *any* interruptions or distractions during termination procedure.

RELATED CARE

1. Assess cannula and site at frequent intervals after terminating hemo-dialysis.
2. Perform cannula and site care (see the next method "Hemodialysis Cannula and Site Care").

COMPLICATIONS

Air embolus   Hemorrhage
Infection   Cannula displacement

SUPPLIERS

B-D Drake Willock (subsidiary of Becton, Dickinson and Company)
Extracorporeal Medical Specialties, Inc.
Gambro, Inc.
Quinton Instruments
Travenol

HEMODIALYSIS CANNULA AND SITE CARE _____

OBJECTIVES

1. To promote integrity of cannula by monitoring and maintaining ad-equate blood flow through cannulas and protecting from trauma or accidental separation.
2. To assess and clean exit sites to prevent and/or detect infection.

SPECIAL EQUIPMENT

Masks
Soap and water
Hydrogen peroxide solution
   (3%)
Sterile cotton swabs
Alcohol prep pads

Sterile gauze pads
Povidone-iodine ointment
Tape
Sterile flexible gauze roll
Telfa pads, if necessary

METHOD

ACTION	RATIONALE
1. Mask all persons in immediate area.	
2. Remove dressing; expose site.	
3. Assess cannula site for: A. Secure connections. B. Proper alignment, no tension at sites. C. Absence of infection at sites. D. Absence of hematoma or clotting problems.	D. Dark color of blood in cannula indicates first stage of clotting. Granular appearance of blood indicates second stage of clotting. Syneresis, an indication of the third stage of clotting, shows separation of blood with clot and clear plasma observed within the cannula.
4. Cleanse extremity with soap and water; rinse and dry well. Carefully lift cannulas to do this but do not wash within immediate area of the exit sites.	4. This avoids contamination of exit sites with skin bacteria.
5. Cleanse each exit site with hydrogen peroxide and sterile cotton swabs. A. Start at exit site. B. Work outward to cover immediate area. Do not go over cleansed area with used applicator stick.	5. This cleanses and gently removes crusts around exit sites. B. This prevents cross contamination from one exit site to another.
6. Dry exit site with cotton swabs, using same technique as in step 5.	6. Dampness predisposes to infection.
7. Cleanse both arterial and venous cannula tubing with alcohol prep pad.	

ACTION	RATIONALE
A. Start at exit site.	
B. Work towards the connection.	B. This prevents contamination of exit sites.
8. Apply povidone-iodine to exit sites, if prescribed.	8. This prevents infection and provides a seal at exit sites.
9. Place a sterile gauze pad over exit sites, touching only side which will be away from skin. (If any drainage or bleeding from exit sites, use Telfa on sites first.)	9. This protects exit sites.
10. Place second sterile gauze pad over cannulas, allowing only a small loop of cannula to be exposed.	10. This allows for ease in checking cannula for signs of clotting.
11. Secure sterile gauze pads to skin with paper tape; do not encircle extremity with tape.	11. This avoids constriction, which may lead to clot formation.
12. Wrap area with soft, flexible gauze roll, wrapping so that dressing is secure but not constrictive; tape end of roll in place.	12. This insures padding and protection of cannula.
13. Put cannula clamps on dressing.	13. This allows for immediate access at all times in case of accidental separation.

PRECAUTIONS

1. Restrict blood pressure determinations on cannulated extremity.
2. Restrict blood drawings or vascular invasive procedures on cannulated extremity above cannulas.
3. Restrict use of constricting device on cannulated extremity over or above cannula.
4. Wash hands well before handling cannulas.

RELATED CARE

1. Perform cannula care every 24 hours, if dressing becomes soiled or wet or if exit sites have been exposed (e.g., after dialysis, after inspection of cannulas).
2. Draw blood from the cannula and administer medications via a heparin infusion T which can be inserted into the cannula. T-connectors may, however, increase the chance of the cannula clotting, due to its small lumen.

COMPLICATIONS

Infection   Disconnection   Clotting

REFERENCES

Gutch, C.F., and Stoner, Martha, H.: Review of Hemodialysis for Nurses and Dialysis Personnel. St. Louis, C. V. Mosby, 1975.

Hansen, Ginny: Caring for Patients with Chronic Renal Diseases: A Reference Guide for Nurses. Philadelphia, J. B. Lippincott, 1972, pp. 53-58.

University of Washington: Renal Learning Modules. Seattle, University of Washington, 1976-1978 (unpublished).

PERITONEAL DIALYSIS

Elaine Larson, R.N., M.A., and
Barbara Fellows, R.N., M.A.

OVERVIEW

Peritoneal dialysis, by the processes of osmosis and diffusion through the peritoneal membrane, removes end products of metabolism and excess fluid which accumulate in acute or chronic renal failure. The dialyzing solution is introduced into and removed from the peritoneal cavity as either a continuous or an intermittent process.

There are three phases to each dialysis exchange.

Inflow Phase.   This is the time required to infuse the exchange volume, as determined by gravity or pump, catheter placement, size of tubing, and volume to be infused. The inflow phase is usually 10 to 15 minutes.

Diffusion Phase (Dwell Time).   This is usually 10 to 25 minutes. Optimal dialysis efficiency is attained with a diffusion time of about 10 to 15 minutes. If dialysate dwells longer than 20 to 25 minutes in the peritoneum, glucose molecules can diffuse, causing potential fluid overload. Patients with peritonitis, however, may have diffusion times as long as 60 minutes to increase antibiotic absorption.

Outflow Phase.   This is the time required to recover the infused dialysate plus any excess fluid from the extracellular fluid space. The outflow phase is usually 10 to 15 minutes. Ideally, outflow volume should be equal to or greater than the inflow volume. Usually the patient being dialyzed has an excess of extracellular fluid volume as manifested by weight gain, hypertension, or peripheral edema, and needs to lose fluid during the dialysis. A *positive balance* (greater total volume than initial volume) means that excess fluid has been removed from the patient. A *negative balance* (greater initial volume than total volume recovered) means that there is excess fluid retained by the patient.

Two methods of peritoneal dialysis are generally used—the single-bottle, manual method, requiring constant nursing surveillance and bottle changes (Fig. 103), and the automated method in which the dialysate (dialysis fluid) is cycled and delivered automatically (Fig. 104). The latter system relieves the nurse of frequent bottle changes, but monitoring the cycles and the effect of therapy on the patient remains a critical component of nursing care. The methods included in this section will be appropriate to both dialysis systems.

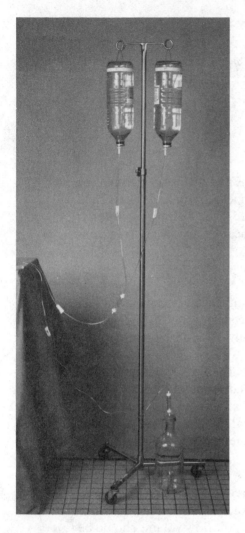

Figure 103. Peritoneal dialysis set-up; single bottle, manual method.

INSERTION OF PERITONEAL DIALYSIS CATHETER (ASSISTING WITH) _____

OBJECTIVES

To monitor and support the patient during this procedure, assisting when necessary.

SPECIAL EQUIPMENT

Sterile surgical gown(s) and glove(s)
Caps
Masks
Sterile plastic draping sheet
Four large draping towels
One split eye drape

Povidone-iodine solution
Heparin 1:1000
Lidocaine 0.5% or 1% without epinephrine
Sterile gauze pads
Towel clips
Needles:
   One 25-gauge, two 20-gauge, 1½" long
   Two No. 20, 4" long
   One stainless steel short bevel, 13- to 15-gauge, 3" or longer
Syringes:
   One 5 ml.
   Two 20 ml.
Four hemostats
One curved Kelly clamp
One blade handle, No. 11 with 15 blades
One toothed thumb forceps
One needle holder
One 00 silk suture with cutting edge needle
One 00 or 000 gut or chromic suture with tapered needle
One large semicurved clamp, 9"
Peritoneal catheter supplies:
   Trocath
   Trocar
   Uterine sound
   Catheter
   2' sterile latex rubber tubing with needle adapter and solution admin-
      istration set attached
Sterile prewarmed dialysate

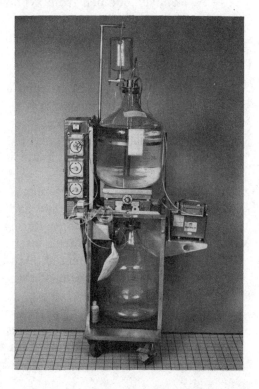

Figure 104.   Peritoneal dialysis set-up; automated system.

METHOD

ACTION	RATIONALE
1. Obtain and record patient's weight, temperature, blood pressure, pulse, respiratory rate, and abdominal girth.	1. This provides a baseline for comparison during dialysis.
2. Assess patient's abdomen for:	
A. Bowel distention; report to physician.	A. With bowel distention there is increased risk of bowel perforation.
B. Urinary bladder distention, empty bladder.	B. This decreases chances of bladder perforation.
C. Abdominal skin integrity for signs of local infection. If present:	C. This prevents introduction of organisms into the peritoneum from locally infected areas.
(1) Clean these sites with povidone-iodine or other antiseptic preparation.	
(2) Cover locally infected sites with a sterile dressing.	
(3) Report these to physician.	
3. Prepare peritoneal catheter insertion site.	3. This helps to control infection.
A. Shave abdomen from xyphoid to symphysis pubis.	
B. Perform a surgical abdominal scrub extending from xyphoid to symphysis pubis, over both flanks, and with particular attention to umbilicus.	B. The umbilicus harbors greater number of organisms.
4. Place patient in supine position.	
5. Employ strict aseptic technique.	
A. Mask all persons in immediate area.	
B. Assist with sterile draping.	
6. Provide desired local anesthesia.	
7. Monitor patient's response during peritoneal dialysis catheter insertion.	
8. Inform patient of potential discomfort during advancement of catheter into the peritoneal cavity.	8. This prevents sudden movement or jerking of the patient.
9. Monitor alteration in comfort level.	
A. Report sudden onset of pressure in bladder, epigastrium, or rectum.	A. Pressure in bladder indicates that the catheter should be pulled back slightly; pressure in the

ACTION	RATIONALE
	epigastrium suggests omental entanglement of the catheter; pressure in the rectal area indicates that the catheter tip is in the proper position.
B. Report continued discomfort in rectal area.	B. Continued rectal pain suggests that the catheter is in too far.
10. Prime patient's abdomen with fluid, as prescribed.	
A. Check priming solution for sterility; warm to body temperature.	
B. If bottle is warmed in a water bath, dry outside of bottle before it is inverted.	B. This prevents contamination of the sterile fluid.
C. Prime the inflow tubing with dialysate.	
D. Connect primed inflow tubing and monitor inflow volume of dialysate.	
E. Assess patient carefully for respiratory distress as well as abdominal discomfort.	E. Large volumes of fluid in the abdominal cavity can cause respiratory insufficiency by limiting lung expansion.
F. Measure amount of fluid instilled accurately.	
11. Place the patient in a 45-degree position.	11. This enhances comfort and facilitates proper drainage.
12. Secure peritoneal dialysis catheter.	
13. Apply dressing.	

PRECAUTIONS

Assess the patient frequently during the procedure for tolerance to supine position, hemodynamic alteration, respiratory status, etc.

RELATED CARE

1. Assess site for hemorrhage.
2. Assess patency of catheter.
3. Assess for fluid leakage at catheter exit; change dressings and clean site when moist.

COMPLICATIONS

Hemorrhage	Bowel perforation
Catheter occlusion	Bladder perforation

PERITONEAL DIALYSIS CATHETER SITE CARE

OBJECTIVES

1. To assess and clean exit site to prevent and/or detect early signs of local and systemic infection.
2. To maintain and assess skin integrity at the peritoneal catheter exit site.

SPECIAL EQUIPMENT

See Figure 105.
Protective bed pad
Tape
Plastic bag
Forceps

Face mask(s)
Povidone-iodine solution
Hydrogen peroxide solution
Sterile gauze pads

METHOD

ACTION	RATIONALE
1. Mask all persons in immediate area.	1. This aids in infection control.
2. Expose catheter site, using forceps to remove dressings around catheter.	
3. Inspect exit site for signs and symptoms of infection (purulence, redness, tenderness, induration).	
4. Remove dried blood with hydrogen peroxide.	4. Dried blood can serve as nutrient for bacteria.

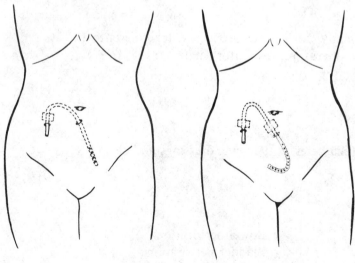

Figure 105. Schematic of peritoneal catheter tract. (From Tenckhoff, H.: Chronic Peritoneal Dialysis Manual. Seattle, University of Washington School of Medicine, 1974, p. 27. Reproduced by permission.)

ACTION	RATIONALE
5. Cleanse exit site gently with povidone-iodine solution. A. Begin around site. B. Work outwards.	
6. Cleanse entire circumference of catheter with povidone-iodine solution; allow antiseptic to dry completely.	6. This prevents gauze dressings from sticking to the skin and allows maximum bacteriostatic effects to occur.
7. Secure peritoneal dialysis catheter on sterile gauze pad.	7. This avoids skin irritation and decreases risk of catheter contamination from skin.
8. Cover area with additional sterile gauze pads.	
9. Secure dressing, keeping areas of gauze exposed.	9. This allows skin to breathe and decreases risk of anaerobic bacterial growth; it also prevents bacterial contamination.

PRECAUTIONS

1. Secure catheter position during site care.
2. Monitor for correct temperature of dialysate.

RELATED CARE

1. Perform peritoneal site care daily after first 48 hours, after each dialysis, whenever dressings are moist, or whenever exit site is exposed or contaminated.
2. Assess skin integrity daily.
3. Vary the position of the taped-down catheter with each dressing change.

COMPLICATIONS

Catheter displacement   Hemorrhage
Infection   Catheter occlusion

MONITORING PERITONEAL DIALYSIS _____

OBJECTIVES

1. To ensure the proper composition and temperature of the dialysate, and proper functioning of equipment.

2. To check proper functioning of equipment during peritoneal dialysis, taking corrective action as necessary.
3. To monitor peritoneal dialysis therapy and to assess the patient's responses during peritoneal dialysis therapy.

SPECIAL EQUIPMENT

Peritoneal dialysis log
Scale
Thermometer
Sphygmomanometer
Stethoscope
Dialysis machine
Warmed fluid (dialysate)
Sterile gauze pads

Sterile gloves
Sterile drapes
Inflow tubing
Two hemostats
Povidone-iodine solution
Mask(s)
Tape
Plastic bag

METHOD

ACTION	RATIONALE
1. Place hemostats and sterile scissors at bedside.	1. These will be used in case of emergency disconnection.
2. Check dialysis machine and temperature of dialysate, which should be warmed to body temperature.	2. Urea clearance is maximized and body heat loss is minimized when dialysate is at body temperature.
3. Check composition of dialysate on label with medical order, noting especially concentrations of potassium and glucose.	3. Glucose in the dialysate increases osmotic pressure, drawing off extracellular fluid from the patient and increasing urea clearance. If too rapid fluid or electrolyte shifts occur, the patient will become symptomatic.
4. Place bed in high position.	4. This provides easy patient access and assists with gravity outflow.
5. Place protective pads under patient.	
6. Obtain patient's weight, blood pressure (supine and standing, if patient is able to detect orthostatic hypotension), pulse, respiratory rate, and temperature.	6. This provides a baseline for comparison during dialysis.
7. Palpate patient's abdomen. A. Note and record degree of any distention. B. Measure abdominal girth with a tape measure.	7. This provides a baseline for comparison during dialysis. Fluid retention is often first noted in increasing abdominal girth.

ACTION	RATIONALE

8. Place dialysis log conveniently at bedside and complete predialysis information (patient's name, hospital number, date and time, vital signs, bath composition, additives, orders for number of cycles).

9. Determine and record on log sheet the ordered time for each phase.
   A. Inflow phase is usually about 10 to 15 minutes.
   B. Diffusion phase (dwell time) is usually 10 to 25 minutes.
   C. Outflow phase is usually about 10 to 15 minutes.

10. Determine and record on log the ordered volume to be infused with each cycle—usually 1500 to 2000 ml. for adults.

10. The amount of fluid tolerated with patient size and tolerance. Exchange volumes of greater than 2 liters increase clearance only minimally. To improve dialysis efficiency, it is preferable to increase the exchange *rate* three cycles per hour rather than to increase the volume infused with each exchange.

11. Prepare machine and connect patient, using strict aseptic technique.

12. Monitor inflow phase.
   A. Ensure that
      (1) All clamps from inflow bottle to peritoneum are released.
      (2) All clamps from peritoneum to outflow bottle are clamped.
      (3) Tubing is free of kinks (or that automated system is functioning properly).
   B. Observe that flow is unobstructed. In severe cases of subcutaneous catheter kinking, outflow will be prevented and the catheter must be replaced. Obstruction can be identified when the tubing pulsates.

   B. Slow inflow can result from external or subcutaneous tube kinking, and should be noted and corrected before the abdomen becomes overdistended.

13. Monitor diffusion phase.
   A. Observe patient's response to fluid volume infused. Note any

   A. Intolerance and discomfort during the diffusion phase may in-

ACTION	RATIONALE
discomfort or respiratory distress.	dicate too much fluid being infused, peritoneal infection, or adhesion formation.
B. Check catheter site for fluid leakage or bleeding.	
14. Monitor outflow phase.	
A. Ensure that	
(1) All clamps from peritoneum to outflow bottle are released.	
(2) Tubing is free of kinks.	
(3) Inflow clamps are secure.	
B. Observe ease and speed of drainage.	B. The dialysate should normally drain by gravity in a steady stream.
C. Check for air in drainage tubing and eliminate it if first outflow is slow in starting; change patient's position to improve gravity, or give another short inflow cycle.	C. The first outflow may be slow due to the presence of air in the tubing, fibrin deposits, or inadequate fluid in the first inflow (some patients, because of a large abdominal cavity, require a larger pool of fluid in the first inflow).
D. Do not continue dialysis if outflow is still slow or poor until problem is resolved.	D. This prevents fluid retention in the peritoneal cavity.
E. Note patient complaints of pain; reassure patient that this sometimes occurs.	E. Pain on outflow is usually due to increased suction during outflow.
F. Observe and record appearance of the outflow fluid.	F. Outflow fluid is normally clear. Cloudy, bloody, or brownish fluid indicates potential complications.
15. Calculate inflow and outflow volumes at end of each outflow cycle.	
A. Add amount of inflow fluid remaining and amount of fluid in outflow bottle to obtain total fluid volume.	
B. Subtract initial dialysate volume from sum of inflow and outflow volumes.	
C. Continue with dialysis inflow if fluid balance is even or positive.	C. A moderately negative fluid balance (100 to 300 ml. in an adult) may result in patients with larger

ACTION	RATIONALE
	abdominal cavities. These patients will not be fluid-overload.
D. Observe patient for symptoms of fluid overload (1) Increasing blood pressure. (2) Distended neck veins. (3) Elevated CVP. (4) Respiratory distress. (5) Especially increased abdominal girth if there is fluid retained in the abdominal cavity.	D. In patients with some extracellular fluid excess, even a slight negative fluid balance can cause symptoms of fluid overload.
E. Continue dialysis cautiously, observing patient carefully if patient is asymptomatic.	E. Negative balance may well be reversed after several cycles.
F. Repeat outflow and, if necessary, notify physician if patient shows symptoms of fluid overload.	F. There may be obstruction due to internal catheter misplacement or obstruction, or the physician may choose to add more glucose to the dialysate to increase the osmotic pressure.
G. Calculate fluid balance at end of each outflow cycle. Under no circumstances should the patient be allowed to retain more than 250 ml.	

PRECAUTIONS

1. Monitor the patient's vital signs, abdominal girth, and mental status throughout the dialysis, since rapid fluid and electrolyte changes can occur during dialysis.
2. Observe patient for symptoms of insulin reaction after the dialysis is terminated, if there was high glucose concentration in the dialysate. High glucose in the dialysate causes hyperglycemia, resulting in increased insulin production. When dialysis is discontinued rapidly, there is less time for the body to reach homeostasis.
3. Maintain sterility when handling the peritoneal catheter.
4. Monitor outflow carefully throughout the dialysis to assure that fluid is not retained in the peritoneal cavity.
5. Assess for shock, since dialysis is hypertonic.
6. Assess for atelectasis, since dialysis encourages hypoventilation.

RELATED CARE

1. Document exact time of infusion initiation and termination, amount of solution infused, recovered, and total balance, color of outflow, and pre- and postdialysis weights.
2. Weigh wet dressings to estimate fluid lost: 1 gram = 1 ml.
2. Obtain a blood chemistry profile, which may include BUN, albumin level (due to protein loss), and electrolyte levels.
4. Utilize effective skin care and range of motion exercises.

COMPLICATIONS

Peritonitis
Bowel, bladder, visceral perforation (mainly at the time of
catheter insertion)
Fluid and electrolyte imbalances

Dysrhythmias
Hemorrhage
Hyperglycemia
Dehydration
Mechanical defects

REFERENCES

Dolan, P., and Greene, H.L.: Renal failure and peritoneal dialysis. Nurs. '75, 5:40, 1975.
Peritoneal Dialysis Procedures. Seattle, University Hospital Nursing Services, 1978.
Standards of Clinical Practice. Section III: Peritoneal Dialysis. Park Ridge, IL, American Association of Nephrology Nurses and Technicians, 1972.
Tenckhoff, H.: Chronic Peritoneal Dialysis. Seattle, University of Washington School of Medicine, 1974.

THE
NEUROLOGIC
SYSTEM

INTRACRANIAL PRESSURE MONITORING

Doreen Gardner, R.N.

OVERVIEW

Intracranial pressure (ICP) is the pressure exerted within the intact skull by the cranial contents—brain tissue, cerebrospinal fluid, and blood. Increased intracranial pressure can cause permanent neurologic damage, impaired cerebral circulation, and brain mass shifts, leading to herniation and death. Clinical signs and symptoms, once the traditional basis of increased intracranial pressure measurement, do not correlate well with the onset or level of increased pressure. Several methods and devices allowing for constant and/or intermittent measurement of ICP have been developed, allowing for earlier detection of increasing intracranial pressure, immediate intervention, and evaluation of treatment.

Intracranial pressure monitoring equipment includes a sensor, an intracranial or extracranial transducer, and a recording device.

Types of ICP Monitoring

Intraventricular. Through a burr hole a small rubber or polyethylene catheter, approximately 7 cm., is inserted usually into the anterior horn of the lateral ventricle. It is connected via a stopcock and pressure tubing to a transducer filled with sterile normal saline or Ringer's lactate solution, and then connected to a recording device or monitor.

Subarachnoid. A ¼-inch twist drill hole is made in the frontal area behind the hairline. The dura is opened, and a hollow subarachnoid screw is inserted and threaded until it is 1 mm. below the dura in the subarachnoid space. It is then connected to a transducer with saline-filled pressure tubing, and then connected to the recording monitor.

Epidural. A burr hole is made and a balloon with an extracranial transducer, a miniature intracranial transducer, or a fiberoptic transducer is placed between the skull and dura. The device may also be placed subdurally. Monitoring equipment depends upon the type of device used.

The advantages and disadvantages of each type of ICP monitoring are given in Table 3.

Table 3. **ADVANTAGES AND DISADVANTAGES OF TYPES OF ICP MONITORING**

	Intraventricular	Subarachnoid	Epidural
Advantages	Ease of CSF drainage and sampling; direct measurement from CSF.	Access for volume-pressure determination.	Less invasive; no outside connections.
Disadvantages	Difficulty in locating ventricles (patients with small ventricles or midline shift).	Risk of infection.	No access for CSF sampling or drainage; questionable reflection of CSF pressure; cannot be calibrated after insertion.

OBJECTIVES

1. To detect increased intracranial pressure (normal values are 0 to 15 mm. Hg or 50 to 200 mm. H_2O).
2. To identify intracranial pressure waves.
3. To allow for early intervention of increased intracranial pressure and for assessment of treatment.
4. To allow for measurement of brain compliance.
5. To measure cerebral perfusion pressure (CPP).
    Mean arterial pressure minus ICP = CPP.
    Normal cerebral perfusion pressure is at least 50 mm. Hg.

SPECIAL EQUIPMENT

Razor
Local anesthetic
Sterile operating room pack for ventriculostomy, including twist drill
Intraventricular catheter, subarachnoid screw, or epidural device
Sutures
Transducer line set-up
Three stopcocks, sterile normal saline solution without preservatives, and tubing
Povidone-iodine solution
Occlusive dressing material
Transfer pack

METHOD ACTION	RATIONALE
1. Fill transducer dome, pressure line tubing, and all stopcocks with sterile normal saline solution; apply caps to maintain sterility.	
2. Position transducer at level of lateral ventricles; connect two stopcocks, flush, and reapply caps (Fig. 106).	2. This maintains accurate readings; prevents excessive drainage of cerebrospinal fluid when line is opened.
3. Open stopcock C to atmosphere; balance and calibrate monitor; close stopcock C to atmosphere (see the method for "Hemodynamic Monitoring Single Pressure Transducer System").	
4. Position patient on back with head raised 30 to 45°.	
5. Hold patient's head firmly during insertion.	
6. Wash area with povidone-iodine solution and apply occlusive dressing after subarachnoid screw or ventricular catheter is inserted.	
7. Maintain sterility of site and line. No ointments should be used on screw site.	
8. Attach a 1-ml. syringe filled with sterile normal saline solution to stopcock A. Do not connect irrigation system to ventricular line or screw system.	

PRECAUTIONS

1. Use 1-ml. syringe on stopcock A if flush of line is ordered; inject 0.25 ml. Record ICP before and after flush.

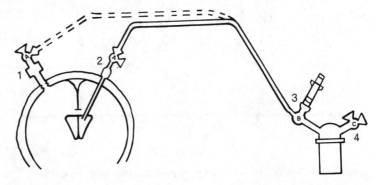

Figure 106. Intracranial pressure monitoring: 1, subarachnoid screw with stopcock A; 2, intraventricular catheter with stopcock A; 3, 1-ml. syringe for flush with stopcock B; 4, transducer stopcock C for calibration.

2. Maintain head of bed at the level ordered, and keep the transducer in alignment with the lateral ventricles. Realign the transducer and recalibrate if the bed level is changed.

3. Monitor the line when turning the patient or when the patient is agitated. Do not reconnect a line that has become disconnected. Cover with sterile dressing, immediately replace with new tubing and stopcocks, notify the physician, and document. Restrain patient.

4. Check the monitoring system regularly for leakage, especially at stopcocks.

RELATED CARE

1. Record ICP readings hourly, depending on the patient's condition. Balance and calibrate the equipment every 4 hours and as needed.

2. Use all known nursing measures to prevent increased ICP.
    A. Preoxygenate before suctioning; suction briefly.
    B. Position the patient with head elevated 30 to 45°; avoid neck flexion.
    C. Avoid the use of the Valsalva maneuver (e.g., straining at stool).

3. Monitor wave patterns (Fig. 107).
    A. "A" or plateau waves—increases in ICP to 50 to 100 mm. Hg for 5 to 20 min. These occur with a mean ICP of 20 mm. Hg and are considered to be an indication of ICP decompensation.
    B. "B" waves—sharp, rhythmic oscillation occurring every ½ to 2 min.; range in amplitude from 0 to 50 mm. Hg. These relate to changes in respirations (e.g., Cheyne-Stokes).
    C. "C" waves—usually occur with a 4 to 8 per minute frequency, with an amplitude from 0 to 20 mm. Hg. They are found to correlate with normal fluctuations of arterial pressure.
    Waves may become flat or dampened if brain tissue occludes the screw. The line may require flushing.

4. Be prepared to intervene in the event of increased ICP. Therapy may include:

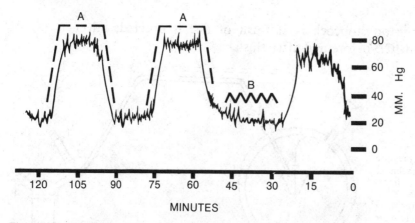

Figure 107.   Ventricular fluid pressure variations: *A,* plateau waves; *B,* "B" waves.

    A.   Fluid restriction.
    B.   Drugs:
        (1)   Steroids.
        (2)   Hyperosmotic agents—mannitol, glycerol.
        (3)   Barbiturates.
    C.   CSF drainage.
    D.   Hyperventilation ($\downarrow pCO_2$).
    E.   Hypothermia.

5. Provide continual supportive care of the patient and family.

6. Drain CSF as prescribed for elevated ICP. Attach IV tubing and transfer pack to stopcock A (see also Fig. 106). Keep transfer pack on bed at ventricle level. Open stopcock and drain CSF until ICP reaches desired level.

7. Change sterile dressing every 24 hours. Watch for redness, swelling, and leakage at insertion site.

8. Measure brain compliance.
    A.   Introduce a small sterile fluid volume and measure pressure.
    B.   A 1-ml. injection over 1 second causing less than 2 mm. Hg increase in ICP is considered normal.
    C.   Response greater than 3 mm. Hg indicates impaired compensatory mechanism.

9. Daily testing of CSF with ventricular catheter, for cells and cultures may be prescribed.

COMPLICATIONS

Infection   Tubing disconnection

REFERENCES

American Association of Neurosurgical Nurses: Core Curriculum for Neurological Nursing. Baltimore, American Association of Neurosurgical Nurses, 1977, pp. 131–134.

Hanlon, Kathryn: Description and uses of intracranial pressure monitoring. Heart Lung, 5:277–282, 1976.

Johnson, Marion, and Quinn, Judith: The subarachnoid screw. Am. J. of Nurs. 77:448–450, 1977.

Johnston, I.H., et al: The place of continuous intracranial pressure monitoring in neurosurgical practice. Acta Neurochir. (Wien), 29:53–64, 1973.

Mauss, Nancy K., et al: Increased intracranial pressure: An update. Heart Lung, 5:919–926, 1976.

Vries, J.K., et al: A subarachnoid screw for monitoring intracranial pressure. J. Neurosurg., 39:416–418, 1973.

LUMBAR AND CISTERNAL PUNCTURES
(ASSISTING WITH)

Marilyn Ricci, R.N., M.S., C.N.R.N.

OVERVIEW

A lumbar or cisternal puncture is the introduction of a hollow needle with a stylet into the subarachnoid space of the spinal canal. It is performed to gain information about the cerebrospinal fluid to help diagnose, treat, or assess the progress of diseases involving the central nervous system.

The lumbar puncture (Fig. 108) is performed at the level of L_{3-4} or L_{4-5} vertebral interspace to avoid damage to the spinal cord, which ends approximately at the L_{1-2} vertebral level. The cisternal puncture (Fig. 109) is the introduction of a short-beveled, hollow needle with a stylet through the midline above the spinous process of the second cervical vertebra and under the posterior rim of the foramen magnum into the cisterna magna (the space between the cerebellum and the medulla). As the needle is correctly placed in the subarachnoid space and the stylet is removed, drops of cerebrospinal fluid will escape. The manometer is then attached to the needle, either directly or by using a three-way stopcock. Care must be taken to avoid sudden loss of the cerebrospinal fluid. Normally the fluid moves up and down on respiration and moves freely upward on straining, coughing, and abdominal compression. After the cerebrospinal fluid pressure measurements are completed, the fluid is allowed to drain off slowly until the desired amount has been obtained.

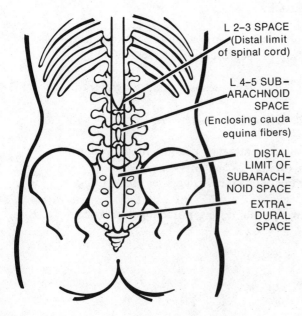

L 2–3 SPACE
(Distal limit
of spinal cord)

L 4–5 SUB–
ARACHNOID
SPACE
(Enclosing cauda
equina fibers)

DISTAL
LIMIT OF
SUBARACH-
NOID SPACE

EXTRA-
DURAL
SPACE

Figure 108. Lumbar puncture.

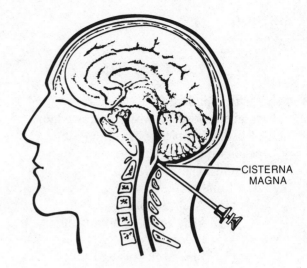

CISTERNA
MAGNA

Figure 109.   Cisternal puncture.

OBJECTIVES

Diagnostic

1. To measure cerebrospinal fluid pressure.
2. To obtain cerebrospinal fluid for visualization and laboratory analysis.
3. To perform "spinal dynamics" tests which could indicate a partial or complete block in the cerebrospinal fluid circulation as a result of a spinal cord or disc lesion.
4. To inject air, oxygen, or radiopaque substances for x-ray visualization.

Therapeutic

1. To remove blood and purulent material from the subarachnoid space.
2. To administer medications.
3. To induce spinal anesthesia (via lumbar puncture only).
4. To drain cerebrospinal fluid for the reduction of intracranial pressure in very select cases.

SPECIAL EQUIPMENT

Sterile gloves
20-gauge hollow needles with
  stylets
Three-way stopcock
Manometer
Drape
Three small test tubes
Needles

Syringes
Sterile gauze pads
Povidone-iodine solution
Local antiseptic
Band-Aid
Razor (for cisternal puncture)

METHOD

ACTION	RATIONALE
1. Position patient in a lateral recumbent position with back at edge of bed. Complete positioning depends upon area of puncture (Figs. 110 and 111).	1. This keeps the plane of the patient's back perpendicular to the plane of the surface on which he is lying.

A. Lumbar:
     (1) Arch the back.
     (2) Flex knees tightly against abdomen.
     (3) Flex neck forward on chest.
     (4) Place small pillow under head.
	A. This position widens the interspinous spaces and promotes easier entry into the subarachnoid space.

B. Cisternal: (1) Place head on small pillow with chin flexed onto chest.	B. This position makes the site accessible by bringing the brain stem and cord forward in the spinal canal.
2. Help patient to maintain desired position during procedure by providing support behind head and knees, and keeping the "up" shoulder from falling forward. Stand on the side of the bed which the patient is facing.	2. Support helps to prevent sudden movements and resultant trauma.
3. Prepare skin site with povidone-iodine solution.	
4. Anesthetize skin.	
5. Monitor patient's status during needle insertion.	5. The patient will feel pressure as the spinal needle is inserted and a stab of pain as the dura is penetrated. Pain radiating down the leg occurs if a spinal nerve root is irritated by the needle.

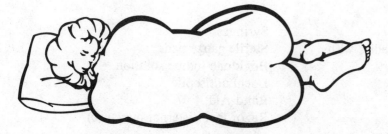

Figure 110. Alignment of vertebral column in a horizontal plane.

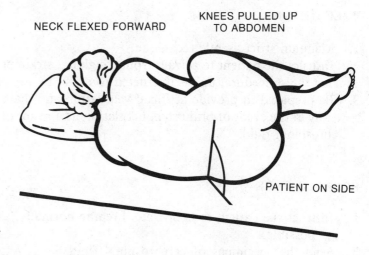

NECK FLEXED FORWARD

KNEES PULLED UP
TO ABDOMEN

PATIENT ON SIDE

Figure 111. Position for lumbar puncture.

ACTION	RATIONALE
6. Help patient to straighten legs slowly after spinal needle is in appropriate position.	6. This prevents a false increase in intraspinal pressure due to muscle tension and abdominal compression.
7. Instruct patient to breathe normally and avoid straining.	
8. Attach manometer to spinal needle and read open pressure.	
9. Perform Queckenstedt test by compressing jugular veins, if requested. Normally there is a rapid rise in pressure in response to compression and a rapid return to normal when compression is released.	9. This aids in determining the patency of the cerebrospinal fluid pathway.

10. Collect specimens of fluid.
  A. Allow it to drip slowly into the test tubes.
  B. Place approximately 1 ml. in each of three test tubes.	

11. Label each test tube with:
  A. Type of specimen.
  B. Specimen number in order of sequence.
	B. The sequence in which the specimens are obtained is essential for interpretation of laboratory results.

C. Patient's name.	
12. Apply a Band-Aid to the puncture site after needle is withdrawn.	

PRECAUTIONS

1. Maintain strict aseptic technique.
2. Instruct the patient to refrain from coughing, straining, or moving during the procedure, unless instructed to do so by the physician.
3. Be prepared to provide artificial ventilation and maintain a patent airway in the event of brain stem herniation as a result of removal of cerebrospinal fluid.

RELATED CARE

1. Instruct the patient to cooperate, breathe normally, and relax as much as possible.
2. Send the specimens of cerebrospinal fluid directly to the laboratory, since the changes which occur if the fluid is allowed to stand will alter the findings.
3. Observe opening and closing pressures, amount and character of the fluid, drugs if administered, tolerance, and patient's reactions.
4. Instruct the patient to lay flat for 1 or more hours following a lumbar puncture.
5. Encourage liberal intake of fluid, if the condition permits.
6. Assess changes in vital signs, neurologic status, headache, nausea/vomiting, and redness, swelling, or drainage from the puncture site.

COMPLICATIONS

Tentorial and brain stem herniation
Respiratory arrest
Headache
Infection
Pain
Paraplegia

REFERENCES

American Association of Neurosurgical Nurses: Core Curriculum for Neurosurgical Nursing. Baltimore, American Association of Neurosurgical Nurses, 1977.

Brunner, Lillian, et al.: The Lippincott Manual of Nursing Practice, 2nd ed. Philadelphia, J. B. Lippincott, 1978.

Luckmann, J., and Sorensen, K.: Medical-Surgical Nursing: A Psychophysiologic Approach, 2nd ed. Philadelphia, W.B. Saunders, 1980.

Skydell, B., and Crowder, A.: Diagnostic Procedures. Boston, Little, Brown and Company, 1975.

HYPOTHERMIA AND HYPERTHERMIA

Marilyn M. Ricci, R.N., M.S., C.N.R.N.

OVERVIEW

Hypothermia and hyperthermia are therapeutic modalities for maintaining total body temperature at a desired level. Hypothermia is utilized to reduce cellular metabolism, which results in a concomitant decrease in the oxygen requirement of the body tissues. Hyperthermia is utilized to increase and maintain body temperature at a normothermic level.

Hypothermia and hyperthermia equipment incorporates both cooling and heating systems. A pump circulates fluid (usually water) from the reservoir through the thermal blanket, which is either warmed or cooled by the circulating fluid. Most control units can regulate the temperature both manually and automatically. The automatic control system monitors the patient's temperature electronically and regulates cycling of the main unit within preset limits. A temperature sensing probe transmits information to the control system, which causes the machine to heat or cool fluid going to the thermal blankets.

Within critical care settings, these units may be portable or built-in. Each unit has a control panel which contains control knobs, indicator lights, and thermometers to indicate the temperature of the circulating fluid and the patient's temperature. Safety features include an alarm system, back-up thermostats, and electrical safeguards. The tubing from the thermal blanket is connected to the unit at two hose couplings. Each unit usually is able to regulate several blankets.

The thermal blankets/pads are made of plastics and synthetic fabrics which are easily cleaned, lightweight to facilitate handling, pliable to fit body contours, firm to resist being pinched off, and smooth enough to avoid causing pressure areas. The blanket/pad may be either reusable or disposable.

OBJECTIVES

To alter body temperature to a prescribed level by means of an elective clinical therapy.

Hypothermia

1. To lower excessively high temperatures secondary to cerebral trauma and febrile diseases.
2. To minimize tissue damage from diminished oxygen delivery when blood flow to vital organs is reduced or interrupted (e.g., in cases of cerebral edema, intracranial surgery, and cardiac surgery).

Hyperthermia

1. To warm a patient to as near normothermia as possible prior to an EEG for the determination of electrocerebral silence.
2. To rewarm the patient to normal body temperature following induced hypothermia.
3. To assist the patient to maintain normal body temperature, such as in cases of spinal cord trauma.

SPECIAL EQUIPMENT

Hypothermia and hyperthermia unit
Thermal blanket/pad
Rectal temperature probe or thermometer
ECG monitor

METHOD

ACTION	RATIONALE
1. Place a single sheet over mattress under thermal pad.	
2. Place one bath blanket on top of thermal pad, under patient. Additional thermal pads may be placed on top of the patient, if increased contact area is needed.	2. Always use a single layer of bath blanket between the patient and thermal pad to facilitate heat exchange and protect the patient's skin.
3. Tuck bath blanket which is on top of pad lightly under mattress.	3. Tight restrictions over the pad or creases in the pad impede the flow of fluid.
4. Place pillows, if needed under head or for positioning, under thermal pad rather than directly under patient.	4. Maximal contact between the patient's skin and the pad increases cooling or heating efficiency.
5. Attach hoses from thermal pad to machine. Be sure the hoses are not kinked or twisted.	
6. Check that reservoir in machine is filled with appropriate solution (distilled water or an antifreeze solution, as recommended by the manufacturer) to level indicated.	
7. Prepare equipment according to manual or automatic mode. Plug into wall outlet.	

ACTION	RATIONALE

A. Manual control:
  (1) Place temperature dial at "start" and push manual button to activate machine.
  (2) Dial desired thermal pad setting.
    (a) Hypothermia:
      (1) Place the temperature dial at 40° F. for approximately 5 minutes.
      (2) Then reset temperature control to a setting of 50 to 60° F.

    (a) Running the machine at the 40° F. setting for long periods of time will increase the possibility of ischemia of the pressure areas and freeze burns of the skin.

      (b) Hyperthermia:
      (1) Place temperature control at 100° F. for approximately 5 minutes.
      (2) Then reset temperature to a setting of 80 to 90° F.
  (3) Adjust temperature setting of thermal pad to attain desired patient temperature.
  (4) Monitor patient's temperature every 15 minutes until desired temperature has been reached.

    (4) Usually it takes 3 to 4 hours to bring a patient's temperature to the desired range when using one thermal pad.

  (5) Adjust temperature setting of thermal pad to maintain a stable body temperature.

    (5) Usually a 20 to 25° F. differential between the pad and body temperatures will maintain a stable hypothermic state.

B. Automatic control. The cooling or heating process is controlled by the patient's body temperature, via a rectal probe.

ACTION	RATIONALE

(1) Place temperature dial at "start" and push manual button to activate machine.

(2) Dial desired thermal pad setting.
    (a) Hypothermia: Place temperature control at 40° F. for 5 minutes.
    (b) Hyperthermia: Place temperature control at 100° F. for 5 minutes.

(3) Reset temperature gauge for desired patient temperature.

(4) Depress automatic control button.

(5) Insert lubricated tip of temperature probe about 4" into patient's rectum and tape it securely in place.

(6) Insert metal jack at other end of probe into patient probe adapter on machine.

        (6) The thermostatic control will heat or cool the fluid circulating through the thermal pad according to the patient's temperature as monitored by the rectal probe.

(7) Obtain rectal temperature of patient by depressing appropriate button on control panel.

(8) Check that electronic control meter is giving accurate readings of patient's temperature.
    (a) Take patient's rectal temperature manually.
    (b) Move temperature control dial to settings 3° F. above and below actual patient temperature. The

ACTION	RATIONALE

"cool" and "heat"
indicators should go
on appropriately.

PRECAUTIONS

1. Prevent shivering which occurs during the initial cooling and rewarming phase, since it can increase metabolic rate, body temperature, oxygen usage, and circulation, cause hyperventilation, and may produce hypoglycemia. Shivering appears first in the masseter muscles, then in the neck or pectoral muscles, and finally in the long muscles of upper and lower extremities. Administer medications to prevent shivering, as prescribed.

2. Reduce or stop the procedure within 1 to 3° F. of the desired level, since temperature may "overshoot" or "drift" 1 to 2° F. after the desired temperature has been reached.

3. Evaluate the patient's clinical status during hypothermia in view of an anticipated depression of sensorium, respirations, cardiac output, renal output, and other vital functions.
    A. Avoid temperature decrease exceeding 1°F. per 15 minutes to avoid PVC's.
    B. Monitor parameters of cardiac dynamics.
    C. Maximal reduction of heart rate usually occurs with the initial temperature drop.

4. Be alert for cardiac insufficiency due to rapid surface rewarming.

5. Be prepared for an alteration in the metabolism of drugs during hypothermic and hyperthermic states. A cumulative effect may occur during rewarming.

6. Avoid any sudden sharp rise in temperature.

7. Avoid puncturing the thermal blanket with pins.

8. Check the equipment for leaks, kinks, twists, and for mechanical and electrical failure.

RELATED CARE

1. Monitor vital signs, neurologic status, color of lips, and capillary refill at least every 30 minutes.

2. Protect skin integrity by repositioning, applying lotion, and massaging bony prominences at least every hour. Wrap distal extremities with towels to decrease incidence of frank shivering and preserve skin integrity.

3. Maintain a patent airway by positioning, suctioning, and avoiding oral intake when the gag and swallow reflexes are depressed.

4. Protect the patient's eyes in the absence of the corneal reflex and when eye secretions are decreased.
5. Reduce circulatory stasis by doing range of motion exercises and avoiding restrictive bands.

COMPLICATIONS

Frostbite/fat necrosis
Focal tissue necrosis
Hypersensitivity to cold
Ventricular fibrillation and
  cardiac arrhythmias
Acidosis (metabolic and/or
  respiratory)

Oliguria
Embolization
Hyperpyrexia
Ileus
Cold diuresis

REFERENCES

American Association of Neurosurgical Nurses: Core Curriculum for Neurosurgical Nursing. Baltimore, American Association of Neurosurgical Nurses, 1977.

Beaumont, Estelle: Hypo/hyperthermia equipment. Nurs. '74, 4:34, 1974.

Hudak, Carolyn, et al.: Critical Care Nursing, 2nd ed. Philadelphia, J. B. Lippincott, 1977.

St. Joseph's Hospital and Medical Center: Nursing Policy and Procedure Manual. Phoenix, St. Joseph's Hospital and Medical Center, 1976.

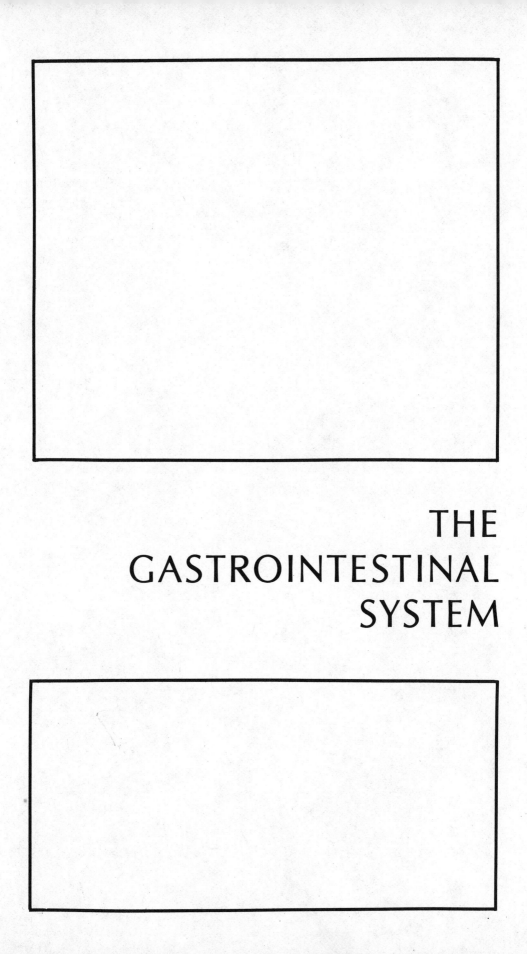

THE
GASTROINTESTINAL
SYSTEM

MANAGEMENT OF UPPER GASTROINTESTINAL HEMORRHAGE

Elaine Brogdon, R.N., B.S.N.
Kathy Mossing, R.N., M.A. and
Barbara Tabor, R.N., B.S.N.

OVERVIEW

Gastrointestinal bleeding can be an insidious process with few manifestations, or it can present with massive hemorrhage. In some cases, it may be necessary to pass a nasogastric tube to observe and test aspirant to determine if bleeding is or has been present. Active bleeding may be nonsurgically controlled by irrigating the gastrointestinal tract with iced saline solution to constrict the arteries by hypothermia, by applying pressure locally with balloon tamponade, or by constricting the bleeding vessels through local or systemic infusion of Pitressin.

NASOGASTRIC TUBE INSERTION

OVERVIEW

Nasogastric tubes are used to assess gastrointestinal function, detect complications, treat problems, administer medications, provide feedings, and decompress the stomach and duodenum. For these purposes the stomach is intubated with either a single-lumen Levin tube or a double-lumen sump tube. The sizes most frequently used for adults are 16 and 18 French.

The Levin tubes are either rubber or plastic, and are approximately 48 inches in length. Marker rings are located at 18-, 22-, 26-, and 30-inch points; lumen size ranges from 10 through 18 French.

Sump tubes are of clear plastic, constructed much the same as Levin tubes. The unique feature of the sump tube is its second lumen, which serves as a decompression vent to prevent blockage of the suction lumen by large particles or gastric mucosa.

OBJECTIVES

1. To determine the site, freshness, and amount of gastrointestinal bleeding.
2. To test aspirant for frank blood (or guaiac) and/or acidity.
3. To administer antacids.
4. To lavage stomach, when necessary.

SPECIAL EQUIPMENT

Nasogastric tube

Water-soluble lubricant

50-ml. irrigating syringe

Emesis basin

Tape

Glass of water/straw

Ice

Suction source

METHOD

ACTION	RATIONALE
1. Position patient, using one of the following:	
A. Left lateral position.	A. This facilitates passage of the tube into the cardia of the stomach.
B. Trendelenburg position.	B. This is indicated for hypotensive, comatose patients.
C. Sitting position.	C. This decreases gag reflex and makes swallowing easier.
D. Hyperextension of the patient's head.	D. This depresses the floor of the nasal passage and facilitates passage of the tube into the nasopharynx.
2. Place red rubber tube on ice (if used).	2. This hardens the tube for easier insertion.
3. Lubricate tube.	3. This lessens irritation of the mucosa.
4. Place 50-ml. irrigating syringe on end of tube.	
5. Measure length of tube to be passed.	
A. Measure from bridge of nose to ear lobe to xyphoid process.	A. This measurement is the approximate length of tube needed to reach the stomach.
B. Indicate this length by placing tape at that point on tube.	
6. Obtain history of nasal trauma to determine appropriate route for tube insertion:	
A. Nasal.	
B. Oral.	B. This is used if nasal obstruction is present.
7. Insert tube.	
A. Pass tube gently into nasopharynx.	
B. If resistance is met rotate tube	

ACTION	RATIONALE
slowly, aiming downward and backward.	
C. Advance tube firmly and steadily while patient is swallowing.	C. Swallowing facilitates passage of the tube.
D. Offer sips of water from a glass when tube reaches posterior nasopharynx.	D. In the alert patient, this minimizes gagging and facilitates passage of the tube.
E. Pass tube until tape mark is reached, and secure to nose with tape.	
8. Withdraw tube immediately if any change in respiratory status is noted.	8. This may indicate placement in the bronchus.
9. Test for tube placement, using one or more of the following techniques.	
A. Obtain gastric content by aspirating with 50-ml. syringe.	
B. Auscultate with stethoscope over gastric area while 50 ml. of air is inserted into tube.	B. If tube is properly placed, a rush of air should be heard.
C. Place end of tube in glass of water to check for bubbling.	C. Bubbling indicates tube is in the bronchus, and immediate withdrawal is necessary.
10. Connect tube to suction, or continue with gastric lavage (see method for "Gastric Lavage").	

PRECAUTIONS

1. Assess for coiling in oral pharynx or esophagus and then for tube patency if patient gags or vomits around the tube.
2. Assess for possible tube placement into the lungs if patient becomes cyanotic or dyspneic.
3. Maintain airway with frequent suctioning if oral secretions persist.

RELATED CARE

1. Maintain patency of the tube by irrigation and repositioning.
2. Observe drainage for changes.
3. Keep a record of the amounts of intake and output.
4. Restrain or sedate patient, if indicated, to prevent removal of the tube and possible aspiration of the gastric contents.

COMPLICATIONS

Aspiration
Electrolyte imbalance
Hyperventilation
Bradycardia

Nasal mucosa erosion
Trauma to gastric mucosa
Reflux esophagitis

REFERENCES

Bockus, Henry L. (ed.): Gastroenterology, 3rd ed. Philadelphia, W. B. Saunders, 1974; Vol. 1, pp. 808–816.

Boedeker, Edgar C., and Dauber, James H. (eds.): Manual of Medical Therapeutics, 21st ed. Boston, Little, Brown and Company, 1974, pp. 245–246.

Brunner, Lillian S., and Suddarth, Doris S. (eds.): Lippincott Manual of Nursing Practice. Philadelphia, J. B. Lippincott, 1978.

Greenberger, N., and Winship, D.: Gastrointestinal Disorders: A Pathophysiologic Approach. Chicago, Year Book Medical Publishers, 1976, pp. 207–208.

Luckmann, J., and Sorensen, K.: Medical-Surgical Nursing: A Psychophysiologic Approach, 2nd ed. Philadelphia, W.B. Saunders, 1980.

McConnell, E.: All about gastrointestinal intubation. Nurs. '75, 5:30–37, 1975.

McConnell, E.: Ten problems with nasogastric tubes and how to solve them. Nurs. '79, 9:78–81, 1979.

Stroup, P.: Recognition and management of GI bleeds. J. Emerg. Nurs., 4:19–25, 1978.

GASTRIC LAVAGE

OBJECTIVES

1. To control upper GI bleeding by vasoconstriction of gastric vessels, using hypothermia.
2. To remove any toxins, large blood clots, or old blood from the stomach.

SPECIAL EQUIPMENT

Large bore (32 Fr.) Ewald tube or 18 Fr. Salem sump tube
Large 2- to 3-liter inflow bottle
Large bore inflow and outflow tubing, connected to the inflow bottle with V-connector
Iced normal saline solution
Outflow bottle
50-ml. aspirating syringe
Lubricant
Large pair of hemostats for clamping tubing

METHOD

ACTION

1. Set up lavage equipment (Fig. 112).
2. Insert Salem sump or Ewald tube (see the method for "Nasogastric Tube Insertion" for details of tube advancement).
3. Obtain gastric specimen.
4. Siphon initial gastric contents into outflow bottle.

RATIONALE

3. This is used for diagnostic purposes.
4. Initial emptying of the stomach decreases chance of vomiting and possible aspiration.

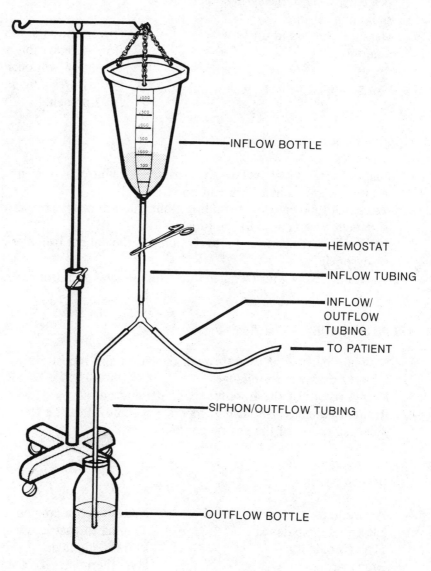

INFLOW BOTTLE

HEMOSTAT

INFLOW TUBING

INFLOW/ OUTFLOW TUBING

TO PATIENT

SIPHON/OUTFLOW TUBING

OUTFLOW BOTTLE

Figure 112.   Gastric lavage equipment.

ACTION	RATIONALE
5. Fill inflow bottle with iced normal saline solution, with inflow tubing clamped.	5. Normal saline solution is isotonic; this prevents decreased osmolarity. Ice is used to cause vasoconstriction in the stomach.
6. Open inflow tubing, starting with 250-ml. inflow rate.	6. An initial 250-ml. amount checks the patient's tolerance for adding extra fluid to the stomach and facilitates emptying the stomach contents.
7. Increase inflow amount to 500 ml. as soon as possible.	7. 500 ml. of fluid are needed to flatten out the rugae of the stomach.
8. Infuse and siphon out solution repeatedly, using large syringe or siphoning set-up.	
9. Measure inflow and outflow amounts.	9. These amounts should be equal; inflow should not exceed outflow or distention will occur.
10. Lavage until clear.	10. This assures adequate "wash-out" of the stomach.

PRECAUTIONS

1. Suction oral cavity frequently during procedure to prevent possible aspiration and enhance patient comfort.
2. Assess for tube patency, including coiling in oral pharynx or esophagus, if patient vomits around the tube.
3. Assess for tube placement into the lungs if the patient becomes cyanotic or dyspneic.
4. Maintain airway with frequent suctioning if oral secretions persist.

RELATED CARE

1. Maintain patency of tube through irrigation and repositioning.
2. Observe drainage for changes.
3. Keep a record of the amounts of intake and output.
4. Restrain patient, if indicated, to prevent removal of the tube and possible aspiration of the gastric contents.

COMPLICATIONS

Aspiration
Electrolyte imbalance
Hyperventilation
Bradycardia

Nasal mucosa erosion
Trauma to gastric mucosa
Reflux esophagitis
Hypothermia, if using iced saline

REFERENCES

Bockus, Henry L. (ed.): Gastroenterology, 3rd ed. Philadelphia, W. B. Saunders, 1974; Vol. 1, pp. 814–815.

Boedeker, Edgar C., and Dauber, James H. (eds.): Manual of Medical Therapeutics, 21st ed. Boston, Little, Brown and Company, 1974, pp. 245–246.

Brunner, Lillian S., and Suddarth, Doris S. (eds.): Lippincott Manual of Nursing Practice. Philadelphia, J. B. Lippincott, 1978, pp. 923–925.

Greenberger, N., and Winship, D.: Gastrointestinal Disorders: A Pathophysiologic Approach. Chicago, Year Book Medical Publishers, 1976, pp. 207–208.

Luckmann, J., and Sorensen, K.: Medical-Surgical Nursing: A Psychophysiologic Approach, 2nd ed. Philadelphia, W.B. Saunders, 1980.

Stroup, P.: Recognition and management of GI bleeds. J. Emerg. Nurs., *4:19*–25, 1978.

SENGSTAKEN/BLAKEMORE TUBE

OVERVIEW

Bleeding from gastric and esophageal varices can be controlled by applying local pressure to the bleeding sites. This is accomplished by the insertion of the triple-lumen, double-balloon, 20 French red rubber Sengstaken/Blakemore tube. One lumen is used for gastric aspiration, one for inflating the esophageal balloon, and one for inflating the gastric balloon (Fig. 113). An additional modification is recommended—that is, the use of an accessory nasogastric tube to remove oral secretions draining into the esophagus and prevent aspiration. After insertion and inflation of the balloons, traction is applied to prevent advancement into the stomach.

OBJECTIVE

To control massive bleeding from esophageal varices via nonoperative management, using esophagogastric balloon tamponade.

SPECIAL EQUIPMENT

Sengstaken/Blakemore tube
Accessory 18 Fr. nasogastric tube
Suction source
Sphygmomanometer
50-ml. aspirating syringe
Lidocaine or cocaine
Topical spray
Oral mouthpiece

Sponge rubber cube
Four rubber-tipped hemostats
Two suction set-ups
2½-ft. rubber tubing (blood pressure tubing size)
Water-soluble lubricating jelly
Catcher's mask, football helmet with mouthguard, or 1 to 2-lb. weights
Scissors
Y-connector
Adhesive tape

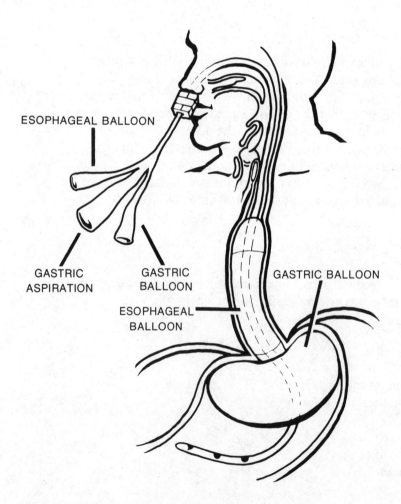

Figure 113.   Sengstaken-Blakemore tube. (Courtesy of Davol, Inc.)

METHOD

ACTION	RATIONALE
1. Place patient in left lateral position.	1. This facilitates gastric balloon introduction into the cardia of the stomach.
2. Prepare tubes.	
A. Hold air-filled balloons under water to test for air leaks.	A. This assures proper function.
B. Lubricate both balloons and lower parts of Sengstaken/Blakemore tube with water-soluble jelly.	B. This decreases trauma to mucous membranes.
C. Tape the 18 Fr. nasogastric tube alongside Sengstaken/Blakemore tube, level with top of esophageal balloon.	
D. Connect accessory esophageal tube to low continuous suction.	D. This prevents secretions from accumulating in the esophagus.
3. Attempt to empty stomach and esophagus with Ewald tube lavage, prior to insertion (see method for "Gastric Lavage").	3. This minimizes the possibility of aspiration.
4. Anesthetize posterior pharynx and nostrils topically.	4. This decreases the discomfort caused by tube passage.
5. Insert tube (see the method for "Nasogastric Tube Insertion").	
A. Pass Sengstaken/Blakemore tube, with balloons deflated, through nasopharynx into stomach to at least 50-cm mark on tubing. (A guide wire into the gastric lumen may facilitate tube insertion.)	A. This decreases the possibility of inflating the gastric balloon in the esophagus.
B. Aspirate gastric tube lumen.	B. This verifies gastric positioning and helps to avoid regurgitation during tube manipulation.
C. Insert plastic bite block or airway, if oral route is used.	C. This prevents biting of the tube.
6. Inflate gastric balloon using 50 to 250 ml. of air, and double clamp inlet immediately distal to opening.	6. This prevents air leaks.
7. Withdraw tube until resistance is encountered.	7. This engages gastric balloon at the cardioesophageal junction.
8. Maintain gentle tension on tube by:	

ACTION	RATIONALE
A. Taping to a cube of sponge rubber as it emerges from the nasal orifice; *or*	A. This fixes position of the tube at the cardioesophageal junction.
B. Applying gentle traction with 1 to 2 lbs. of pull and small sponge taped on tube; *or*	
C. Fixing the tube to a baseball catcher's mask or a football helmet with mouthguard worn by patient.	
9. Obtain x-ray.	9. This confirms proper placement of the gastric balloon.
10. Lavage stomach (see the method for "Gastric Lavage"). A. Irrigate until clear through gastric inlet. B. Then connect gastric end to continuous or intermittent suction.	10. This prevents clotted blood from plugging tube. Immediate evacuation of stomach contents allows for subsequent evaluation of gastric tamponade effectiveness.
11. Inflate esophageal balloon if bleeding is not controlled by gastric tamponade.	
A. Connect 2½-ft. rubber tubing from esophageal inlet via Y connector to sphygmomanometer (Fig. 114). Observe baseline pressure and *not* transient peak pressure.	A. This permits periodic checking of esophageal balloon pressure. With proper position, pressure will vary with respirations and esophageal contractions.
B. Inflate to 30 to 45 mm. Hg pressure.	B. The lowest pressure necessary to stop bleeding is used.
C. Double clamp with rubber-tipped hemostat.	C. This prevents air leaks.
D. Check to see if patient complains of substernal pressure.	D. Complaint of substernal pressure as higher pressures are reached is not an uncommon sensation.
12. Switch accessory nasogastric tube suction from constant to low intermittent suction.	
13. If bleeding continues after esophageal balloon pressure is maintained at 45 mm. Hg, inflate gastric balloon with air gradually up to 400 ml.	13. Prolonged maintenance of high pressure causes mucosal ulceration within a few hours.
14. Maintain tamponade for 72 hours.	

ACTION   RATIONALE

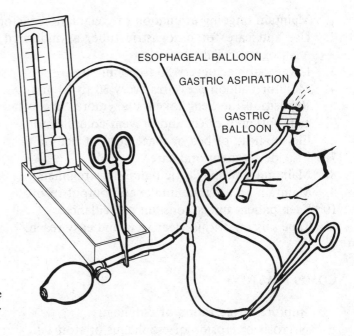

ESOPHAGEAL BALLOON

GASTRIC ASPIRATION

GASTRIC BALLOON

Figure 114. Sengstaken-Blakemore tube connected to a sphygmomanometer. (Courtesy of Davol, Inc.)

A. Release esophageal balloon pressure and relax traction on gastric balloon 12 to 24 hours prior to withdrawal.

B. Observe for rebleeding and should bleeding recur, re-establish esophageal pressure.

C. Transect tube with scissors and remove Sengstaken/Blakemore tube if there is no rebleeding.

C. This ensures balloon deflation prior to removal.

PRECAUTIONS

1. Observe for persistent gastric bleeding; this indicates possible gastric erosions or peptic ulcer.

2. Maintain balloon pressures and tube position to prevent persistent bleeding or pulling up of the balloon to the trachea.

3. Suction pharyngeal secretions frequently to prevent aspiration. If alert and able to cooperate, the patient may be provided with a dental suction tip to suction his/her own secretions.

4. Observe for ineffective gastric lavage and stomach emptying that may result in regurgitation.

5. Restrain the patient if agitated or confused to prevent removal of the tube.

RELATED CARE

1. Maintain ongoing evaluation of coagulation factors.
2. Use and care for nasogastric tube, as indicated, in the method for "Nasogastric Tube Insertion."
3. Lavage stomach every 30 to 60 minutes.
4. Monitor balloon pressures every 30 to 60 minutes.
5. Reposition the Sengstaken/Blakemore tube, when necessary, to maintain optimum effect and prevent complications.
6. Elevate head of bed or place head of bed on 6- to 8-inch blocks.
7. Provide frequent oral care.
8. Maintain a prophylactic pulmonary regimen.
9. Maintain an accurate intake and output record.
10. Keep patient under constant surveillance.
11. Tape scissors within clear view and easy reach.

COMPLICATIONS

Rupture or laceration of esophagus
Necrosis or erosion of esophagus or stomach
Aspiration
Asphyxiation
Prolonged bleeding

SUPPLIER

Davol, Inc.

REFERENCES

Blakemore, A.H., (ed.): Instructions for Passing the Esophageal Balloon for Control of Bleeding from Esophageal Varices. New York, Davol, Inc.

Hermann, Robert E., and Traul, Don: Experience with the Sengstaken/Blakemore tube for bleeding esophageal varices. Surg. Gynecol. Obstet., *130*:879, 1970.

Pitcher, J.L.: Safety and effectiveness of using the modified Sengstaken/Blakemore tube: A prospective study. Gastroenterology, *61*:291, 1971.

Smith, Gardner W., Maddrey, Willis C., and Zuidema, George D.: Portal hypertension as we see it. In Child, Charles G., 3rd (ed.): Portal Hypertension as Seen Today by Seventeen Authorities. Philadelphia, W. B. Saunders, 1974, p. 22.

LINTON TUBE

OVERVIEW

Compression of the submucosa venous network in the cardia of the stomach may control bleeding esophageal varices by preventing blood flow into them. This is accomplished by insertion of a triple-lumen, x-ray-opaque tube with a single intragastric balloon. The three ports are used for gastric suction, esophageal suction, and inflation of the gastric balloon (Fig. 115).

OBJECTIVE

To control massive bleeding from esophageal varices via nonoperative management using gastric balloon tamponade.

SPECIAL EQUIPMENT

Linton tube
Two suction set-ups
Topical anesthetic spray
Oral mouthpiece
Cube of sponge rubber

Water-soluble lubricating jelly
Two rubber-tipped hemostats
Pulley set-up
1-kg. weight, or baseball catcher's mask, or football helmet with mouthguard

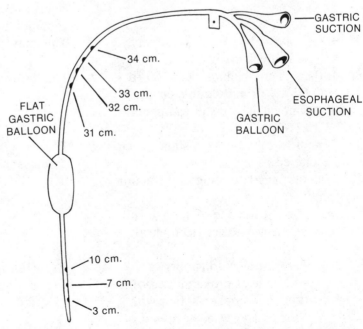

Figure 115. Linton tube. (Courtesy of Davol, Inc.)

METHOD

ACTION	RATIONALE
1. Position the patient in left lateral position or upright sitting position.	1. This facilitates gastric balloon introduction into cardia of stomach and facilitates swallowing.
2. Prepare tube.	
A. Test air-filled balloon under water for air leaks.	A. This ensures proper function.
B. Lubricate balloon and lower part of tube with water-soluble jelly.	B. This decreases trauma to mucous membranes.
3. Empty stomach and esophagus with Ewald tube lavage prior to insertion (see method for "Gastric Lavage").	3. This minimizes possibility of aspiration.
4. Anesthetize posterior pharynx and nostrils, using topical anesthetic spray.	4. This decreases discomfort of tube passage.
5. Pass the Linton tube, with balloon deflated, through either naso- or oropharynx into stomach to pre-measured mark (see method for measurement for "Nasogastric Tube Insertion").	5. This decreases the possibility of inflating the gastric balloon in the esophagus.
6. Aspirate gastric tube lumen.	6. This verifies gastric positioning and helps avoid regurgitation during tube manipulation.
7. Insert plastic bite block or airway, if oral route is used.	7. This prevents biting of tube.
8. Inflate gastric balloon with 700 to 800 ml. of air and double clamp inlet immediately distal to opening (Fig. 116).	8. This prevents air leaks.
9. Withdraw tube until resistance is encountered.	9. This engages the gastric balloon at the cardioesophageal junction.
10. Maintain gentle tension and traction on tube.	
A. Tape it to cube of sponge rubber as it emerges from nasal orifice.	
B. Attach pulley to rubber tab, with hole at proximal end of tube, and apply traction with either a 1-kg. weight at end of pulley on end of bed, a base-	B. This fixes position of the tube at the cardioesophageal junction.

ACTION	RATIONALE

ball catcher's mask, or a football helmet with mouthguard.

11. Apply suction to esophageal lumen and irrigate frequently.

12. Obtain an x-ray.

13. Lavage stomach through gastric inlet (see method for "Gastric Lavage").
    A. Irrigate until clear.
    B. Then connect gastric end to continuous or intermittent suction.

14. Maintain tamponade for maximum of 48 hours.
    A. Relax traction on gastric balloon 12 to 24 hours prior to withdrawal.
    B. Observe for rebleeding and re-establish firm gastric traction, should bleeding recur.
    C. Transect tube with scissors and remove if there is no rebleeding.

11. This eliminates possibility of aspiration.

12. This confirms proper placement of gastric balloon.

13. This prevents clotted blood from plugging the tube. Immediate evacuation of stomach contents allows for subsequent evaluation of gastric tamponade effectiveness.

C. This ensures balloon deflation prior to removal.

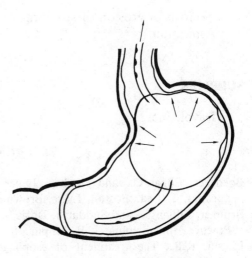

Figure 116. Linton tube in place, inflated with 700 to 800 ml. of air. (Courtesy of Davol, Inc.)

PRECAUTIONS

1. Observe for persistent gastric bleeding; this indicates possible gastric erosions or peptic ulcer.
2. Maintain balloon pressure and tube position to prevent persistent bleeding or pulling up of the gastric balloon to the trachea.
3. Suction pharyngeal secretions frequently to prevent aspiration. If alert and able to cooperate, the patient may be provided with a dental suction tip to suction his/her own secretions.
4. Observe for ineffective gastric lavage and stomach emptying that may result in regurgitation.
5. Restrain the patient if agitated or confused to prevent removal of the tube.

RELATED CARE

1. Maintain ongoing evaluation of coagulation factors.
2. Irrigate esophageal suction lumen every hour.
3. Lavage stomach every 30 to 60 minutes.
4. Reposition tube, when necessary, to maintain optimum effect and prevent complications.
5. Elevate head of bed or place head of bed on 6- to 8-inch blocks.
6. Provide frequent oral care.
7. Maintain a prophylactic pulmonary regimen.
8. Maintain an accurate intake and output record.
9. Keep patient under constant surveillance.
10. Tape scissors in place within clear view and easy reach.

COMPLICATIONS

Necrosis or erosion of stomach   Asphyxiation
Aspiration   Prolonged bleeding

SUPPLIER

Davol, Inc.

REFERENCES

Boedeker, Edgar C., and Dauber, James H. (eds.): Manual of Medical Therapeutics, 21st ed. Boston, Little, Brown and Company, 1974, pp. 248–249.
Brunner, Lillian S., and Suddarth, Doris S. (eds.): Lippincott Manual of Nursing Practice. Philadelphia, J. B. Lippincott, 1978.
Linton, R.R.: The treatment of esophageal varices. Surg. Clin. North Am., 46:485–498, 1966.
McConnell, E.: All about gastrointestinal intubation. Nurs. '75, 5:30–37, 1975.

MESENTERIC ARTERY LINE AND PITRESSIN INFUSION _____

OVERVIEW

Portal vascular system bleeding may be identified and located by angiography. Pitressin infusion may be selected as the treatment of choice; it may be administered systemically via a peripheral intravenous line or, preferably, by a local infusion. The latter is accomplished by catheterizing the superior mesenteric artery or one of its branches through the femoral artery under fluoroscopy.

OBJECTIVE

To induce splanchnic arteriolar vasoconstriction and decreased portal blood flow by use of Pitressin in patients with esophageal varices.

SPECIAL EQUIPMENT

Infusion pump and administration tubing
500 ml. normal saline solution, or 500 ml. 5% dextrose in water
Pitressin, 20 units/vial

METHOD

ACTION	RATIONALE
1. Monitor patient response while line is inserted via femoral artery, under fluoroscopy.	1. Visualization is necessary for accurate placement in superior mesenteric, celiac, left gastric, or gastroduodenal artery.

2. Prepare solution.
  A. Add 100 units Pitressin to 500 ml. 5% dextrose in water or to 500 ml. normal saline solution (provides 0.2 units /ml.).
  B. Label admixture.	

3. Prime intravenous administration tubing and infusion pump tubing, removing all air.	3. This prevents infusion of air and possible air embolism.
4. Prepare infusion pump. Guidelines for infusion rates are:	4. An infusion pump is necessary to maintain a constant accurate flow

ACTION	RATIONALE

A.   Intra-arterial: 0.1 to 0.4 units/minute (60 drops/ml. = 30 to 120 drops/minute with 6 to 24 units/hour).

B.   Peripheral intravenous: 20 units/100 ml. 5% dextrose in water infused over 10 to 20 minutes every 3 to 4 hours (approximates 5 units/hour).

5.   Assess effectiveness of infusion by decreased or stoppage of bleeding.

6.   Wean patient from pitressin infusion.

A.   Taper off over 24 hours and then infuse plain 5% dextrose in water for 24 hours at a keep open rate;

B.   Administer Pitressin at a rate of:

(1)   0.2 units/ml./min. for 24 hours.

(2)   0.1 units/ml./min. for 48 hours.

(3)   0.05 units/ml./min. for 12 hours.

(4)   Plain 5% dextrose in water or normal saline solution, 1 ml./min. for 24 hours.

C.   Remove catheter the fifth day.

Rationale column:

rate and, in the case of arterial infusion, to overcome arterial pressure.

6.   Immediate withdrawal of the drug may precipitate hemodynamic instability and/or renewed bleeding.

PRECAUTIONS

1.   Use extreme care to prevent dislodging the arterial catheter, as arterial bleeding and hemorrhage may result. In addition, clotting or compromised circulation of the leg used for catheter insertion may occur.
2.   Stabilize the intravenous catheter securely. If the solution infiltrates, immediately remove the intravenous line to avoid tissue sloughing.
3.   Keep the leg used for arterial line insertion straight, restrain if necessary.

RELATED CARE

1.   Assess for infection or clot formation at the cutdown site.
2.   Assess frequently for IV patency (systemic) and possible infiltration.

3. Assess the leg used for insertion of the arterial catheter for changes in pulses, temperature of extremity, and mottling.
4. Evaluate frequent blood pressures for trends indicating development of hypertension.
5. Place the patient on a cardiac monitor and observe for development of dysrhythmias and myocardial ischemic changes.
6. Secure line with tongue blade and keep in direct vision.

COMPLICATIONS

ADH effect; water and sodium retention
Decreased splanchnic blood flow, including hepatic artery and renal artery vasoconstriction and subsequent damage
Coronary artery vasoconstriction in systemic administration

REFERENCES

Bockus, Henry L. (ed.): Gastroenterology, 3rd ed. Philadelphia, W. B. Saunders, 1974; Vol. 1, pp. 829–845.

Boedeker, Edgar C., and Dauber, James H. (eds.): Manual of Medical Therapeutics, 21st ed. Boston, Little, Brown and Company, 1974, p. 248.

Malt, R.A.: Current concepts: Control of massive upper GI hemorrhage. N. Engl. J. Med., *286*:1043, 1972.

Sedwigk, Cornelius, and Reale, Vincent, F.: Upper GI bleeding: Diagnosis and treatment. Surg. Clin. North Am., *56*(No. 3):695-707, 1976.

GASTRIC LAVAGE IN OVERDOSE

Elaine Brogdon, R.N., B.S.N.
Kathy Mossing, R.N., M.A., and
Barbara Tabor, R.N., B.S.N.

OBJECTIVES

1. To remove poisons, life-threatening overdoses of medication, and irritating substances from the stomach quickly and efficiently.
2. To obtain a specimen for analysis.

SPECIAL EQUIPMENT

Large 2- to 3-liter inflow bottle
Large bore inflow and outflow
   tubing connected to inflow
   bottle with V connector
Large bore 32 Fr. Ewald tube
Outflow bottle
50-ml. aspirating syringe
Lubricant
Hemostats
ECG recorder
Cardiac monitor
Intravenous line with 5% dextrose in water
Saline irrigating solution
Charcoal tablets (10 to 15)
Magnesium citrate (340 ml.)
Restraints

METHOD

ACTION	RATIONALE
1. Obtain vital signs.	1. This is done to detect hypotension and/or cardiac dysrhythmias.
2. Place patient on cardiac monitor.	2. This monitors for dysrhythmias and bradycardias.
3. Start intravenous line with 5% dextrose in water at a keep open rate.	3. This provides access for emergency drug administration.
4. Draw samples for blood work (usually electrolyte levels and toxicology screen; in addition, determinations of alcohol and arterial blood gas levels may be indicated).	4. These are used for baseline studies, to detect levels of toxins in the blood stream, and to document respiratory status.
5. Obtain ECG.	5. This will detect any cardiac abnormalities.
6. Assess for gas reflex.	6. If absent, the patient may need to be intubated to prevent aspiration.
7. Place patient in left lateral, Trendelenberg, or sitting position.	7. See rationales under the method for "Nasogastric Tube Insertion."

ACTION	RATIONALE
8. Assess heart rate prior to insertion of Ewald tube.	8. If it is below 100, atropine 0.4 mg. IV is given to block vagal response and prevent bradycardia during passage of the tube.
9. Place padded tongue blade in mouth.	9. This prevents the patient from biting on the tube.
10. Place lubricated Ewald tube in mouth and pass tube to black ring (approximately 20 inches) into stomach. See method for "Nasogastric Tube Insertion" for specifics of tube advancement.	
11. Lavage stomach (see method for "Gastric Lavage").	
12. Administer the following, if prescribed, after lavage is completed:	
A. Charcoal (10 to 15 tablets), liquefied and instilled into tube.	A. Charcoal helps to absorb any remaining toxins.
B. Magnesium citrate (340 ml.).	B. This encourages peristalsis and elimination.

PRECAUTIONS

1. Maintain suicide precautions (e.g., remove any remaining pills from patient area; keep in restraints after lavage) if patient is suicidal.
2. Maintain airway by suctioning excess oral secretions if the patient is comatose.
3. Insert a nasogastric tube after the Ewald tube is removed as a precaution against vomiting if the patient is comatose and not intubated.
4. Place the patient in four-point restraints and a waist restraint, if necessary. Restraint is necessary for most patients to prevent them from pulling out the Ewald tube.

RELATED CARE

1. Maintain a clear oral airway throughout procedure.
2. Assess neurologic, respiratory, and cardiovascular status.
3. Observe for any sign of trauma to the patient.
4. Obtain medical history regarding pharmacologic profile.
5. Obtain samples for repeat electrolyte determinations to monitor for electrolyte imbalance, especially potassium depletion, if over 20 liters of normal saline solution are used.
6. Catheterize the patient during the procedure, if comatose, to monitor output more closely.
7. Request a psychiatric consultation as part of follow-up care.

COMPLICATIONS

Aspiration	Hypertension
Respiratory arrest	Hypotension
Cardiac arrhythmias	Acidosis
Renal failure	Coma
Hepatic failure	Delirium
Seizures	Pulmonary edema
Urinary retention	Bleeding disorders
Hyperthermia	

REFERENCES

Bird, Thomas, and Copass, Michael: The House Officers' Guide to Common Drug Intoxication in Adults. Seattle, Harborview Medical Center, 1973, pp. 2–3.

King, Eunice, Wierck, Lynn, and Dyer, Marilyn: Illustrated Manual of Nursing Techniques. Philadelphia, J. B. Lippincott, 1977, pp. 159–165.

PARACENTESIS (ASSISTING WITH)

Elaine Brogdon, R.N., B.S.N.
Kathy Mossing, R:N., M.A., and
Barbara Tabor, R.N., B.S.N.

OVERVIEW

Withdrawal of fluid from the abdominal cavity may be required for diagnostic or therapeutic purposes. After a history of trauma, this may help to determine intra-abdominal bleeding. In other cases, samples of ascitic or abdominal fluid may be obtained for composition analysis. Paracentesis may also be necessary to relieve dyspnea and/or urinary frequency caused by large amounts of accumulated fluid, which places pressure on the diaphragm and bladder, respectively.

OBJECTIVE

To introduce a needle or catheter into the peritoneum to remove accumulated fluid for laboratory studies and/or to decompress the abdomen.

SPECIAL EQUIPMENT

Sterile gauze pads
Povidone-iodine solution
Tape
Cotton swabs
Local anesthetic
2-ml. syringe and 25-gauge needle
Scalpel blade and handle
Normal saline solution for injection
Paracentesis needle and/or catheter

50-ml. syringe
Sterile collection container
Sterile drapes
Ringer's lactate solution
Sterile specimen container(s)
Sterile gloves
Foley catheterization tray (if needed)
Suture material
Suction source

METHOD

ACTION	RATIONALE
1. Have the patient void (or catheterize patient, if necessary) before procedure is begun.	1. This prevents bladder distention and possible nicking of bladder with needle.

ACTION	RATIONALE

2. Position the patient:
  A. Upright, on side of bed, supported; *or*
  B. Flat in bed.	

3. Prep area with povidone-iodine solution.	3. The procedure should be performed under sterile technique.
4. Provide local anesthetic for introduction at puncture site.	4. This eliminates some of the pain of large-bore needle introduction.

5. Assist with insertion of trocar.
  A. A needle trocar with obturator is introduced, with sterile precautions, through a stab incision in midline below the umbilicus.
  B. Obturator is removed.
	
	B. This allows introduction of drainage tube and removal of fluid.

6. Introduce solution and drain fluid.
  A. Inject small amount of saline.
  B. Apply small amount of suction.
  C. Drain blood or ascitic fluid through tube into sterile container by gravity.
  D. Obtain only as much fluid as necessary to decrease abdominal pressure or to obtain samples for lab studies.
  E. Lavage peritoneum with 1 liter of Ringer's lactate solution, in trauma.
	
	A. This maintains patency.
	
	D. Removal of 1 to 1.5 liters can cause hypotension and shock.
	
	E. This enables the color of the return to be determined for assessing intra-abdominal injury.

7. Reposition patient side-to-side (optional).	7. This helps to obtain extra fluid that may be accumulated in pockets on either side.
8. Monitor patient response during trocar removal.	
9. Apply sterile dressing to incision site.	

10. Send fluid for:
  A. Lab studies (WBC's, bile, intestinal or pancreatic juices, proteins, and cultures).
  B. RBC determination. Test for RBC's and blood is negative if newsprint can be read through solution.	

PRECAUTIONS

1. Remove fluid slowly to prevent hypovolemia and hypotension.
2. Catheterize the patient or have him void prior to procedure. If bladder is distended it may be punctured.

RELATED CARE

1. Monitor blood pressure, pulse, and respiratory status preparacentesis and frequently postparacentesis for indications of developing hypotension.
2. Observe the size of the trocar wound; if it is large, it may require suturing.
3. Assess incision site for bleeding several times during the first 30 minutes after paracentesis.
4. Measure abdominal girth to identify possible internal bleeding and/or further accumulation of ascitic fluid; do this at least once daily.

COMPLICATIONS

Hypotension   Protein depletion
Hemorrhage   Encephalopathy
Infection

REFERENCES

Bockus, Henry L. (ed.) Gastroenterology, 3rd ed. Philadelphia, W.B. Saunders, 1976, Vol. 4, pp. 15-16.

Brunner, Lillian S., and Suddarth, Doris S. (eds.): Lippincott Manual of Nursing Practice. Philadelphia, J. B. Lippincott, 1978.

Flint, Lewis M., Jr.: Intraperitoneal injuries. Heart Lung, 7(No. 2): 273-277, 1978.

STOMA/FISTULA MANAGEMENT

Carolyn A. Tamer, R.N., E.T.

OVERVIEW

Ostomy or fistula management has three aims: skin care, containment, and odor control. Because many variables are present in the acute care setting, a basic method of practice is described in handling each ostomy/fistula, and will usually be different from that taught to the patient for self-care.

The three major types of procedures — colostomy, ileostomy, and urostomy — require specific stoma care. The stoma is created by the part of the ileum or colon that is brought out to and made flush with or raised above the abdominal wall. The nature of the discharge depends upon the portion of the intestinal tract that is used to create the stoma.

Colostomies may involve a surgical opening of the colon through the abdominal wall. Placement may be made in the ascending, transverse, descending, or sigmoid colon. The stoma may be a temporary measure, involving loop or double-barreled procedures, or may be permanent. Care of the descending or sigmoid colostomy is contingent upon the expected discharge from the stoma. Under normal conditions only flatus is passed, and drainage will be absent for approximately 1 week postoperatively. A transverse colostomy is generally a loop ostomy or, less commonly, a double-barreled ostomy. The loop ostomy stoma is maintained postoperatively outside the abdomen for approximately 2 weeks by a stomal support consisting of either a rod or an X-shaped bridge (Figs. 117 and 118). Opening of the loop ostomy may be delayed for several days and, in that case, will only require a dressing. The double-barreled ostomy allows complete separation of the healthy bowel from diseased or injured portions. Occurrence of fecal discharge is unpredictable and may be liquid to soft in nature, depending upon oral intake.

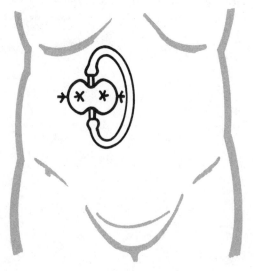

Figure 117. Transverse colostomy with rod and tubing.

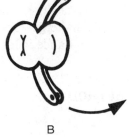

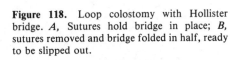

Figure 118. Loop colostomy with Hollister bridge. *A,* Sutures hold bridge in place; *B,* sutures removed and bridge folded in half, ready to be slipped out.

A   B

An ileostomy is usually a permanent procedure which discontinues use of the colon and rectum (which may be removed). The terminal ileum is everted and sutured, usually on the right side of the abdomen, to make a spout-type stoma. The discharge is liquid to paste-like and has a high enzyme content that is caustic to the peristomal skin.

Urostomies may involve ileal or colon loop procedures (ileal conduit, ileal bladder, and Bricker pouch) or cutaneous ureterostomies. These urinary diversions are generally permanent. They function immediately and require containment beginning in the operating room.

Fistulas or drain sites do not always have caustic drainage, but do often require frequent dressing changes. Drainage containment can be effectively and efficiently accomplished by application of a skin barrier and bag. In addition, the skin is protected, patient comfort is improved, and output can be measured.

Ostomy/fistula care is a clean procedure, not usually sterile. After cleansing the skin, a skin barrier should be applied for protection before placing the bag. Examples include Skin Prep Spray, Stomahesive, Colly-Seel, Crixilline, or karaya. The ostomy bag to be applied over the skin barrier should be drainable, adhesive-backed, transparent, and odorproof. Adhesive-backed bags are more reliable, will not shift, and may not require the use of an appliance belt.

OSTOMY/FISTULA CONTAINMENT _____

OBJECTIVES

1. To contain the discharge efficiently and effectively.
2. To permit observation of the stoma/fistula.

SPECIAL EQUIPMENT

Ostomy bag   Soap and water
Skin barrier   Face cloth and towel

Appliance deodorant
Bag closure, elastic or clamp
Nonallergic tape—2''
Appliance belt (if needed)

Protective bed pad
Clean gauze pads
Straight drainage collection set

METHOD

ACTION	RATIONALE

Colostomy/Ileostomy/Urostomy

1. Place protective bed pad under
   patient.
2. Prepare skin.
   A. Wash peristomal skin gently
       with mild soap and warm
       water.
   B. Rinse thoroughly and pat dry.
   C. At this point, if bagging a
       urostomy, apply gauze pads as
       wick.
3. Measure stoma diameter.
4. Select and prepare most appropriate
   skin barrier.
   A. Cut hole in wafer, washer, or
       gasket to fit stoma.
   B. Cut separate holes in a large
       piece of skin barrier (and
       ostomy bag) if there is 2 to

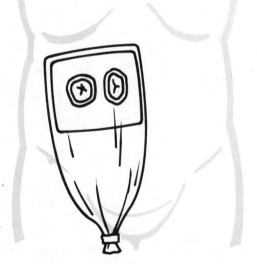

Figure 119. Double-Barreled Colostomy stomas, both
stomas covered by pouch.

ACTION	RATIONALE

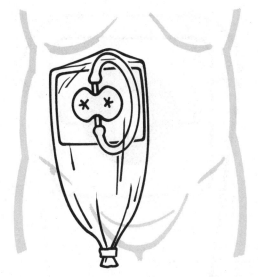

Figure 120. Ease the pouch over rod and tubing, being careful to have opening cut to fit closely over stoma.

8 cm. of skin between double-barreled colostomy stomas.

   C. Then, using a spray, apply twice, allowing to dry between applications (Fig. 119).

5. Stretch karaya ring (if used) enough to hug base of stoma securely; moisten one side, allow to become tacky, and then apply around stoma.

5. These substances adhere best in moist areas and protect the skin while permitting healing.

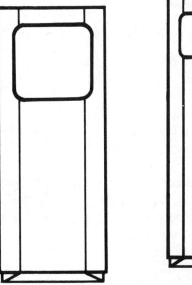

Figure 121. Postoperative appliances. *A,* Extra width and length; *B,* extra length average width; *C,* fistula drain.

A   B   C

ACTION   **RATIONALE**

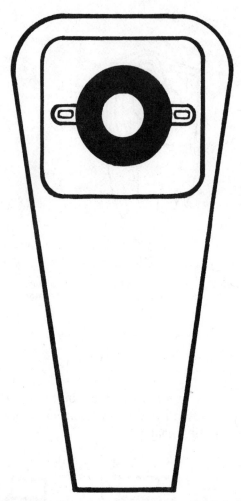

Figure 122.   Example of presized, open-ended drainable pouch. Must be ordered according to size of stoma.

    A.   Apply ring under double-barreled colostomy stomas with rod stomal support. Both stomas and rod support are covered by pouch (Fig. 120).

    B.   Apply over an X-shaped stomal bridge.

6. Draw stoma size onto adhesive backing of ostomy bag, and cut out an opening approximately 1/8'' to 1/4'' larger than karaya ring (Fig. 121). Choose bag with precut hole, if available (Fig. 122).

7. Remove protective backing of adhesive portion of ostomy bag, cut

6. This provides leeway for skin barrier to melt away without exposing adhesive backing of the bag.

ACTION   **RATIONALE**

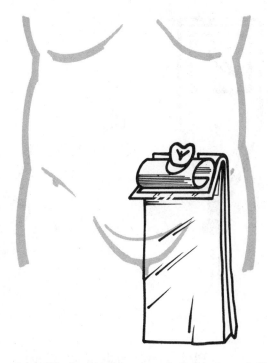

Figure 123. Applying large piece of adhesive. Lower half is already adhering; upper half is ready for removal of paper backing.

into half- or quarter-sections, and
replace (Fig. 123).
8. Apply bag.

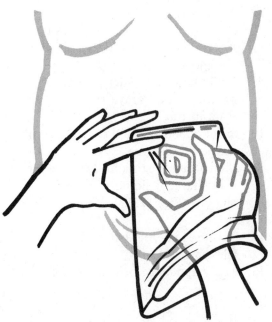

Figure 124. Sealing adhesive around stoma.

ACTION   **RATIONALE**

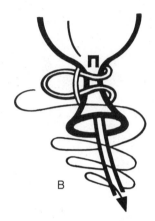

A   B

Figure 125. Attaching drainage bag to constant drainage when dealing with large quantity of liquid. *A,* Pouch attached to constant drainage tube; *B,* method for attaching tube using a rubber band around junction of pouch and tube—pull rubber band tightly, securing it with a small piece of tape.

A. Place hand inside ostomy bag and apply sideways over skin barrier.	A. Sideways application permits increased ease of drainage and emptying.
B. Remove protective backing in half- or quarter-sections, starting with bottom side, and secure each section to skin barrier (Fig. 124).	B. This permits seal-tight adherence and prevents leakage.
C. Hold clean gauze pads in hand over stoma, if discharge is liquid in nature.	
9. Apply karaya powder around edge of stoma and karaya ring, and to seam in ring.	9. This helps to protect exposed skin and may strengthen weak areas in karaya seal.
10. Instill deodorant and close bag with elastic or clamp.	
11. Attach bag to straight drainage set, if discharge is liquid in large amount (Fig. 125).	11. This allows accurate output measurement, eliminates the need for frequent emptying, and lessens the chance of bag leaking from overfill.
12. Picture-frame the bag with non-allergic tape.	12. This provides additional support.
13. Apply appliance belt, if needed.	13. This may add an increased sense of patient security and aid in maintaining the seal.

PRECAUTIONS

1. Observe for deviations of stoma color from characteristic dark pink to red.
    A.   Blanching or lightening of color may indicate interference with circulation.
    B.   A dark red to purple color may indicate damage to the stoma's blood supply.
2. Observe for stomal edema as well as for bleeding from the peristomal area or the stoma.
3. Use a bag that can be emptied, cleaned, resealed, and left in place for several days. Repeated removal of appliances increases the risk of skin irritation or damage.
4. Exercise care when removing an appliance from a suture line. Avoid pulling the sutures and do not contaminate the incision with the bag contents.
5. Do not tape a leak from beneath the adhesive backing. Leaking discharge will be trapped, resulting in excoriation of the skin.
6. Assess for tension on the stoma due to edema, mesenteric pull, position of skin folds, or position of the patient. Extra tension on the stomal support could damage the bowel nerve or blood supply. The patient may have to sit in a reclining position to avoid placing tension on the stoma.
7. Never twist or turn a stomal support; this puts torsion on the bowel.
8. Insure that the appliance belt is applied correctly. It must remain even with the bag tabs. If it rides up or down the bag may cut the stoma or pull up from the skin, causing leakage. Tight belts may cause cutaneous or stomal pressure ulcers. If applied improperly, a belt can predispose a patient to a prolapsed stoma or parastomal hernia.
9. Press the bag adhesive gently but firmly to form a seal, and be especially careful that it has no wrinkles.
10. Do not allow mucus or drainage to get under the skin barrier, since this will prevent a good seal.

RELATED CARE

1. Use warm water or a mild solvent to permit easier removal of the appliance. Wash any solvent used from the skin to avoid irritation. Expose the skin to the air for several minutes before applying additional adhesive.
2. Measure intake and output accurately in case of potential electrolyte imbalances.
3. Use two or three appliances if there is a wide area of skin between stomas or fistulas. If the margins of skin between sites are narrow, apply one large bag over the openings (Fig. 126).
4. Attach the bag to a straight drainage collection set at night to avoid having to wake the patient.

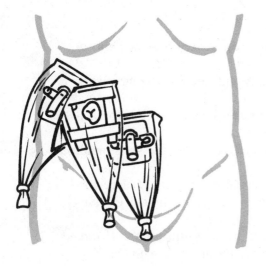

Figure 126. Ileostomy appliance flanked by two fistulas that have drains and pouches. This prevents excoriation by containing the fistula drainage.

5. Use a template as a pattern for cutting the adhesive-backed opening in the bag.
6. Change the bag every 1 to 2 days if no skin protection is used, or every 4 to 5 days if a skin barrier is used and/or whenever leakage is noted.
7. Apply the appliance belt loosely enough so that two fingers can be easily inserted under it.
8. Apply an additional karaya ring around the stoma if the stoma recedes into the skin folds when the patient stands or sits.

COMPLICATIONS

Edema   Parastomal hernia
Lacerations   Excoriated skin
Pressure ulcers   Infection
Prolapsed stoma

FISTULA/DRAIN SITE CARE

OBJECTIVES

1. To cleanse the skin surface surrounding the fistula/drain.
2. To prevent skin irritation, excoriation, and infection from drainage material.
3. To measure drainage output accurately.

SPECIAL EQUIPMENT

See equipment for "Ostomy/Fistula Containment"

Sterile gauze pads
Sump tube
Optional:
    Thoracic catheter
    15-gauge needle
    Gastric suction pump

METHOD

ACTION	RATIONALE
1. Place protective pad under patient.	
2. Wash peristomal skin gently with mild soap and warm water; rinse thoroughly and pat dry.	
3. Apply Skin Prep Spray or Skin Prep Wipe and a sterile dressing to a site when drainage is less than 200 ml./ day.	3. Skin Prep is an excellent skin barrier that can be applied under dressings to prevent irritation, when bagging is not necessary.
4. Apply adhesive-backed bag and a skin barrier, if drainage is greater than 200 ml./day (see method for "Ostomy/Fistula Containment").	4. This provides accurate output, protects the skin, and eliminates dressing changes.
5. Attach bag to constant drainage if fistula or drain site drains over 800 ml./day.	5. The bag is less likely to fall off or leak from weight and permits measuring the output.
6. Attach bag.	
A. Attach bag to sump suction (e.g., Shirley or Salem) if fit is precarious and if bagging around an existing tube; or	A. Suction improves fluid flow away from the fistula/drain and reduces reflux while the air vent in the sump tube reduces the force being exerted on the site, allows an elastic closure to be put around the existing tube or bottom of the bag while the suction tube picks up the drainage, and eliminates the need to empty the bag frequently.
B. Attach drainage bag to suction system using a 28 Fr. thoracic catheter with a 15-gauge needle, inserted as an air vent, if drainage is too thick for sump tube.	B. The thoracic tube has a single large chamber that is less likely to become obstructed or require flushing.

PRECAUTIONS

Same as precautions for "Ostomy/Fistula Containment."

RELATED CARE

Same as related care for "Ostomy/Fistula Containment."

COMPLICATIONS

Same as complications for "Ostomy/Fistula Containment."

COLOSTOMY IRRIGATION

OVERVIEW

A sigmoid colostomy is generally the only ostomy to be irrigated regularly. It is generally ordered in the acute setting, to relieve constipation or to prepare the patient for radiologic studies or surgery. If the patient in the acute care setting has not been regulated previously with this technique, the nurse may have to assume the responsibility for providing this care.

OBJECTIVES

1. To empty the colon.
2. To cleanse the lower gastrointestinal tract.
3. To prevent intestinal obstruction.

SPECIAL EQUIPMENT

Colostomy irrigation set
Irrigation reservoir
1000 ml. tepid tap water
  or other ordered solution
Cone-tip or catheter
Irrigation sleeve
Belt
Bag closure or elastic
Lubricant
Bed pan or commode
Toilet paper

Protective bed pad

Equipment for colostomy care (see special equipment for "Ostomy/Fistula Containment").

METHOD

ACTION	RATIONALE
1. Fill irrigating reservoir with 1000 ml. tepid water or other solution prescribed.	1. Using too little solution does not stimulate a good evacuation.
2. Hang irrigating reservoir with solution 45 to 50 cm. (18 to 20 inches) above stoma.	
3. Remove existing bag from patient, if irrigation sleeve is provided.	
4. Attach irrigation sleeve snugly to patient with belt from set.	4. This helps to control odor and splashing.
5. Lubricate irrigating tip; allow some solution to flow through catheter.	
6. Instill irrigation fluid using cone tip method or catheter.	
A. Insert cone tip 1 to 2 cm. (½ to ¾ inch) into stoma and hold with firm, gentle pressure; *or*	A. The cone tip shape acts as a natural dam, holding the water in the colon until its removal.
B. Insert catheter gently about 10 to 15 cm. (4 to 6 inches); move it in and out slowly while allowing solution to flow.	B. This cleanses and clears the terminal end of the colon up to 15 cm. (6 inches). The slowly-flowing solution helps to relax the bowel and facilitates passage of the tube.
7. Allow long drainage sleeve to hang in bed pan or commode during evacuation, which may take up to 1 hour.	7. This prevents soiling of the patient or bed linen.
8. Remove sleeve, rinse, and dry for reuse (if reusable).	
9. Wash and dry skin; apply clean bag (see method for "Ostomy/Fistula Containment").	

PRECAUTIONS

1. If cramping occurs stop the flow of solution, and allow the patient to

rest before progressing. Painful cramps may be caused by too rapid flow or too much solution.

2. Do not finger-dilate any stoma. Dilation may cause tearing of mucosa and skin leading to infection, fibrosis, and stricture formation.
3. Be sure the belt fits snugly to prevent leakage.

RELATED CARE

1. Insert the catheter 10 to 15 cm. (4 to 6 inches) through a baby bottle nipple to develop a cone tip. Insert the tube into the stoma up to the nipple hub, and hold firmly against the stoma while running the fluid in.
2. If all fluid is not evacuated, insert catheter and siphon off the remainder.
3. Place the patient on a bed pan or commode if the distal limb of a loop, or double-barreled ostomy is to be irrigated, since the fluid will exit through the rectum.

COMPLICATIONS

Colon perforation   Retention of irrigation fluid
Lacerations

OSTOMY/FISTULA SKIN CARE

OBJECTIVES

1. To prevent peristomal tissue damage caused by stomal/fistula discharges.
2. To treat damaged peristomal tissue effectively and promote healing.

SPECIAL EQUIPMENT

Mild soap   Antacid
Warm water   Telfa gauze
Face cloth and towel   Karaya powder
Skin barrier

METHOD

ACTION	RATIONALE

Prevention of Leakage

1. Cleanse skin, using mild soap and warm water; rinse and pat dry thoroughly.
2. Apply skin barrier (e.g., Stomahesive or Skin Prep Spray) as preventative measure.
   A. Only when it leaks; *or*
   B. If using Stomahesive, by the seventh day; *or*
   C. If using a karaya substance (e.g., Colly-Seel), every 2 to 4 days.
4. Shave area before applying ostomy appliance, if body hair is present.

2. This provides protection between the skin and adhesive.

B. Change by the seventh day as a hygienic measure.
C. Karaya substances are water-soluble and do not always last as long as Stomahesive.

Treatment of Mild Irritation (skin not broken, only reddened)

1. Cleanse skin, using mild soap and warm water; rinse, and pat dry thoroughly.
2. Use skin barrier that ensures a good seal.
   A. Use Sween skin care cream daily prior to application of bag, instead of spray or water; *or*
   B. Use Skin Prep Spray or Wipes.
3. Keep an adequate supply of nonsterile sponges at hand to soak up drainage.

2. This prevents the skin from being disturbed for several days.

Treatment of Moderate Irritation (skin red with some broken areas)

1. Wash skin with mild soap and warm water; rinse thoroughly and expose to air for a few minutes.
2. Paint area with thin coat of decanted antacid. (Note: Do not shake the bottle.)
   A. Allow hydroxide suspension (e.g., Amphojel or Maalox) to settle in bottle.
   B. Pour off thin liquid on top.

2. This soothes the irritated skin and helps prevent the karaya powder from stinging.

ACTION	RATIONALE
C. Use pasty liquid on bottom.	
D. Fan painted area dry.	
3. Sprinkle karaya powder lightly over antacid, applying additional coats if it darkens as it soaks up moisture from weeping skin.	3. This dries the skin.
4. Spray lightly with Skin Prep Spray, let dry, spray again.	4. This provides a new surface on which to apply a clean bag.
5. Apply clean bag over Skin Prep Spray.	
6. Change daily, and repeat skin treatment until healed.	

Treatment of Severe Irritation (skin weeping, may have small ulcerated spots)

1. Follow steps 1 to 4 under method for "Treatment of Moderate Irritation." Step 4 may need to be repeated several times as skin continues to weep.	1. This allows the skin to become as dry as possible.
2. Use Skin Prep Spray when karaya no longer darkens.	
3. Cover ulcerated spots with small amount of karaya powder and tiny piece of Telfa gauze.	3. This helps to absorb the moisture.
4. If skin is severely injured perform treatment every 12 hours until condition improves, then every 24 hours.	
5. Omit steps 3 through 5 when condition sufficiently improves; use only Stomahesive.	

PRECAUTIONS

1. Avoid the use of normal saline solution, alcohol, or hydrogen peroxide as these agents can irritate and cause drying of the skin.
2. If the skin barrier or adhesive cannot be removed easily do not scrub the skin, as this can irritate the skin severely and provide a site for infection.
3. *Never* use benzoin or benzoin compounds on irritated skin to improve the adhesiveness of the bag. Benzoin compounds contain aloes that are

harmful to the skin and, since benzoin doesn't dry, it can cause continued damage.

4. Do not miss a treatment, since the skin can quickly become more irritated than previously if it is neglected.
5. Avoid using creams or ointments because they prevent the bag from adhering.

RELATED CARE

1. See related care for "Ostomy/Fistula Containment."
2. Treat for *Monilia* by spreading a very light coat of Mycostatin powder to the affected area with a fingertip daily until the skin clears. Then spray the area with Skin Prep, and apply the bag.

OSTOMY/FISTULA ODOR CONTROL

OBJECTIVE

To control odors caused by containment of stomal/fistula discharges.

SPECIAL EQUIPMENT

Air freshener
Appliance deodorant
Warm water

Mouthwash
Distilled vinegar

METHOD

ACTION	RATIONALE
1. Rinse open-ended bags with: A. Lukewarm water and mouthwash solution; *or* B. Distilled vinegar solution—60 ml. vinegar to 1 liter water.	1. This cleans and deodorizes the bags.
2. Use new bag, if necessary.	
3. Use room air freshener spray.	3. This reduces embarrassment.
4. Use an appliance deodorant after emptying and cleaning the bag.	4. This continuously deodorizes the bag contents during use.
5. Carefully wash and dry the skin between changes of the appliance. (See Ostomy/Fistula Containment.)	

ACTION	RATIONALE
6. Do not make holes in the bag.	6. This defeats the use and purpose of the bag.
7. Use a disposable bag.	7. This reduces all aspects of maintenance.

PRECAUTIONS:

1. Excessive rinsing and cleaning the bag can weaken the skin seal resulting in leakage.
2. Follow manufacturer's directions for use of appliance deodorants.

OBTAINING URINE SPECIMEN FOR CULTURE AND SENSITIVITY FROM ILEAL LOOP STOMA

OBJECTIVE

To obtain a sterile urine specimen for culture and sensitivity.

SPECIAL EQUIPMENT

Catheterization set
Protective bed pad
Culture container
Urostomy bag
Containment equipment (see equipment for "Ostomy/Fistula Containment")

METHOD

ACTION	RATIONALE
1. Place protective bed pad under patient.	
2. Remove urostomy bag.	
3. Don sterile gloves and cleanse stoma site with same solution and technique used for catheterizing a urinary meatus; drape accordingly.	
4. Put drainage end of catheter in culture container.	

ACTION	RATIONALE
5. Insert catheter tip gently into stoma 10 to 15 cm. (4 to 6 inches).	
6. Hold culture container lower than stoma.	6. This facilitates urine flow by gravity.
7. Have patient cough if no urine flows.	
8. Pinch catheter with fingers and remove from stoma.	
9. Release pinch, thus siphoning a few drops.	
10. Record on the patient's chart if there was a residual greater than 5 to 10 ml.	10. Higher residuals indicate poor function.
11. Indicate that specimen was obtained by catheter.	
12. Apply clean bag.	

PRECAUTIONS

Use caution when catheterizing the urostomy stoma so as not to injure the stoma site. Do not force the catheter.

RELATED CARE

See related care for "Ostomy/Fistula Containment."

COMPLICATIONS

Perforation
Injury to anastomosis leading to internal urine leak

SUPPLIERS

E. R. Squibb and Sons, Inc. (Stomahesive; Mycostatin powder)
Hollister, Inc. (Disposable pouches; skin gel; deodorizer and germicide)
Mason Laboratories (Colly-Seel)
Perma-Type Company, Inc. (Fresh Tabs deodorant)
Pettibone Labs, Inc. (Ostobon deodorant)
Sween Corporation (Sween cream; Hex-On spray)
United Surgical Corporation (Skin Prep Spray and Wipes; Bongort bags; Banish deodorant)

REFERENCES

Broadwell, Debra C., and Sorrells, Suzanne L.: Loop transverse colostomy. Am. J. Nurs., *78*:1029–1031, 1978.

Brunner, Lillian S., et al.: The Lippincott Manual of Nursing Practice. Philadelphia, J. B. Lippincott, 1978.

Mahoney, Joanne M.: Guide to Ostomy Nursing Care. Boston, Little, Brown and Company, 1976.

Mahoney, Joanne M.: What you should know about ostomies. Nurs. '78, *8*:74–84, May, 1978.

THE
HEMATOLOGIC
SYSTEM

BLOOD AND BLOOD COMPONENT
ADMINISTRATION

Ruth DeLoor, R.N., M.S.N. and
Mary Jo Schreiber, R.N., M.S.N.

OVERVIEW

Improved diagnostic techniques and increased knowledge of transfusion therapy have enabled specific blood components needed by the patient, such as platelets, clotting factors, plasma, and granulocytes, to be identified. With sophisticated equipment available for separating blood into its cellular and fluid parts, it is now possible to obtain these components in large quantities. An understanding of blood and blood component therapy, together with nursing responsibilities when transfusion therapy is prescribed, is important to the critical care nurse. The classification of blood and blood components for clinical use, a brief description, and some important uses are as follows.

Whole Blood

Whole blood may be either stored or fresh. In either case, it is drawn from a donor and collected in plastic bags (usually polyvinylchloride) containing citrate compounds to prevent coagulation (ACD—acid citrate dextrose [rarely used], or CPD—citrate-phospate-dextrose). If CPD-adenine (CPDA-1) is used, whole blood may be stored for 35 days after collection. Fresh whole blood is infused within 24 hours. Whole blood may be kept at 1° to 6° C. for up to 21 days after collection; when stored properly it contains all the normal constituents of fresh whole blood. Both fresh and stored blood must be typed and cross-matched before transfusing.

Stored Whole Blood (SWB). SWB is used to increase the oxygen-carrying capacity and circulating volume of the blood. The most common clinical indication for its use is the replacement of acute blood loss to avoid hypovolemic shock. Due to the increased complexity of blood component therapy and a limited supply of SWB, both indications should be present when SWB is ordered.

Fresh Whole Blood (FWB). The use of FWB is indicated for the infusion of platelets and clotting factors in addition to the indications for SWB if blood components are not available. Due to severe limitations in the availability of FWB, other blood component therapy is used more frequently.

Red Blood Cells (RBC's)

RBC's constitute the blood component remaining after most of the plasma is removed from whole blood. RBC's provide the same oxygen-carrying capacity as whole blood, but in smaller volume. Therefore, RBC's reduce the risk for circulatory overload. There are three general types of RBC's, and all require typing and cross-matching.

Packed Red Blood Cells. Packed RBC's are prepared by removal of supernatant plasma sedimentation from or centrifugation of whole blood; this results in a unit containing 250 to 300 ml., with a hematocrit of 70%. When RBC's are prepared from a single plastic bag they should be used within 24 hours. RBC's prepared in double plastic bags, using a closed system, are viable for as long a period as an original container of whole blood.

The use of packed RBC's is indicated to increase oxygen-carrying capacity, or for correction of anemia by transfusion. Increased use can allow effective production of other blood components through fractionization of plasma.

Fresh-Frozen Red Blood Cells. The technique of fresh-freezing RBC's prolongs the shelf life of RBC's and is used for storage of rare blood types, autotransfusion, patients who are a high risk for transfusion reactions, and immunodeficient patients.

The cells are frozen within 6 days of a phlebotomy and stored for long periods. Fresh-frozen RBC's must be deglycerolized (washed) before administration; they are essentially free of WBC's, plasma proteins, and irregular antibodies.

Leukocyte-Poor Red Blood Cells. Leukocyte-poor RBC's are prepared from whole blood by the removal of supernatant plasma, and the "buffy coat" of leukocytes, which results in 80 to 90 percent removal of total leukocytes. Leukocyte-poor RBC's are also called "buffy"-poor RBC's. Washed RBC's are also considered leukocyte-poor. Patients who have repeated transfusions, febrile reactions to transfusions, and demonstrable leukocyte antibodies are considered for leukocyte-poor RBC transfusion. Proper screening is required, due to the difficulty in preparation, as are typing and cross-matching.

Platelet Concentrate

Platelets should be type-compatible with the individual patient. Three methods of preparation produce: (1) single-donor platelets; (2) random pool platelets; and (3) a single-donor platelet pool. Single-donor platelets are prepared by centrifugation of fresh whole blood within 4 hours after collection and contain approximately 30 ml. of platelet concentrate, with an average number of 5×10^{10} platelets. Random pool platelets are prepared with platelet concentrates obtained from multiple donors (usually 4 or 8 units per bag) and pooled into a single unit. A single-donor platelet pool is obtained from a single donor by manual pheresis (2 to 4 units) or cell separation (4 to 8 units). Four to eight units are usually prescribed.

Platelets are used in cases of thrombocytopenia caused by lack of platelet production. The frequency of use depends upon the half-life of the transfused platelets, which can be 2 days or less. In transfusion reactions due to HL-A antigen formation, platelet survival may be only a few hours. When infusing multiple units of platelets, either single-donor or in a random pool, the risk of side effects such as chills, fever, and allergic reactions is increased. Hepatitis risk is the same as for whole blood. HL-A-matched platelets can be obtained if multiple transfusions and reactions are anticipated.

Fresh-Frozen Plasma (FFP)

Fresh-frozen plasma is obtained from whole blood containing albumin, globulins, coagulation factors, water, and electrolytes. The plasma is collected by plasmapheresis or separated from a unit of whole blood and frozen within 4 hours after initial donation. The exact amount of plasma is recorded on each unit bag; each unit contains approximately 200 ml. plasma. Fresh-frozen plasma is used primarily for plasma coagulation deficiencies and antibodies and must be used for infusion of viable factors V and VIII. Viability of the factors in fresh frozen plasma is 1 year. Plasma must be typed specifically for each patient; however, cross-matching and Rh compatibility testing are not necessary. Because fresh-frozen plasma requires 30 minutes to thaw, the Blood Bank must be notified early to facilitate preparation.

Factor VIII

Factor VIII (antihemophilic globulin) is a component of fresh plasma that has been processed and frozen to prevent denaturation. Preparations include:

Cryoprecipitate Antihemophilic Factor (Cryo). Cryo is prepared from FFP; traces of all plasma constituents are present and it contains factors VIII and I (fibrinogen). The exact amount of factor VIII varies in each unit. Multiple units are usually administered, with an average of 100 units per bag. Cryo may be stored frozen for 1 year. It is used in classical hemophilia or in von Willebrand's disease as prophylaxis against spontaneous hemorrhage and treatment of hemorrhage. Cryo must be typed specifically for the patient, and the risk of hepatitis is present.

Antihemophilic Factor (AHF)

AHF is prepared in dried form and contains an assayed amount of AHF. Indications for use are the same as for cryo but, because the amount of AHF is known precisely and it is easier to prepare, its use may be preferred. There is a risk of hepatitis.

Granulocyte Transfusion (WBC)

WBC's are obtained by plasmapheresis from an HL-A-compatible donor. With proper refrigeration WBC's may be stored for 24 hours without loss of effectiveness. WBC's are indicated for patients with decreased WBC count, usually secondary to radiation therapy or chemotherapy for malignancies.

25% Normal Serum Albumin

25% normal serum albumin is prepared from pooled human plasma and heat-treated at 60° C. for 10 hours to decrease hepatitis risk. It contains 25% protein, with approximately 96% albumin, 135 mEq. sodium, and small amounts of chloride and potassium. Indications for use include shock, burn therapy, and hypoproteinemia. Normal serum increases intravascular volume by increasing colloid osmotic pressure, and is therefore not indicated for the treatment of overall dehydration. It is available in 20-, 50-, and 100-ml. vials, and does not require typing and cross-matching.

Plasma Protein Fraction

Plasma protein fraction is prepared from pools of human plasma, and is heated at 60° C. for 10 hours to decrease the risk of hepatitis. Situations such as shock or burns, in which the patient needs replacement of the intravascular volume, are examples of cases indicating the use of plasma protein fraction. Each vial contains 250 to 500 ml., composed of approximately 5% protein, 83% albumin, 17% alpha and beta globulins, 110 mEq. sodium, 50 mEq. chloride, and a small amount of potassium.

Advances in procuring, processing, storing, and infusing blood and blood components are constantly being made. This overview is intended as a basis for encouraging continued learning and respect for the properties of human blood, and its safe handling and administration. One method is offered as a useful approach for blood and blood component administration, and technical details specific to each blood component are presented in Table 4.

Table 4.   BLOOD AND BLOOD COMPONENT ADMINISTRATION GUIDE

Blood Component	Action(s)	Administration Set	Infusion Rate	Select Instructions
Whole blood (WB)				
Stored WB	Increases blood volume and oxygen-carrying capacity of the blood.	Blood filter	2 to 4 hours	Gently but thoroughly mix WB by inverting bag several times to give a uniform suspension before administration. Infuse very slowly for first 15 minutes; observe patient for adverse reactions. Adjust infusion rate to infuse in 2 hours, unless patient's condition warrants slower infusion. Infusion should not take longer than 4 hours.
Fresh WB	Same as for stored WB; also provides platelets and clotting factors.	Component filter	2 to 4 hours	Same as for stored WB. If FWB is being used for viable platelets, use a component/platelet infusion administration set so that platelets will be adequately maintained and transfused.
Red Blood Cells (RBC's)				
Packed RBC's	Increases oxygen-carrying capacity of the blood.	Blood filter	2 to 4 hours	Same as WB, except *do not* mix. When RBC's are prepared from a single plastic bag, they must be transfused within 24 hours. RBC's prepared in double plastic bags using a closed system have the same dating period as an original container of whole blood.
Fresh-frozen RBC's	Same as for packed RBC's.	Blood filter	2 to 4 hours	Same as for packed RBC's.
Leukocyte-poor RBC's	Same as for packed RBC's.	Blood filter	2 to 4 hours	Same as for packed RBC's.
Platelet Concentrate	Increases platelet count; aids clot formation.	Component filter	Rapidly	Store at room temperature, and administer within 24 to 72 hours of preparation. Infuse concentrate rapidly, within 15 to 30 minutes. Check label on container, which specifies the number of units.
Fresh Frozen Plasma (FFP)	Raises clotting factor level.	Blood or component filter	Rapidly	Requires 30 minutes to thaw; notify Blood Bank early to facilitate preparation. This must be given within 6 hours of thawing.

Table continued on following page

Table 4. BLOOD AND BLOOD COMPONENT ADMINISTRATION GUIDE   (continued)

Blood Component	Action(s)	Administration Set	Infusion Rate	Select Instructions
Factor VIII				
Cryoprecipitate antihemophilic factor (cryo)	Raises factor VIII and XIII levels; prevents and controls bleeding in hemophilia A, hypofibrinogenemia.	Component filter	Rapidly	May not be refrozen. Administer rapidly, approximately 4 units (60 ml.) in 15 minutes.
Antihemophilic factor (AHF)	Same as for cryo.	Component filter	Rapidly	Refrigerate with diluent until used. Use within 60 minutes of preparation; administration should be completed 3 hours after mixing.
Granulocyte Transfusion (WBC)	Raises leukocyte level.	Platelet filter	2 to 6 hours (varies with each bag)	May be refrigerated for up to 24 hours without loss of effectiveness. Clear only with sodium chloride. Infuse over a 2- to 6-hour period; this depends upon the number of units in bag. Assess for infusion reaction; decrease infusion rate and call physician for orders. (Elevated temperature, rash, and chills are expected reactions.)
25% Normal Serum Albumin	Increases intravascular volume.	Special administration set with vial	Adjusted according to clinical response	Considered compatible with common IV solutions. Infuse carefully; adjust rate according to clinical response. This should be used cautiously in patients who are susceptible to volume overload. Due to the high osmotic power of this preparation, it can increase intravascular volume rapidly and result in congestive heart failure or pulmonary edema. Also, patients with trauma or postoperative wounds may increase their bleeding with the rise in intravascular pressure.
Plasma Protein Fraction	Increases intravascular volume and protein level.	Component filter	Adjusted according to clinical response	Compatible with most parenteral IV solutions. Infuse carefully, according to clinical response.

OBJECTIVES

1. To ensure preservation of blood and select blood components during transfusion therapy.
2. To provide safe transfusion therapy through select patient assessment and nursing interventions.

SPECIAL EQUIPMENT

Venipuncture equipment:
    Tourniquet
    18-gauge or 19-gauge needle or catheter
    Sterile gauze dressing
    Povidone-iodine swab applicators
    Povidone-iodine ointment
    Tape
250 ml. normal saline solution, isotonic, for IV administration
IV administration set, appropriate for blood or blood component being infused
Transfusion requisition
Blood or blood product
IV standard
Blood pressure cuff
Stethoscope
Thermometer

METHOD

ACTION	RATIONALE

1. Collect the specimen for cross-matching.
  A. Draw blood in tubes according to Blood Bank instructions.
  B. Label tubes carefully with:
    (1) Patient's full name.
    (2) Date.
    (3) Hospital identification number.
	B. An error in the proper labelling of the specimen or in the completion of the requisition form could result in the patient receiving the wrong blood or blood component unit.

2. Order prescribed blood or blood component.
  A. Validate for physician's order.
  B. Complete appropriate requisition form with such information as:	

ACTION	RATIONALE

(1) Patient's first and last name.

(2) Patient's identification number.

(3) Name of requesting physician.

(4) Blood or blood component to be administered.

(5) Amount of blood or blood component to be administered.

(6) Date and time of administration.

(7) Previous transfusion reaction history.

C. Facilitate specimen transport to Blood Bank with completed blood requisition.

3. Prepare patient.
   A. Obtain vital signs.   A. This provides baseline data.
   B. Position patient comfortably.
   C. Secure patent venous route for administration of blood or blood component.

(1) Use 18- or 19-gauge needle or intracatheter.

(1) This allows easy flow of blood and causes less destruction of RBC's.

(2) Use only isotonic saline solution IV before, during, and following administration of blood or blood components.

(2) Certain IV solutions, including 5% dextrose in water, contain no electrolytes and can cause hemolysis of the erythrocytes.

(3) Use sterile, pyrogen-free transfusion filter set with pore size of approximately 170 to 180 micrometers. (Special filters, with approximately a 20-micrometer pore size for microaggregates may be required for certain patients; this is specified on the transfusion label of the blood or blood component unit.)

(3) Blood, RBC's, platelets, granulocytes, fresh-frozen plasma, and cryoprecipitate administration require a filter to prevent fibrin clots and particulate debris from infusing. Pore size of the filter and surface area, arrangement of the filter, and drip chamber affect the infusion rate. Microaggregates can develop in stored blood; they have been im-

ACTION	RATIONALE
	plicated as a possible cause of shock lung. Patients who are massively transfused or who are undergoing cardiopulmonary bypass may warrant the use of special filters.
(4) Prime transfusion administration system; check system for absence of air.	(4) The entire filter should be completely covered and the ball should be free-floating to preserve blood components during the filtration process.
(5) Maintain slow infusion of isotonic saline solution IV.	(5) This secures a patent venous route.
4. Obtain blood or blood component.	
A. Match patient identification form to unit of blood or blood component supplied by Blood Bank personnel. Note that only one unit is issued at a time, unless handling more than one unit concurrently on the same patient.	A. Improper refrigeration increases the risk of complications; monitored Blood Bank unit refrigerators are used to store blood at a constant temperature.
B. Sign proper form for release of blood or blood component.	B. This certifies that information is accurate and blood is released for transfusion to the appropriate patient.
5. Check blood or blood component, verifying identification data. A. Check chart for physician's order. B. Inspect the blood or blood component unit for abnormal color or appearance. C. Check unit of blood or blood component, requisition form, and patient's identification band to match: (1) Patient's name. (2) Patient's identification number. (3) Unit number. (4) ABO and Rh type. (5) Expiration date.	5. The majority of hemolytic transfusion reactions (HTR's) are due to errors in giving the wrong blood or blood component to a patient.

ACTION	RATIONALE

    D. Ask patient to identify himself.

    E. Check all data at patient's bedside. Two staff members should check data together; one of these should be an R.N. or physician.

    F. Sign blood requisition form.

    G. Return blood or blood component to Blood Bank immediately if any discrepancy is noted.

6. Administer blood or blood component, as prescribed by physician:

    A. Read blood or blood component unit label for general and specific cautions and instructions.

          RATIONALE: A. This ensures safe administration; individualized cautions and instructions may be required.

    B. Assess clinical condition of patient.

          RATIONALE: B. This serves as baseline data.

    C. Attach blood or blood component unit to primed solution administration system, maintaining sterility of system.

    D. Infuse slowly for first 15 minutes, observing patient for adverse reactions.

    E. Adjust infusion rate based on clinical condition of patient and blood product being transfused (see Table 4).

    F. Assess patient closely for 15 minutes after transfusion begins, and thereafter as appropriate.

7. Discontinue blood or blood component after completion of transfusion.

    A. Flush line with sodium chloride solution IV.

    B. Resume parenteral infusion, as ordered, or discontinue IV.

8. Complete transfusion form.

          RATIONALE: 8. The transfusion record is a legal document, and copies must be retained in the chart and Blood Bank.

    A. Indicate presence or absence of suspected reaction.

    B. Return laboratory copy of transfusion record with blood

ACTION	RATIONALE

bag to Blood Bank.

C. File one copy of transfusion record in patient's medical record.

PRECAUTIONS

1. Use fresh blood; monitor for hyperkalemia with blood nearing the end of a 21-day expiration period.
2. Monitor serum calcium levels. Multiple blood transfusions offer potential risk for hypocalcemia, since citrate binds calcium. Calcium gluconate is often prescribed after every second or third unit of blood.
3. Warm blood to body temperature or use a blood warmer during massive transfusion therapy, or as instructed specifically on the blood unit label (see the method for "Blood Warming").
4. Do not add medication directly to the blood or blood component prior to or during a transfusion; if needed, it may be given separately. Medications in high concentrations or with a wide range in pH may in themselves cause hemolysis when injected into the blood tubing.
5. Do not allow the blood or blood components to stand longer than 30 minutes at room temperature prior to administration. The risk of complication increases with the length of time blood is out of the refrigerator.
6. Infuse blood and blood components in less than 4 hours because the longer the blood is left at room temperature the greater is the danger of bacteria proliferation and RBC hemolysis. If the blood must be infused for longer than 4 hours, many Blood Banks split the unit into two smaller units to be infused consecutively. If the unit is split the blood must be infused within 24 hours.

RELATED CARE

1. Monitor changes of vital signs taken periodically during blood and blood component administration, and for the effect of changes on the patient.
2. Monitor the infusion rate and the patient's response to therapy. As the filter becomes saturated with debris and microaggregates, the infusion rate is slowed.
3. Assess for symptoms and signs of early transfusion reactions. Monitor the patient closely during the first 15 minutes of 50 ml./per minute infusion. Hemolytic reactions can occur early in the transfusion; the reaction may be proportional to the amount of blood infused (see the method for "Transfusion Reaction").

4. Assess for oliguria, hemoglobinuria, shock, and jaundice as late transfusion reactions (see the method for "Transfusion Reaction").

5. Perform site care, as prescribed by physician (see method for "Invasive Site Care").

6. Change the blood administration set after every unit of blood is infused, or every 24 to 48 hours if the administration set is not used for blood or blood component administration.

COMPLICATIONS

Air emboli	Hemolytic transfusion reactions
Allergic reactions	Hyperkalemia
Alloimmunization	Hypocalcemia
Bacterial contamination	Hypothermia
Bleeding diathesis	Microemboli
Circulatory overload	Shock
Death	Viral hepatitis
Febrile nonhemolytic transfusion reactions	

REFERENCES

American Association of Blood Banks: The Technical Manual of the American Association of Blood Banks, 7th ed. Philadelphia, J. B. Lippincott, 1977.

American National Red Cross: Blood and Blood Components. American Red Cross, 1974, ARC 1751.

Becker, G.A.: Therapeutic use of blood components. In Conn, H.F. (ed.): Current Therapy. Philadelphia, W. B. Saunders, 1976.

Greenwalt, T.J. (ed.): General Principles of Blood Transfusions. Chicago, American Medical Association, 1973.

Grindon, A.J.: Therapeutic use of blood components. In Conn, H.F. (ed.): Current Therapy. Philadelphia, W. B. Saunders, 1975.

Guyton, Arthur C.: Textbook of Medical Physiology, 5th ed. Philadelphia, W. B. Saunders, 1976.

Tikian, S.M., and Conover, M.H.: Clinical Implications of Laboratory Tests. St. Louis, C. V. Mosby, 1975.

Wintrobe, M.M., Lee, G.R., Boggs, D.R., et al.: Clinical Hematology, 7th ed., Philadelphia, Lea and Febiger, 1974.

TRANSFUSION REACTION

Ruth DeLoor, R.N., M.S.N. and
Mary Jo Schreiber, R.N., M.S.N.

OBJECTIVES

1. To recognize and facilitate prompt nursing interventions should a transfusion reaction be suspected.
2. To enhance prompt determination of a potential transfusion reaction by providing specimens for analysis and maintaining collaboration with support services during which critical changes might occur.

SPECIAL EQUIPMENT

Transfusion reaction form
Thermometer
Blood pressure cuff
Stethoscope
IV administration set
Urine specimen container
Blood specimen containers (one each for clotted and anticoagulated blood samples)

METHOD

ACTION	RATIONALE
1. Monitor patient closely while first 50-ml. are being transfused. Assess patient for apprehension, headache, back pain, chills, fever, dyspnea, cyanosis, urticaria, hypotension, nausea/vomiting, or rash.	1. Hemolytic reactions can occur early in the transfusion.
2. Monitor for changes of vital signs taken periodically during transfusion administration, and effect of changes on patient.	
3. Assess for oliguria and jaundice posttransfusion therapy.	3. These are late signs.
4. Facilitate prompt nursing interventions.	
A. Stop blood immediately.	A. The transfusion reaction may be proportional to the amount of blood infused.

ACTION	RATIONALE
B. Maintain patent IV route using a slow infusion of normal saline solution IV.	B. This provides a route for further IV medications or fluids.
C. Notify physician immediately of potential transfusion reaction.	C. The physician will decide whether the symptomatology warrants a follow-through with the subsequent steps of this procedure. The physician should specify if the IV is to be left in place and what fluids are to be infused.
D. Notify Blood Bank immediately of potential transfusion reaction.	D. The blood bank will outline the lab tests necessary for evaluating and defining the reaction.
E. Take the following to Blood Bank. (1) Partially used blood container and IV administration set. (2) Posttransfusion clotted and anticoagulated blood specimen. (3) Posttransfusion urine sample. (4) Completed copies of transfusion and transfusion reaction records.	E. Grouping, typing, and crossmatching procedures using both pre- and posttransfusion specimens of the recipient's blood will be repeated. A direct Coombs' test on the recipient's blood will be performed immediately and may be repeated in 24 hours. Bilirubin studies are also usually done. A gram stain and culture are done on the blood container and tubing.
F. Perform clinical check of labels for potential errors.	F. This ensures that the correct blood unit has been given to the correct patient.
G. Start the patient on 24-hour urine collection.	G. Urine is collected for the determination of heme pigments, granular casts, and presence or absence of RBC's.
H. Monitor patient's vital signs immediately and every 15 minutes, or as often as indicated by severity of reaction.	H. The patient presents a potential risk for hypotension and shock.
I. Assess for oliguria or anuria, using continuous intake and output.	I. Hemoglobin may precipitate in kidney tubules and offer high risk for renal failure.

PRECAUTIONS

1. Clarify acceptable parameters with the physician regarding reaction

symptomatology. If a transfusion reaction is anticipated, such as in a leukemia patient, prophylactic antihistamines or antipyretics may be given prior to administration, or as needed with the occurrence of symptoms, as prescribed by the physician.

2. Administer oxygen, epinephrine, and sedation therapy, as prescribed by the physician for hemolytic transfusion reaction.
3. Monitor for circulatory overload, especially in patients with a medical history of cardiac dysfunction or anemia.
4. Monitor for bacterial transfusion reactions and/or allergic reactions.

RELATED CARE

1. Maintain accurate documentation regarding blood or blood component administration, amount infused, and sequence of symptomatology for ongoing clinical investigation.
2. Monitor for delayed hemolytic transfusion reactions.
3. Note that transfusion reactions must be reported to the Bureau of Biologics of the Food and Drug Administration.

COMPLICATIONS

Hypotension	Alloimmunization
Delayed hemolytic reaction	Allergic reaction
Shock	Sepsis
Viral hepatitis	Respiratory arrest
Renal dysfunction	Cardiac arrest

REFERENCES

American Association of Blood Banks: The Technical Manual of the American Association of Blood Banks, 7th ed. Philadelphia, J. B. Lippincott, 1977.

Greenwalt, T.J. (ed.): General Principles of Blood Transfusion. Chicago, American Medical Association, 1973.

Grindon, A.J.: Therapeutic use of blood components. *In* Conn, H.F. (ed.): Current Therapy. Philadelphia, W. B. Saunders, 1975.

Wintrobe, M.M., Lee, G.R., Boggs, D.R., et al.: Clinical Hematology, 7th ed., Philadelphia, Lea & Febiger, 1974.

AUTOTRANSFUSION

Ruth DeLoor, R.N., M.S.N. and
Mary Jo Schreiber, R.N., M.S.N.

OVERVIEW

Autotransfusion is used to reduce the risk of transfusion reactions, delayed hemolysis, and isoimmunization. It is often indicated for cases involving high frequency antigen states, rare cell types, or difficult cross-matching due to multiple antibodies.

OBJECTIVE

To remove, preserve, and transfuse blood or blood components from/to the original donor as a prescribed therapy for select patients.

SPECIAL EQUIPMENT

Sterile blood recovery system, with suction device
Filters, with pore size 170 micrometers
Sterile collecting container with anticlotting agent
Blood administration set

METHOD

ACTION	RATIONALE
1. Determine appropriate method for autotransfusion. A. Follow select protocols by Blood Bank and as prescribed by physician. These include: (1) Phlebotomy with anti-coagulating agent in vacuum container. (2) Modified blood recovery system during surgery or postoperative with mediastinal drainage after open heart procedures. B. Ensure that blood is collected with sterile system in less than a 4-hour period.	B. This reduces the potential for bacterial growth.

370

ACTION	RATIONALE
2. Facilitate transport of blood or blood components for storage/freezing, as prescribed by physician.	2. Storage of blood in the liquid state is utilized on a short-term basis. If a large volume of blood is needed, red cells are preserved by freezing for long-term storage.
3. Administer patient's reclaimed blood or blood components as prescribed (see the method for "Blood and Blood Component Administration").	
4. Assess patient's hemodynamic status closely before, during, and after autotransfusion.	

PRECAUTIONS

1. See precautions for "Therapeutic Phlebotomy," "Blood and Blood Component Administration," and "Transfusion Reaction."
2. Monitor closely for prevention of air emboli and microemboli; use filters as prescribed.
3. Do not transfuse blood that has been collected over a period longer than 4 hours.

RELATED CARE

1. Check that the informed consent of the patient has been obtained and check for the physician's order when autotransfusion involves blood collection.
2. See related care for "Therapeutic Phlebotomy," "Blood and Blood Component Administration," and "Transfusion Reaction."

COMPLICATIONS

Potassium intoxication   Emboli
Sepsis   Circulatory overload
Vascular trauma

REFERENCES

American Association of Blood Banks: The Technical Manual of the American Association of Blood Banks, 7th ed. Philadelphia, J. B. Lippincott, 1977.
Autotransfusion. Assoc. Operating Room Nurses, 24(No. 6):12, 1976.

Grindon, A.J.: Therapeutic use of blood components. *In* Conn, H.F. (ed.): Current Therapy. Philadelphia, W. B. Saunders, 1975.

Guyton, A.C.: Textbook of Medical Physiology, 5th ed. Philadelphia, W. B. Saunders, 1976.

Wintrobe, M.M., Lee, F.R., Boggs, D.R., et al.: Clinical Hematology, 7th ed. Philadelphia, Lea & Febiger, 1974.

BLOOD WARMING

Ruth DeLoor, R.N., M.S.N. and
Mary Jo Schreiber, R.N., M.S.N.

OVERVIEW

Blood warming is used in such unusual circumstances as massive transfusions, rates above 50 ml./min., more than two units of blood given consecutively, exchange transfusions of the newborn, patients with potent cold agglutinins, or patients whose body temperature is 35 to 38°C (95 to 100°F).

OBJECTIVE

To administer blood safely by a blood warming technique.

SPECIAL EQUIPMENT

Blood warming coil   Blood
Water bath   Blood administration set
Water bath thermometer   Normal saline solution, IV

METHOD

ACTION	RATIONALE
1. Prime blood warming coil after blood unit and administration set have been attached; close distal clamp.	
2. Submerge blood coil into a 37° C. (99° F.) water bath (Fig. 127).	2. This procedure applies to a blood warming coil using heated water; devices are also available for controlled water baths or dry heat warmers. Note that dry heat warmers, microwaves, and radiowaves may cause gross hemolysis; their use requires close temperature monitoring and quality control measures.

3. Perform blood transfusion as usual.
  A. Obtain patient's temperature prior to blood transfusion.
  B. Assess patient's status continuously.	

ACTION	RATIONALE
4. Monitor water bath temperature range; maintain between 35 and 38° C (95 and 100°F).	4. Hemolysis may occur if blood is subjected to temperatures greater than 40° C (104°F).
5. Flush blood coil thoroughly with normal saline posttransfusion. The coil holds approximately 50 ml. of blood.	

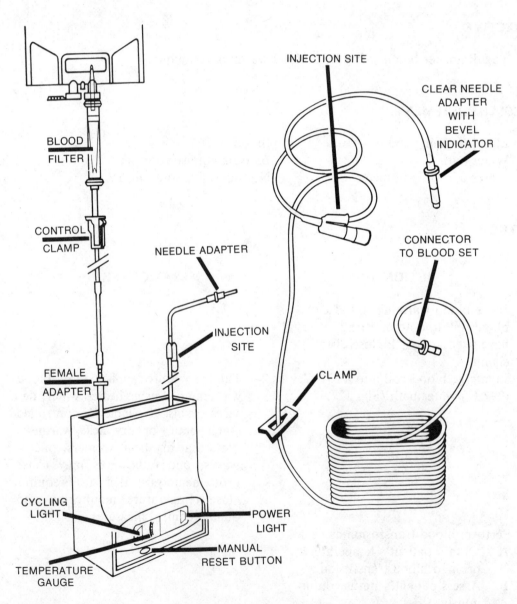

Figure 127.   Water bath and blood-warming coil. Courtesy of McGaw Laboratories, Irvine, Cal.

PRECAUTIONS

1. Ascertain that the warming device has undergone a preventive maintenance check within the institution.
2. Do not submerge Y adapter when immersing blood coil into water bath.

RELATED CARE

1. See related care for "Blood and Blood Component Administration."
2. Maintain records appropriately, indicating use of blood warming therapy, temperature of water bath, and patient's temperature.
3. Follow additional protocols as recommended by the manufacturer for the specific blood warming device used.

COMPLICATIONS

Activation of cold agglutinins   Sepsis
Hemolysis   Equipment malfunction
Microshock

REFERENCES

Grindon, A.J.: Therapeutic use of blood components. *In* Conn, H.F., (ed.): Current Therapy. Philadelphia, W. B. Saunders, 1975.

St. Joseph's Hospital: Critical-Care Procedure Manual. Milwaukee, St. Joseph's Hospital, 1979.

USE OF A BLOOD PUMP

Ruth DeLoor, R.N., M.S.N. and
Mary Jo Schreiber, R.N., M.S.N.

OBJECTIVE

To infuse whole blood or packed RBC's rapidly when blood volume and oxygen-carrying capacity need to be increased immediately.

SPECIAL EQUIPMENT

Blood pump
Blood and blood administration set

METHOD

ACTION	RATIONALE
1. Prepare blood for administration (see the method for "Blood and Blood Component Administration").	
2. Invert and insert a plastic, non-vented blood or solution container, with recipient set attached, through lower opening of mesh panel on blood pump apparatus.	
3. Check security of connections and complete insertion of total solution container into blood pump apparatus; suspend infuser by fabric strap.	
4. Inflate to desired pressure on gauge for pressure infusion; do not exceed 300 mm. Hg.	4. Over inflation may damage infuser.
5. Adjust infusion rate by recipient set clamp.	
6. Maintain pressure infusion by squeezing bulb pump as blood is infused.	
7. Remove empty blood container by opening air valve to deflate infuser rapidly.	

PRECAUTIONS

1. Check for blood bag rupture due to instrumentation.
2. Check for blood contamination due to leak in system.
3. Determine if air is trapped in the system. This could result from pumping blood when there is air in the bag. To prevent this, the pump should be deflated before the bag is completely empty.

RELATED CARE

1. Monitor patient's status and effect of rapid transfusion continuously.
2. Check accuracy of the blood pump. Failure of the needle gauge to return to zero may indicate that the accuracy of the gauge has been impaired. Accuracy of the gauge may diminish with extensive use or age.
3. See related care for "Blood and Blood Component Administration."

COMPLICATIONS

Air embolism   Infiltration
Volume overload

REFERENCES

Grindon, A.J.: Therapeutic use of blood components. *In* Conn, H.F. (ed.): Current Therapy. Philadelphia, W. B. Saunders, 1975.
St. Joseph's Hospital: Critical-Care Procedure Manual. Milwaukee, St. Joseph's Hospital, 1979.

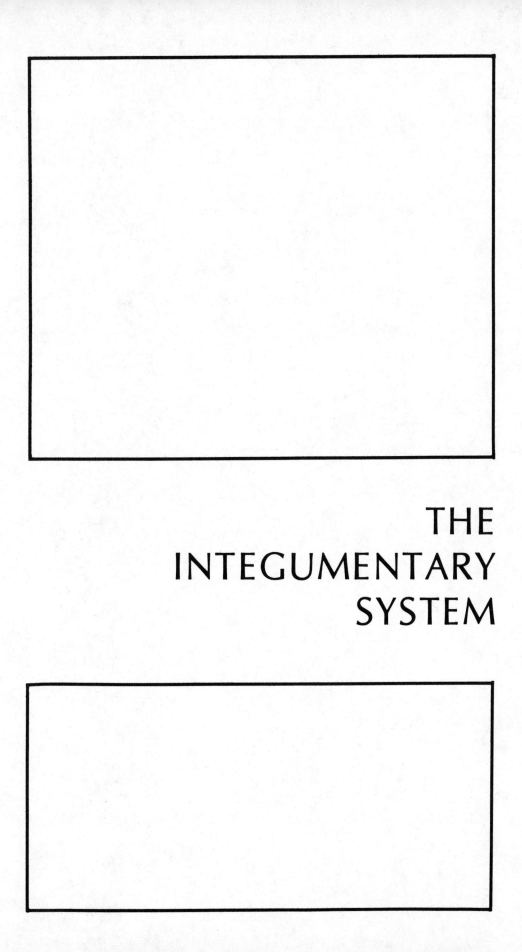

THE
INTEGUMENTARY
SYSTEM

WOUND MANAGEMENT: CLEAN WOUNDS

Sandra J. Pfaff, R.N., B.S.N.

OVERVIEW

Wound healing is a three-phase process of re-establishing the continuity of cellular and anatomic structures, and may be characterized as follows:

I inflammatory phase: Leaking of circulating blood substances into wound; migration of polymorphonuclear neutrophil leukocytes, lymphocytes, macrophages, and antibodies into wound; bacterial proliferation in wound.

II proliferative phase: Development of granulation tissue; migration and proliferation of epithelial and endothelial cells.

III remodeling phase: Cell production and death; collagen production and absorption; capillary formation and obliteration; filling in by fat cells.

Factors which affect wound healing may be classified as intrinsic (host) and extrinsic (iatrogenic). Intrinsic factors may include nutritional status, shock, acidosis, hepatic or renal failure, remote infection, and bacterial flora. Extrinsic factors may include surgical technique, devitalized tissue, hematoma, seroma, dehiscence, steroid therapy, chemotherapy, and irradiation.

Nursing responsibilities extend beyond the wound and dressing, encompassing all the intrinsic and extrinsic factors affecting wound healing. Cognizance of these factors, early recognition of alterations in the patient's condition, and prompt intervention are vital for wound healing.

OBJECTIVES

1. To promote wound healing through nursing management of factors which affect wound healing.
2. To reduce the risk of delayed wound infection through aseptic wound cleansing and dressing changes.
3. To assess the condition of the wound, and intervene appropriately when alterations or problems occur.

SPECIAL EQUIPMENT

Mineral or baby oil	Gloves
Acetone	Plastic bag
3% hydrogen peroxide solution	Sterile gauze pads
Sterile normal saline solution	Tape
Tincture of benzoin	Cotton swabs

METHOD

ACTION	RATIONALE
1. Loosen tape with mineral or baby oil if extremely adherent to skin.	1. This decreases trauma to skin and pain.
2. Remove tape by pulling it straight away from skin and toward wound.	2. This decreases pain and injury to new tissue and substrata.
3. Don clean glove over dominant hand.	
4. Remove dressing slowly, pulling gently from side to side.	4. This prevents injury to new tissue and substrata.
5. Discard dressing and glove in plastic bag.	
6. Remove tape residue with acetone, as needed.	6. This helps to prevent skin breakdown.

7. Assess and record:
  A. Wound condition (note erythema, bruising, pain, swelling).
  B. Drainage (note color, odor, consistency, amount).
  C. Skin condition (note erythema, pain, blistering, turgor).	

8. Cleanse the wound.
  A. Dry wounds:
    (1) Cleanse wound and surrounding skin with mild soap and warm water, using gentle circular motion.
	(1) This cleanses and stimulates circulation.

(2) Rinse and dry.
    (3) Assess wound and skin condition.
  B. Draining wounds:
    (1) Don sterile glove on dominant hand.
    (2) Cleanse wound.
	(2) This loosens and removes organic debris.

(a) Use sterile gauze pad saturated with hydrogen peroxide solution.
      (b) Start at incision and work outward.
    (3) Cleanse deep narrow areas and suture sites with cotton swabs saturated with	

ACTION	RATIONALE

hydrogen peroxide
solution.

(4) Rinse with saline-soaked
sterile gauze pad; dry with
sterile gauze pad.

(5) Assess and record wound
and skin condition, and
drainage; differentiate between hard and fluctuant
swelling.

9. Dress the wound.

   A. Don sterile glove on dominant
   hand, or hold sterile forcep in
   dominant hand.

   B. Apply dressings, touching them
   only with glove or forcep.
   Avoid dragging dressing across
   skin to wound.

   C. Apply tincture of benzoin to
   skin around dressing, as needed.

   C. This toughens and protects
   damaged or fragile skin and pro-
   motes tape adherence.

PRECAUTIONS

1. Use solutions in unit dose or small capacity containers supplied to each
individual patient.
2. Never use cotton balls, since loose fibers can act as foreign bodies.
3. Use unpowdered gloves, since powder particles can act as foreign bodies.

RELATED CARE

1. Integrate the following concepts into clean wound care.
   A. Dressings are used to support, immobilize, protect from trauma
   and contamination, absorb drainage, promote granulation and
   debridement, and provide an esthetic appearance. After the first
   24 to 48 hours, dressings should be used only for esthetic
   reasons and/or protection from trauma.
   B. Wet dressings enhance wicking of organisms; therefore, dry dressings are preferred.
   C. The choice of dressing supplies and the size of the dressing are
   based on wound size, drainage, and protection needs. They must
   be secure enough to immobilize but loose enough to promote air
   circulation. Tape should be selected according to skin condition,
   allergies, frequency of dressing changes, and anticipated length of
   time dressings will be needed.

D. Wound cleansing and dressing changes should occur when particulate matter in the air is at a low level, before or well after cleaning (i.e., housekeeping) activities, and with a limited number of persons present.

E. Removal of rings and watches and careful hand washing prior to any procedure are esssential.

2. Monitor nutrition and hydration.

3. Perform dressing changes of other wounds (surgical, decubitus, intravascular or intra-arterial puncture sites, tracheostomy) as separate procedures, using separate supplies.

COMPLICATIONS

Wound infection
Wound dehiscence

REFERENCES

American College of Surgeons: Manual on Control of Infection in Surgical Patients. Philadelphia, J. B. Lippincott, 1976.

Castle, M.: Wound care—clear-cut ways to speed healing. Nurs. '75, 5(No. 8):40, 1975.

Schilling, J.A.: Wound healing. Surg. Clin. North Am., 56(No. 4):859, 1976.

WOUND MANAGEMENT: CONTAMINATED WOUNDS

Sandra J. Pfaff, R.N., B.S.N.

OVERVIEW

All wounds, both clean and contaminated, are colonized by the patient's endogenous resident dermal and transient epidermal flora. The terms "clean-contaminated" or "contaminated" apply when organisms other than endogenous skin flora are likely to be present—e.g., in cases involving surgery of the gastrointestinal, pulmonary, or reproductive tracts, presence of drains, open or traumatic wounds, or colonization by exogenous organisms. The risk and incidence of infection and dehiscence in contaminated wounds exceeds that of clean wounds.

The terms "pathogenic" and "nonpathogenic" are misleading: *any* organism present in numbers greater than 10^5 is a potential cause of infection. Prevention depends upon controlling both the numbers of organisms which reach the wound and factors which enhance microbial growth. Infected wounds are much more likely to dehisce than are noninfected wounds.

Direct transmission by the hands of personnel is the primary source of cross-contamination. Hand washing is the single most important aspect of prevention. Adjuncts to control of cross-contamination are proper patient placement, and proper handling and disposal of contaminated fomites.

Methods for the management of wounds with drains, open wounds, wound irrigation, and wound cultures are presented. Because the objectives, precautions, related care, and complications are similar for all four methods they will be presented only once, identified as "general."

OBJECTIVES: General

1. To promote wound healing and reduce the risk of infection through nursing management of the contaminated wound.
2. To contain and manage infected and noninfected wound drainage, thereby reducing the risk of cross-contamination.
3. To intervene promptly and appropriately when infection is suspected.

SPECIAL EQUIPMENT: General

Tape
Sterile gauze pads

DRESSING WOUNDS WITH DRAINS

SPECIAL EQUIPMENT

Drainage bags
Karaya blanket
Montgomery straps
3% hydrogen peroxide solution
Sterile normal saline solution and/or iodophor solution
Mask (if wound is infected)
Sterile safety pin
ABD pads

METHOD

ACTION	RATIONALE
1. Remove soiled dressing (see method for "Clean Wounds"), and replace Montgomery straps, as needed. Avoid dislodging drains, drainage bags, or drainage suction tubing.	
2. Replace crusted or rusty safety pin in Penrose drains.	
3. Cleanse wound and drain site. A. Use separate, hydrogen peroxide-soaked, sterile gauze pads, and cotton swabs. B. Follow with normal saline and/or iodophor cleansing.	3. This reduces the risk of cross-contamination and removal of organic debris stimulates circulation.
4. Change sterile gloves.	
5. Apply slit gauze around drain, or apply or replace drainage bag (based upon amount of drainage and skin condition). Ensure that hole in karaya blanket and/or adhesive backing of drainage bag is large enough to prevent occlusion of drain but small enough to expose a minimum of skin to drainage.	5. This draws drainage away from skin.
6. Apply sterile gauze pads separately to incision and drain site.	6. This wicks drainage up into ABD pads.
7. Apply ABD pad over both sites; or overlap two or more ABD's to cover both sites. Apply so that air can circulate (Fig. 128).	
8. Secure dressing with tape or Montgomery straps.	

ACTION   RATIONALE

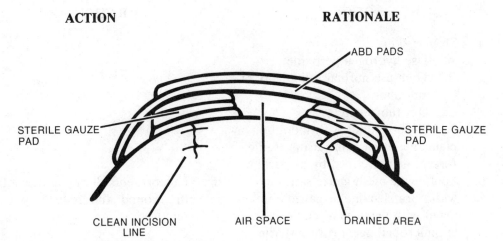

ABD PADS

STERILE GAUZE
PAD

STERILE GAUZE
PAD

CLEAN INCISION   AIR SPACE   DRAINED AREA
LINE

Figure 128. Clearcut ways to speed healing. (Reprinted with permission from *Nursing 75* © 1975, Intermed Communications, Inc., Horsham, PA. 19044.)

9. Assess and record:
    A. Wound, drain site and skin
        condition.
    B. Amount and characteristics of
        drainage.

DRESSING OPEN WOUNDS

SPECIAL EQUIPMENT

Wide mesh gauze (plain or impregnated)
Iodophor or plain fine mesh gauze packing
Sterile forceps or gloves
3% hydrogen peroxide solution
Sterile normal saline solution
Petroleum jelly
Antimicrobial cream

METHOD

ACTION	RATIONALE
1. Remove soiled dressing slowly, pulling gently from side to side.	1. This provides gentle debridement.
2. Remove soiled packing slowly with sterile forcep.	2. This provides gentle debridement.
3. Irrigate wound gently with hydrogen peroxide, followed by sterile normal saline.	3. This removes organic debris.

ACTION	RATIONALE

4. Cleanse skin.
   A. Use hydrogen peroxide.
   B. Then use normal saline and/or iodophor.
   C. Dry thoroughly.
5. Pack deep wounds with iodophor or plain fine mesh gauze using sterile forcep, as prescribed by physician.	

6. Apply wide mesh gauze saturated with normal saline or gauze impregnated with petroleum jelly or an antimicrobial agent, using sterile forceps or sterile glove, as prescribed by physician.	6. This prevents drying and scabbing of the wound and reduces pain when removed.

7. Apply dry, nonocclusive dressing; secure in place.
8. Change dressing every 4 to 6 hours, if using saline method.
9. Assess and record:
   A. Condition of wound edges, subcutaneous and granulation tissue, and skin.
   B. Amount and characteristics of drainage.	

WOUND IRRIGATION

SPECIAL EQUIPMENT

Small plastic barrier drape with adhesive backing
No. 8 French red rubber catheter
Gown and mask (if wound is infected)
Protective bed pads
Bulb syringe
Safety pin
Irrigation solution
Sterile gauze pads

METHOD

ACTION	RATIONALE
1. Protect bed linens. 2. Apply plastic barrier drape.	

ACTION	RATIONALE

A. Remove a 1″ strip of paper backing from one edge of adhesive plastic barrier drape.

B. Secure barrier drape to patient's skin between wound and Montgomery straps so that drape covers straps.

                    B. This protects the Montgomery straps.

3. Position patient so solution will flow in desired direction.

4. Place free end of barrier drape into solution receptacle.

5. Don sterile glove on nondominant hand.

6. Attach red rubber catheter to tip of bulb syringe while holding bulb with dominant hand.

    5 and 6. The dominant hand controls the pressure of solution instillation; the gloved hand manipulates sterile items.

7. Aspirate irrigation solution, warmed to body temperature, into bulb syringe.

    7. Aspirating through the catheter removes air and lubricates it for less traumatic insertion.

8. Irrigate wound.

A. Insert tip of catheter or bulb syringe gently into wound; inject irrigation solution.

B. Use sterile gauze pad in gloved hand to help direct flow of effluent.

C. Direct flow of solution from cleanest to most contaminated for multiple wounds.

9. Cleanse wound and skin; remove barrier drape, and dress wound.

10. Assess and record:

A. Condition of wound and skin.

B. Amount and characteristics of drainage.

WOUND CULTURES

SPECIAL EQUIPMENT

Aspiration technique:
  Syringe
  Large bore needle

Swab technique:
  Aerobic culture tube
  Anaerobic culture tube

Polyethylene tubing
Small cork
Sterile normal saline or
   iodophor solution

Sterile normal saline or iodophor
   solution

METHOD

ACTION	RATIONALE
1. Remove surface debris and drainage with sterile normal saline or iodophor solution.	1. This removes surface contaminants which might alter culture results.
2. Milk wound gently.	2. This helps to obtain fresh drainage.
3. Select technique for obtaining wound culture.	
A. Aspiration technique:	A. This is the preferred technique for recovery of both aerobic and anaerobic organisms.
(1) Attach polyethylene tubing or large bore needle to syringe.	
(2) Insert tubing or needle into wound and aspirate fresh drainage.	
(3) Evacuate air from syringe.	(3) This facilitates recovery of anaerobic organisms.
(4) Cork needle, if using large bore needle. If using polyethylene tubing replace with a needle, expel air, and cork needle.	
B. Swab technique:	
(1) Remove swab from aerobic culture tube and insert swab into wound.	
(2) Replace swab in tube, insuring contact with transport media.	
(3) Repeat with anaerobic culture tube.	
4. Transport specimens to laboratory immediately to facilitate recovery of fastidious organisms.	

PRECAUTIONS: General

1. Use solutions in unit dose or small capacity containers supplied to each individual patient.

2. Never use cotton balls, since loose fibers can act as foreign bodies.
3. Use unpowdered gloves, since powder particles can act as foreign bodies.
4. Avoid dislodging drains, drainage bags, or drainage suction tubing.

RELATED CARE: General

1. Integrate the following concepts into wound care.
    A. Fluid collection, nonviable tissue, and/or drains diminish the ability of normal host defense mechanisms to rid a wound of organisms.
    B. An already infected wound can be invaded by other organisms and develop a secondary infection or superinfection. An infected wound can seed other sites and cause secondary infections.
    C. Open drainage systems are a portal of entry for organisms from skin, dressings, and the air. Closed suction drainage systems utilizing small diameter tubes greatly reduce the incidence of wound infection.
    D. Drainage bags should be used over open drains in the presence of heavy drainage to protect healthy skin and/or other nearby wounds.
    E. Montgomery straps should be used when frequent dressing changes or increased air circulation is needed. Straps should be periodically moved to new sites to prevent skin breakdown.
2. Ascertain whether plain gauze should be left dry or moistened with sterile normal saline solution when dressing open wounds.
3. Utilize wound precautions, as needed.

COMPLICATIONS

Primary, secondary, or superinfection of wound
Secondary infection in other sites
Secondary septicemia, with or without endotoxic shock
Wound dehiscence

SUPPLIERS

Bard Hospital Division (wound drainage bags)
BBL, division of Becton Dickinson (Port-a-Cul—anaerobic culture tubes)
Hollister (wound drainage bags)
Marion Scientific Corporation (Cepti-Seal Culturette—aerobic culture tubes; Silvadene—antimicrobial cream)
Orthopaedic Equipment Company (Redi-vacette—closed suction wound drains)
Parke Davis and Company (Vi-Drape—adherent barrier drapes)

Schering Corporation (Garamycin—antimicrobial cream)
3M Company (Steri-Drape—adherent barrier drapes)
Winthrop Labs (Sulfamylon—antimicrobial cream)
Zimmer U.S.A. (Hemovac—closed suction wound drains)

REFERENCES

Alexander, J.W., Korelitz, J.K., and Alexander, N.S.: Prevention of wound infections—a case for closed suction drainage to remove wound fluids deficient in opsonic proteins. Am. J. Surg., *132*:59, 1976.

American College of Surgeons: Manual on Control of Infection in Surgical Patients. Philadelphia, J. B. Lippincott, 1976.

Castle, M.: Wound care—clear-cut ways to speed healing. Nurs. '75, 5(No.8):40, 1975.

Cruse, P.J.E., and Foord, R.: A five-year prospective study of 23,649 surgical wounds. Arch. Surg., *107*:206, 1973.

Krizek, T.J., and Robson, M.C.: Biology of surgical infection. Surg. Clin. North Am. *55*(No. 6):1261, 1975.

Levine, N.S., et al.: Comparison of coarse mesh gauze with biologic dressings on granulating wounds. Am. J. Surg., *131*(No. 6):727, 1976.

Sandra J. Pfaff, R.N., B.S.N.

OVERVIEW

There are a number of intrinsic and extrinsic factors which predispose to decubiti. Intrinsic (host) factors include diabetes, malnutrition, dehydration, coma, paralysis, incontinence, and fever. Extrinsic (iatrogenic) factors include immobilization (casts, traction) and sedation-induced insensitivity to pain.

Prevention of decubiti focuses on four basic nursing approaches: (1) recognition of high risk patients (those with one or more predisposing factors); (2) monitoring for early signs of decubitus development; (3) nursing intervention, such as positioning, hygiene, and nutrition; and (4) patient protection, such as padding and/or the use of turning frames. Methods for both the prevention and management of decubitus ulcers are presented. Objectives, precautions, related care, and complications are similar for both and are identified as "general."

OBJECTIVES: General

1. To prevent the development of decubiti through nursing management of the high risk patient.
2. To promote healing and prevent infection when a decubitus ulcer occurs.

PREVENTION OF DECUBITI

SPECIAL EQUIPMENT

Karaya powder
Adhesive foam padding
Polyurethane foam padding

METHOD

ACTION	RATIONALE
1. Cleanse site with soap and water and dry thoroughly.	1. Sites to focus on are areas over bony prominences, areas experiencing undue or chronic pressure (intrinsic or extrinsic), and/or chronic reddened areas.

ACTION	RATIONALE
2. Gently massage site.	2. This stimulates circulation.
3. Sprinkle karaya powder liberally onto center of sticky side of adhesive foam padding.	
4. Apply adhesive foam padding to site and seal edges to skin.	
5. Cut a hole in polyurethane foam padding to fit it around adhesive foam padding.	
6. Apply to skin; add second layer if patient is very thin.	6. This prevents pressure on the site by distributing body weight more evenly around it.

7. Replace foam paddings:
    A. Immediately if they become wet, dislodged, or soiled.
    B. At least every 10 days.
	7. This prevents discomfort and/or skin maceration.

8. Assess for skin turgor, erythema, and pain and record findings.	

MANAGEMENT OF DECUBITI

SPECIAL EQUIPMENT

Karaya powder
Karaya ring
Polyurethane foam padding
3% hydrogen peroxide solution
Sterile normal saline for irrigation
Iodophor solution

METHOD

ACTION	RATIONALE

1. Irrigate decubitus with:
    A. Hydrogen peroxide.
    B. Then normal saline.
    C. Then iodophor solution.
	A. This removes organic debris.

2. Cleanse surrounding skin with soap and water and dry thoroughly. Avoid removing karaya residue that adheres after irrigation.	

ACTION	**RATIONALE**
3. Massage area around decubitus gently.	3. This stimulates circulation.
4. Mold karaya ring to fit closely around edge of ulcer.	

5. Apply karaya powder. Use syringe to apply in hard to reach or very deep areas.
   A. Sprinkle karaya powder into decubitus.
   B. Allow it to absorb moisture in wound.
   C. Reapply until wound appears "dusty."	

6. Apply foam padding.
   A. Cut hole in polyurethane foam padding so it fits snugly around karaya ring.
   B. Apply to skin.
   C. Apply second layer, if needed, and extend 1″ to 2″ beyond perimeter of first layer for better pressure distribution.
	C. This prevents pressure by distributing body weight more evenly.

7. Place plastic film from karaya ring over opening in ring.	7. This protects the wound from bed linens and insures easy observation.
8. Add karaya powder every 8 to 9 hours to maintain "dusty" appearance.	
9. Irrigate and apply karaya powder daily.	

10. Change entire system:
   A. Immediately, if loose or soiled.
   B. At least every 10 days.	

11. Assess for infection; intervene as necessary.	

12. Assess and record:
   A. Size, depth, and condition of decubitus.
   B. Condition of surrounding skin.
   C. Amount and characteristics of drainage.	

PRECAUTIONS: General

1. Use individual supplies for each patient.

2. If gloves are worn during care of extensive decubiti, use unpowdered gloves, since powder particles can act as foreign bodies.

RELATED CARE: General

1. Integrate the following concepts into wound care.
    A. Nursing management centers on prevention of decubiti.
    B. Remote infection increases the risk of infection in decubiti and, therefore, requires early recognition and prompt intervention.
    C. Karaya is a vegetable gum that is slightly water-soluble. It is effective for gentle debridement of ulcers and promotion of the development of granulation tissue.
2. Support nutrition and hydration measures.
3. Turn and/or ambulate the patient routinely.

COMPLICATIONS: General

Infection

SUPPLIERS

Squibb and Sons, E.R. (Stomahesive—adhesive foam padding)
3M Company (Reston—adhesive foam padding)

REFERENCES

Kavchak-Keyes, M.A.: Four proven steps for preventing decubitus ulcers. Nurs. '77, 7(No. 9):58, 1977.
Wallace, G., and Hayter, J.: Karaya for chronic skin ulcers. Am. J. Nurs., 74(No. 6):1094, 1974.

WOUND MANAGEMENT: BURNS

Sandra J. Pfaff, R.N., B.S.N.

OVERVIEW

Physiologic abnormalities in burns alter normal healing processes. These include: (1) altered neutrophilic antibacterial activity, in which bacteria multiply and are protected from antibiotics while inside the burn neutrophils; (2) occluded vascular supply, which reduces the delivery of humoral and cellular defense mechanisms; (3) bacterial invasion by gram-positive organisms during the first 3 post-burn days, and by gram-negative organisms from beneath eschar by the fifth post-burn day; (4) edema, which neutralizes protective fatty acids; and (5) tissue necrosis, which enhances the growth of a bacterial population.

Medical therapy includes: (1) debridement by means of dressings and/or hydrotherapy; (2) surgical debridement with the application of heterografts; and (3) surgical debridement with the application of biologic dressings (cadaver skin or porcine xenografts).

Many critical care areas have a "resident" flora of multiply-resistant organisms. Prevention of patient colonization by these organisms is accomplished through rigid adherence to strict technique by all health care team members. Endogenous patient flora must be controlled to keep their total numbers below the infection threshold. Fluid and electrolyte losses through wounds must be adequately replenished.

Methods for the management of open, intact second-degree, non-intact second-degree, and third-degree burns (also referred to as full-thickness burns) are presented. Because the objectives, precautions, related care, and complications are similar, they are presented only once, identified as "general."

OBJECTIVES: General

1. To promote healing of burns through wound care appropriate to the type of burn.
2. To prevent infection through inhibition of burn colonization by endogenous and exogenous flora.

CARE OF FIRST-DEGREE BURNS

METHOD

ACTION	RATIONALE
1. Elevate and immobilize affected area.	1. This reduces pain and swelling.
2. Apply cold.	2. This provides comfort.
3. Keep area clean and dry; avoid application of ointments, creams, or lotions.	
4. Assess and record condition of burn and surrounding skin.	

CARE OF OPEN BURNS

SPECIAL EQUIPMENT

Sterile cotton swabs   Bed cradle
Iodophor solution   Infrared lamp
Antimicrobial cream

METHOD

ACTION	RATIONALE
1. Cleanse with iodophor and sterile water.	
A. Use all sterile supplies, gown, and gloves.	A. This stimulates circulation and provides gentle debridement.
B. Wear mask.	
2. Apply antimicrobial cream (if prescribed by physician) with sterile cotton swab or sterile gloved hand.	
3. Use bed cradle to elevate top bed sheet.	3. This provides comfort and prevents adherence to burns.
4. Position infrared lamp above bed; position lamp carefully to prevent additional burning or pain to patient.	4. This helps to maintain body temperature.
5. Assess and record:	
A. Condition of blisters or eschar.	
B. Amount and characteristics of drainage.	
C. Signs of maceration.	

CARE OF INTACT SECOND-DEGREE BURNS (UNBROKEN BLISTERS)

SPECIAL EQUIPMENT

Sterile nonadherent surgical
  dressings
Stretch gauze

Iodophor solution
Sterile water

METHOD

ACTION	RATIONALE
1. Cleanse skin around burns with iodophor and sterile water; avoid any cleansing or manipulation of blisters.	
2. Apply sterile nonadherent pads *around* burns which are on bony prominences and pressure areas; secure with stretch gauze.	2. This protects blisters, relieves pressure, and enhances air circulation.
3. Assess and record condition of blisters and surrounding skin.	

CARE OF NONINTACT SECOND-DEGREE BURNS (BROKEN BLISTERS)

SPECIAL EQUIPMENT

Sterile, nonadherent surgical
  gauze roll
Sterile bulky gauze
Stretch gauze or net

Iodophor solution
Sterile water or sterile normal
  saline solution
Antimicrobial cream
Sterile gloves

METHOD

ACTION	RATIONALE
1. Cleanse with iodophor and sterile water or normal saline.	1. This stimulates circulation and provides gentle debridement.
2. Air-dry for 20 minutes.	

ACTION	RATIONALE

3. Apply antimicrobial cream, if prescribed by physician.
4. Apply sterile, nonadherent surgical dressing.
5. Apply bulky gauze dressings.
6. Wrap with stretch gauze or net.
7. Change dressings:
   A. Twice a day on deep wounds.
   B. Every 2 to 4 days on superficial wounds.
8. Assess and record:
   A. Condition of wound and surrounding skin.
   B. Presence of any odor.
   C. Amount and characteristics of drainage.

CARE OF THIRD-DEGREE BURNS (FULL-THICKNESS BURNS)

SPECIAL EQUIPMENT

Sterile nonadherent surgical gauze roll
Sterile bulky gauze
Stretch gauze or net
Antimicrobial cream

Bed cradle and heat lamp (if needed)
Iodophor solution
Sterile water or sterile normal saline solution
Sterile gloves

METHOD

ACTION	RATIONALE
1. Cleanse with iodophor and sterile water or normal saline.	1. This stimulates circulation and provides gentle debridement.
2. Air-dry 20 minutes.	
3. Apply antimicrobial cream, if prescribed by physician.	
4. Apply sterile, nonadherent surgical dressing; use bed cradle and heat lamp, if needed.	4. The heat lamp helps to maintain body temperature.

ACTION	RATIONALE

5. Apply bulky gauze and stretch gauze *only* if large amounts of drainage are present.
6. Change dressings as needed, depending upon amount of drainage.
7. Assess and record:
    A. Condition of wound, granulation tissue, and skin.
    B. Amount and characteristics of drainage.

PRECAUTIONS: General

1. Use antimicrobial creams rather than ointments, since they are easier to apply and remove and are less occlusive.
2. Reduce the potential of cross-contamination from personnel and equipment. Personnel with an infection in *any* site should not care for burn patients. Masks should be worn when caring for second-degree burns with broken blisters or for third-degree burns.
3. Utilize a private room with positive air pressure. Cleaning should be done with wet cloths and mops, and with minimal agitation of air currents. Burn care should be performed before or well after cleaning.

RELATED CARE: General

1. Integrate the following concepts into wound care:
    A. Blisters on second-degree burns act as protective barriers for both fluid loss and the development of infection. They should not be cleansed or manipulated so that they are maintained intact as long as possible.
    B. Local application of moist compresses should be utilized, rather than hydrotherapy, if infection exists on another area of the body.
    C. Antimicrobial therapy should be instituted when the possibility of remote infection exists. Prophylaxis may be instituted if the blisters on second-degree burns break or after the eschar on third-degree burns is no longer intact.
    D. If used, dressings should be individualized according to the type and depth of the wound. They should absorb fluid to prevent maceration, protect from trauma, and be comfortable. Non-adherent dressings are used for healing wounds; adherent dressings are used to debride infected wounds.
    E. Sterile bed linens and bed clothing should be used for all except first-degree burns.
    F. All patients should be checked for remote infection, and appropriate intervention taken.

    G.   Change only bulky and stretch gauze on nonintact second-degree burns (blisters broken) if superficial wounds are clean and dry. Change dressings on superficial wounds more often if:

        (1)   Any odor is detected;

        (2)   Patient complains of discomfort; or

        (3)   Stretch gauze becomes soiled.

2.   Utilize protective isolation precautions, as necessary.

3.   Maintain optimal fluid and electrolyte balances.

4.   Monitor and assess the patient's nutritional status.

5.   Utilize effective wound management of any infected wounds.

COMPLICATIONS: General

Infection, local or systemic	Hypothermia
Dehydration	Electrolyte imbalance

SUPPLIERS

The Kendall Company (Telfa—nonadherent surgical dressings)

Marion Scientific Corporation (Silvadene—antimicrobial cream)

Schering Corporation (Garamycin—antimicrobial cream)

3M Company (Micropad—nonadherent surgical dressings)

Winthrop Labs (Sulfamylon—antimicrobial cream)

REFERENCES

Jacoby, F.G.: Individualized burn wound dressings. Nurs. '77, 7(No. 6):62, 1977.

Jones, C.A., and Feller, I.: Burns—what to do during the first crucial hours. Nurs. '77, 7(No. 3):22, 1977.

Judith Henderson, R.N., M.S.N.

OVERVIEW

Effective site care for venous and arterial indwelling catheters is imperative to preserve the patient's skin integrity and to prevent any complications resulting from improper site care. The catheters referred to in these methods may include:

1. Arterial:
   A. Peripheral.
   B. Left atrial.
2. Venous:
   A. Peripheral, steel needle, and short catheter.
   B. Central.
   C. Pulmonary artery.
   D. Right atrial.

Whether these catheters are inserted by puncture, surgical cutdown, or transthoracically, the methods for their care are quite similar. The precautions, related care, and complications apply to both short and long venous and arterial indwelling catheter site care, and are identified as "general."

SHORT VENOUS INDWELLING CATHETER SITE CARE

OBJECTIVES

1. To decrease the incidence of phlebitis and infection at the catheter insertion site and catheter-related sepsis.
2. To assess the patient for phlebitis, infection, infiltration, and leakage of fluid at the catheter insertion site and catheter-related sepsis and, if present, to take appropriate nursing measures.
3. To preserve skin integrity at the insertion site.

SPECIAL EQUIPMENT

Sterile gloves
Sterile gauze pads and sterile solution (e.g., normal saline)
Iodine and 70% alcohol, *or* iodophor solution (for sensitive skin), *or* 70% alcohol (when patient has allergy to iodine)
Povidone-iodine ointment
Adhesive tape

METHOD

ACTION	RATIONALE
1. Wash hands thoroughly.	

2. Expose site:
  A. Remove old dressings and tape from catheter insertion site.
  B. Leave one piece of tape in place to secure catheter.	

3. Don sterile gloves.	
4. Remove residual ointment or dried blood and secretions from site with sterile gauze pad or sterile solution (e.g., normal saline) as appropriate.	4. Dried blood and secretions could neutralize iodine's germicidal activity.

5. Assess insertion site for signs of inflammation, phlebitis, infection, infiltration, and/or leakage of fluid.
  A. If any of these is present, remove catheter.
  B. If infection at the site and/or sepsis are suspected, obtain appropriate cultures; see "Related Care" further on.
  C. Insert new catheter at another site with entirely new apparatus.	

6. Scrub skin around insertion site and catheter with antiseptic solution, using a circular motion from cannula outward to periphery.	6. Working from the cleanest area of the wound, the insertion site, to the less clean area, the periphery, prevents wound contamination and infection.
7. Apply povidone-iodine ointment to insertion site, and emerging catheter.	7. Iodine ointment is bacteriocidal, fungicidal, virucidal, and amebicidal. The clinical advantages and safety of antiseptic ointments remain to be established by controlled clinical trials.

8. Dress site and anchor needle or catheter.
  A. For a winged steel needle:
    (1) Apply short piece of ¼-inch adhesive tape across each wing parallel to needle.
    (2) Apply piece of ¼-inch tape across both wings, at
	8. To-and-fro motion of the needle or catheter may facilitate entry of cutaneous microorganisms into the wound and increase the risk of phlebitis by traumatizing the cannulated vessel.

ACTION   **RATIONALE**

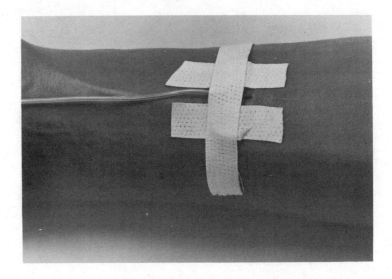

Figure 129.

right angle to needle (Fig. 129).

(3) Place sterile gauze pad over insertion site and tape.

(3) Use of occlusive dressings remains optional, since there are no controlled investigative studies to warrant a definitive recommendation. An occlusive dressing is warranted at a site that could easily be contaminated.

(4) Make loop of intravenous tubing near to wings and tape it to skin; do not cross tubing over itself (Fig. 130).

(4) Compression of line may hinder flow.

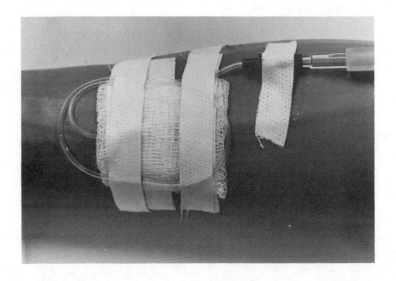

Figure 130.

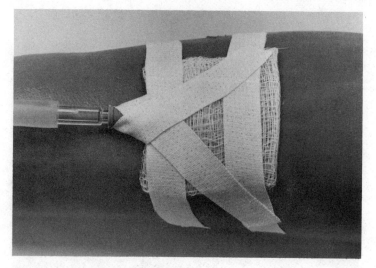

Figure 131.

B. For a short catheter:
   (1) Place small sterile gauze pad over insertion site, and tape.
   (2) Place piece of ¼-inch tape under hub of catheter, adhesive side up, crisscross it over hub, and secure it to dressing (Fig. 131).
   (3) Place piece of 1-inch tape across crisscrossed tape.
   (4) Place 1-inch strip of tape lengthwise over intravenous tubing and hub. To allow for easy removal of the tape, fold tape onto itself, making a tab at the distal end.

   (4) This helps to avoid disconnection of the tubing and hub.

   (5) Make loop of intravenous tubing and tape it to arm (Fig. 132).
9. Label new dressing with:
   A. Type and size of needle or catheter in place.
   B. Date and time of insertion.
   C. Date of site care.
10. Document site care and catheter and skin integrity, as appropriate.

LONG VENOUS AND ARTERIAL INDWELLING CATHETER SITE CARE

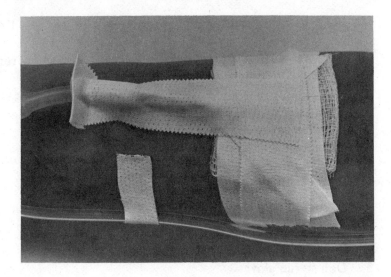

Figure 132.

OBJECTIVES

1. To decrease the incidence of phlebitis and infection at the catheter insertion site and catheter-related sepsis.
2. To assess the patient for phlebitis, infection, infiltration, and leakage of fluid at the catheter insertion site, and catheter-related sepsis and, if present, to take appropriate nursing measures.
3. To preserve skin integrity at the insertion site.

SPECIAL EQUIPMENT

Face mask
Sterile gloves
Sterile drapes
Acetone
Sterile gauze pads and sterile solution (e.g., normal saline)
Iodine and 70% alcohol, *or* iodophor solution (for sensitive skin),
  or 70% alcohol (when patient has allergy to iodine)
Povidone-iodine ointment
Sterile scissors
Tincture of benzoin
Adhesive tape

METHOD

ACTION	RATIONALE
1. Mask all persons in immediate area.	1. Optimum sterile technique is recommended, since many of these

ACTION	RATIONALE
	catheters remain in place longer than 48 hours.
2. Wash hands thoroughly.	
3. If catheter is in patients's arm or shoulder, abduct arm and have patient turn his face away from site or place a mask over patient's face.	
4. Expose site:	
A. Remove old dressings and tape from catheter insertion site.	
B. Leave one piece of tape in place to secure catheter.	
5. Don sterile gloves.	
6. Place sterile drapes around exposed site.	
7. Remove residual ointment or dried blood and secretions from site with sterile gauze pad or sterile solution (e.g. normal saline) as appropriate.	7. Dried blood and secretions could neutralize iodine's germicidal activity.
8. Assess insertion site for signs of inflammation, phlebitis, infection, infiltration, and/or leakage of fluid.	
A. If present, remove catheter after consultation with physician.	
B. If infection at the site and/or sepsis are suspected, obtain appropriate cultures (see "Related Care," further on).	
C. When new catheter is inserted at another site, use entirely new apparatus.	
9. Defat skin surrounding insertion site with acetone, working from catheter to periphery in circle of about 3 inches.	9. Acetone removes cellular debris and oil.
10. Scrub skin around insertion site, any sutures, and catheter with antiseptic solution, working in circles from catheter out to periphery.	
11. Apply povidone-iodine ointment to insertion site, emerging catheter, and sutures.	11. Iodine ointment is bacteriocidal, fungicidal, virucidal, and amebicidal. The clinical advantages and safety of antiseptic ointments remain to be established by controlled clinical trials.

ACTION   RATIONALE

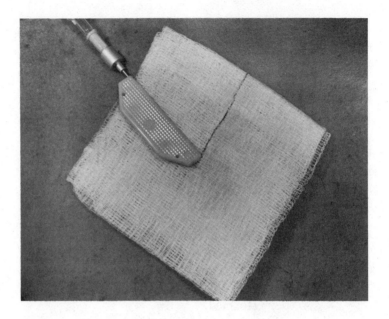

Figure 133.

12. Dress site and anchor catheter.
   A. For a central catheter:
      (1) Cut to center of sterile
           gauze pad with sterile scis-
           sors.
      (2) Place sterile gauze pad   (2) Gauze under the catheter
           over insertion site, with   prevents it from pressing
           catheter exiting in center   directly onto the skin.
           (Fig. 133).
      (3) Place another sterile gauze
           pad over insertion site and
           catheter.
      (4) Apply tincture of benzoin   (4) Tincture of benzoin pro-
           to skin surrounding gauze;   tects the skin and promotes
           allow it to dry.   adherence of the adhesive
                                                  tape.
      (5) Discard first layer of wide   (5) Exposure of connection al-
           adhesive tape and apply   lows the intravenous tubing
           fresh layer of tape over   to be changed, if needed,
           gauze, leaving connection   without   disturbing   the
           of catheter to intravenous   dressing.
           tubing exposed.
      (6) Secure all edges of dress-
           ing with 1-inch tape.
      (7) Place 1-inch strip of tape   (7) This avoids disconnection
           lengthwise over intraven-   of the tubing and con-
           ous tubing and connection.   nection.

ACTION	RATIONALE

To allow for easy removal of the tape, fold tape onto itself, making a tab at the distal end.

  (8) Make loop of intravenous tubing and tape it on top of dressing (Fig. 134).

B. For a right or left atrial line:

  (1) Cut to center of sterile gauze pad with sterile scissors.

  (2) Place sterile gauze pad over insertion site, with catheter exiting in center. Suturing of line may not permit steps (1) and (2) to be performed.

  (3) Place another sterile gauze pad over insertion site and line.

  (4) Discard first layer of wide adhesive tape and apply fresh layer of tape over gauze, cutting to center of tape.

                      (4) Cutting to the center of the tape enables it to fit snugly around the catheter.

  (5) Anchor exposed catheter to top of dressing or skin with tape.

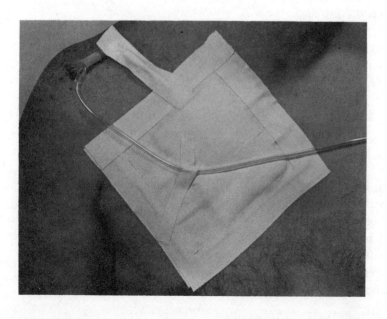

Figure 134.

ACTION	RATIONALE

13. Label new dressing with:
    A. Type and size of catheter in place.
    B. Date and time of insertion.
    C. Date of site care.
14. Document site care and catheter and skin integrity, as appropriate.

PRECAUTIONS: General

1. Maintain strict asepsis during site care, since contamination of the insertion site could progress to phlebitis or infection.
2. Do not leave short intravenous catheter in place longer than 72 hours, and preferably change them at 48-hour intervals. If an intravenous catheter is not replaced after 72 hours, the nurse or physician should:
    A. Document in patient's medical record the rationale for leaving it in place longer than 72 hours.
    B. Ensure adherence to aseptic methods for the care of the line and site.
    C. Observe the site frequently for inflammation, phlebitis, infection, infiltration, and leakage of fluid, or any possibility of catheter-related sepsis.

RELATED CARE: General

1. Perform site care once daily for short venous indwelling catheters and every other day for long-term arterial and venous indwelling catheters and when the dressing becomes contaminated. These recommendations arise from standard practice across the country, since there are no controlled studies to indicate frequency of site care.
2. Change intravenous tubing and solution at the same time site care is performed.
3. Remove hair from the site only if needed to facilitate the placement or removal of adhesive tape. Remove hair with a depilatory or scissors, because razor shaving produces microabrasions of the skin, with resultant bacterial access and growth. The presence of hair bears little relation to the bacterial flora of skin, and methods used to clean the skin also suffice to clean hair.
4. Use iodine solution when scrubbing the skin with antiseptic solution. Allow the tincture to dry for 30 seconds and then wash it off with 70% alcohol. Alcohol is used to decrease further the risk of burns from iodine. If the patient has sensitive skin, an iodophor solution is used instead. It is allowed to dry in place and is not to be removed, because its

germicidal action is augmented by the sustained release of iodine. If the patient has an allergy to iodine, scrub with 70% alcohol for at least 1 full minute.

5. Assess for signs of phlebitis plus purulent drainage if infection is suspected at the site. Collect any purulent material for culture and Gram stain. The catheter may then be cultured in the following manner.

    A . If the patient has no allergy to iodine, scrub the skin around the catheter with iodine and 70% alcohol, working from the catheter out to the periphery. Allow the iodine to dry for 30 seconds and then wash it off with 70% alcohol, working in a similar manner as above. Applying an antiseptic to the skin decreases the chance of contaminating the catheter with skin flora as it is removed.

    B . If the patient has an allergy to iodine, scrub the skin around the cannula with 70% alcohol solution, working in a similar manner as above.

    C . Remove the catheter, applying pressure with dry sterile gauze to the artery or vein, as needed.

    D . Clip the tip of the catheter off with sterile scissors, letting it fall into appropriate tube for culture.

    E . Send specimens to the laboratory for culturing.

6. Monitor the temperature of the patient regularly when a catheter is in place; an unexplained fever or chills may indicate catheter-related sepsis. If sepsis is present and thought to be related to infection from the catheter, blood may be drawn through the catheter. The catheter is then removed and cultured, as above.

COMPLICATIONS: General

> Phlebitis
> Infection at insertion site
> Cannula-related sepsis
> Emboli
> Mechanical separation of lines
> Displacement and/or accidental removal of cannula
> Impairment of circulation

SUPPLIERS

> Clinipad Corporation (standard dressing change kits)
> Pharmaseal Inc. (sterile dressing trays)
> Shield Laboratories, Inc. (central venous catheter dressing change set)

REFERENCES

Goldmann, D.A., Maki, D.G., Rhame, F.S., Kaiser, A.B., Tenney, J.H., and

Bennett, J.V.: Guidelines for infection control in intravenous therapy. Ann. Intern. Med., *79*:848, 1973.

Jarrand, M.M., and Freeman, J.B.: The effects of antibiotic ointments and antiseptics on the skin flora beneath subclavian catheter dressings during intravenous hyperalimentation. J. Surg. Res., *22*:521, 1977.

Maki, D.G.: Preventing infection in intravenous therapy. Hosp. Pract., *11*(No. 4):95, 1976.

Maki, D.G., Goldman, D.A., and Rhame, F.S.: Infection control in intravenous therapy. Ann. Intern. Med., *79*:867, 1973.

Retailliau, Henry F.: Personal communications. Atlanta, Center for Disease Control, Hospital Infections Branch, 1978

Seropian, R., and Reynolds, B.M.: Wound infections after preoperative depilatory versus razor preparation. Am. J. Surg., *121:*251, 1971.

NUTRITIONAL SUPPORT

TOTAL PARENTERAL NUTRITION

Rita Colley, R.N.

OVERVIEW

Administration of total nutrition by vein has evolved into a specialty with its own nomenclature — total parenteral nutrition (TPN), hyperalimentation, or intravenous hyperalimentation (IVH). The object of TPN is to provide sufficient nutrients by vein to achieve anabolism and to promote weight gain, when necessary.

The solutions are made with hypertonic glucose, amino acids, electrolytes, minerals, vitamins, and trace elements. Often, intravenous fat is also needed to prevent essential fatty acid deficiency and/or supply calories. (IV fat is administered separately; see the method for "Lipid Therapy—Administration of Intravenous Lipids.")

Indications for TPN are varied and include patients who have inflammatory bowel disease, draining fistulas, hypermetabolic demands, often from major trauma, inadequate gastrointestinal (GI) tracts as a consequence of malabsorption, and short bowel syndrome. TPN is also used as adjunctive therapy with some cancer treatment modalities that affect the GI tract. The common factor that should always be present in a patient before this therapy is instituted is the inability of the GI tract to function in a manner that allows achievement of anabolism. This point is made because the therapy is not without risk and use of the GI tract (for feeding) is easier, safer, and more economical.

The solutions must be prepared daily in the pharmacy under a laminar airflow (LAF) unit. Using a closed transfer method and in-line filtration during admixture, the pharmacist is able to provide the highest degree of quality control. When a LAF unit is not available, the solution should be prepared in a clean area, free from traffic and air turbulence, that has been set aside for IV admixture. The manufacturer's instructions for closed transfer, using a special kit, should be followed exactly to guarantee asepsis. Extreme preoccupation with asepsis is necessary, because sepsis is the most dreaded complication of TPN therapy; yet, it may almost always be avoided when proper technique is used in every aspect of its delivery.

The solutions should be refrigerated until use and should expire within 24 hours of preparation time. The expiration date and time should be placed on the solution bottle label, along with all other necessary identifying information.

Although it is desirable to have total admixture done in the pharmacy under a LAF unit, some institutions find it necessary to add to the solutions after they have been obtained from the pharmacy. It is prudent to delegate this responsibility only to a qualified IV nurse therapist. Substances would then be added by the IV nurse therapist in a specifically designated place in the clinical area. Compatibility of any additive with the basic TPN mixture should be authorized by the pharmacy department. After supplementing the

TPN infusion solution with prescribed additives, the IV therapist should cover the infusion bottle with a new, sterile, airtight, waterproof cap (unless the bottle is to be used immediately).

INSERTION OF A TOTAL PARENTERAL NUTRITION CATHETER (ASSISTING WITH)

OVERVIEW

The usual intracatheter for TPN infusion is 8 inches long, made of polyvinylchloride (PVC). There are many brands available, and choice is dependent upon the physician and institutional availability. Recently the advantages of Silastic over PVC intracatheters have been reported. Many physicians now theorize that this less reactive catheter will not irritate the vein wall as easily as PVC catheters seem to do. It has also been reported that Silastic catheters have far less fibrin sheath formation on them; theoretically, this reduces the possibility of bacterial seeding upon the catheter. Because Silastic is more flexible than PVC, it must be secured to the skin with great care in order to avoid kinking of the catheter.

Placement of a catheter for infusion of TPN solution is a sterile procedure, usually performed in the patient's room. Before infusion begins, the patient should be clean, with all wound dressings freshly changed to decrease the chance of contamination. The patient's blood volume should be or have been restored to normal so that an adequate venous pressure exists. This prevents the physician from attempting to puncture the collapsed vein of a dehydrated hypovolemic patient.

OBJECTIVE

To monitor and support the patient during insertion of a TPN catheter, assisting at crucial moments.

SPECIAL EQUIPMENT

This consists of a sterile catheter placement kit, containing:
  Four sterile drapes
  Three towel clips
  Ten sterile gauze pads
  Two 3-ml. syringes
  One 000 silk suture with autraumatic straight needle
  Two hemostats
  One pair scissors
  One 10-ml. vial 1% lidocaine
  Povidone-iodine ointment

One 16-gauge 8-inch intracatheter
One gown
Two pairs sterile gloves
Two masks
One bottle acetone
One bottle 1% tincture of iodine ⎫
One bottle 70% isopropyl alcohol ⎬ New unopened bottles
One can tincture of benzoin ⎭
One 6″ × 8″ plastic sterile adhesive backed drape
One role 1″ plastic nonallergic tape
One 500-ml. bottle 5% dextrose in water for intravenous infusion
One adult drip intravenous tubing
One towel (to be used as a towel roll)

METHOD

ACTION	RATIONALE
1. Wash hands thoroughly and rinse with surgical scrub solution.	
2. Prepare site for catheter insertion by washing and shaving area of catheter insertion. It is preferable to shave the area the night before catheter insertion in case surface abrasions occur in the skin.	2. This is done to eliminate pain during adhesive removal at future dressing changes, as well as to facilitate aseptic technique.
3. Place catheter insertion implements on clean, alcohol-scrubbed bedside table; prime IV tubing.	
4. Place patient in supine position with towel roll (12″ long and 3″ in diameter) along thoracic vertebrae (Fig. 135).	4. The towel roll elevates the clavicle, facilitating location of the subclavian vein and separating it from the apex of the lung.
5. Place bed in Trendelenburg position at approximately 45°. If the patient has difficulty tolerating this position, do not implement it until the procedure actually begins.	5. This position aids in filling the subclavian veins.
6. Instruct patient to turn head away from insertion site.	
7. Mask all persons in immediate area, except patient. (Gowning and gloving is required for the person performing the invasive procedure.)	7. The patient's face will be draped and doesn't require a mask.
8. Assist in surgical preparation of skin and surgical draping.	

ACTION   **RATIONALE**

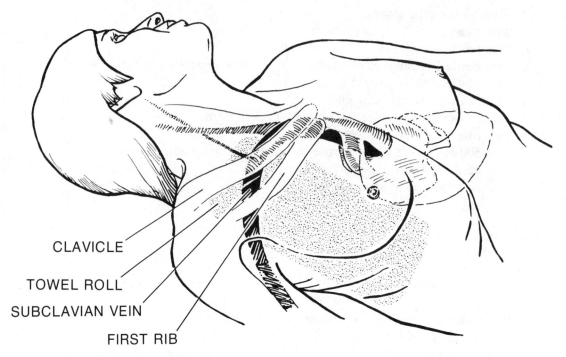

CLAVICLE

TOWEL ROLL

SUBCLAVIAN VEIN

FIRST RIB

Figure 135. Positioning of patient for subclavian cathether insertion.

   A. Prep is similar to dressing
      change scrub: acetone, iodine,
      and alcohol.

   B. Do not cover eyes or nose with   B. This panics some patients.
      drape.

9. Ensure patient comfort.

   A. Explain that area will sting as
      it is infiltrated with local anes-
      thetic (similar to a bee sting),
      that it will subside, and that
      medication will be given time to
      take effect.

   B. Hold patient's hand—enor-
      mous comfort and security
      usually provided by this simple
      gesture is immeasurable.

   C. Make sure anesthetic is given
      time to take effect.

10. Inform patient that there will be a   10. This should not be extremely painful
      feeling of pressure as catheter nee-   or anxiety-provoking if the patient
      dle penetrates skin.   is prepared.

11. Instruct patient to perform Valsalva   11. The Valsalva maneuver must be
      maneuver after venous blood has   maintained until the intracatheter is

ACTION

been aspirated into syringe and before syringe is disconnected to allow catheter introduction.

A. Compress abdomen if patient is unable to perform Valsalva maneuver.

B. Effect Valsalva maneuver in intubated patient by maintaining inspiratory phase of Ambu bag (effective approximately 3 to 5 seconds after inspiration is initiated).

12. Encourage a single suture at insertion site and placement of catheter straight down on chest as intracatheter is sutured (Fig. 136).

13. Instruct patient to perform Valsalva maneuver as catheter hub plug is removed and isotonic IV infusion is hooked up.

RATIONALE

threaded to the needle hub, occluding it. Failure to do this invites air embolism. Remember to tell the patient when it is all right to breathe again!

12. This allows cleaning of the catheter beneath it (during dressing changes) and prevents kinking.

13. This is done so that the catheter is not open to the air unnecessarily.

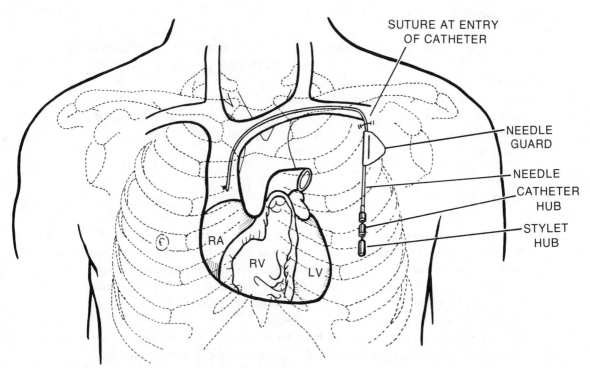

Figure 136. Anatomic cathether placement.

ACTION	RATIONALE
A. Set rate at 20 cc/hour. B. Maintain this rate until catheter tip location is verified by x-ray.	
14. Lower IV bottle below heart level to observe venous backflow of blood into tubing.	14. This helps to verify venous placement of the catheter; it is also the reason a filter has not yet been connected—it could clog with venous blood.
15. Remove drapes and towel roll and reposition patient comfortably; prepare patient for chest x-ray.	
16. Bring patient out of Trendelenburg position and apply dressing (see method for "Total Parenteral Nutrition Catheter Site Care").	
17. Initiate the first bottle of TPN upon verification of catheter tip location by x-ray (Fig. 136). Correct catheter tip location is the mid-superior vena cava or the innominate vein. The right atrium is not an acceptable location.	

PRECAUTIONS

1. *Never* use anything other than TPN—e.g., central venous pressure monitoring, blood withdrawal, bolus or piggy back infusions—through the TPN catheter. It is an inviolate system!
2. Observe the patient carefully for signs and symptoms of respiratory distress (e.g., dyspnea, decreased breath sounds, chest pain, cyanosis or shock) and/or a slowly growing hematoma following catheter placement.

RELATED CARE

1. Clean the tracheostomy wound of tracheostomy patients prior to catheter insertion and cover with povidone-iodine sponges as part of the surgical preparation. A sterile, adhesive, waterproof plastic drape should be placed between the tracheostomy tube and the insertion area as an additional barrier. The catheter insertion site should be located as far away from the tracheostomy as possible.
2. Place the catheter on the side with a thoracostomy tube, if applicable, because the tube often prevents pleural space complications during catheterization.

3. Place the catheter on the side opposite the planned surgical incision if patients are preoperative for head, neck, or upper thorax surgery.
4. Monitor IV solution administration; the IV tubing should be double-clamped.
5. Maintain catheter asepsis. The patient should have routine temperatures taken every 6 hours, and any elevation should be reported. There seems to be no single febrile pattern associated with TPN catheter sepsis; it can be manifested by a low grade temperature, either constant or intermittent, by daily temperature spikes, or by a dramatic elevation accompanied by clinical signs of septicemia. Glucose intolerance is often an early warning of catheter sepsis in the TPN patient. If this develops suddenly for an unexplained reason, catheter sepsis should be suspected. If a TPN patient has a single dramatic temperature spike the total IV system (down to the catheter hub) should be removed and cultured, including the solution from the bottle and from the IV tubing, both proximal and distal to the filter, if one is used. Any TPN patient with a fever should have a complete history and physical examination, and thorough culturing, followed by serologic diagnostic monitoring. If the fever remains unexplicable, the catheter should be removed and cultured (see the method for "Culturing a Total Parenteral Nutrition Subclavian Venous Catheter"). If blood cultures are positive and recurrent, or if the patient is in septic shock, the catheter should also be removed.

COMPLICATIONS

Sepsis	Lymphatic leak
Pneumothorax	Air embolism
Hemothorax	Catheter embolism
Hydrothorax	Myocardial irritability
Extravasation	Myocardial perforation
Nerve damage	Thrombosis

REFERENCES

Dudrick, S.J., MacFadyen, B.V., Souchon, E.A., Englert, D.M., and Copeland, E.M., III: Parenteral nutrition techniques in cancer patients. Cancer Res., 37:2240–2250, 1977.

Ryan, John A., Jr.: Complications of total parenteral nutrition. In Fischer, J.E. (ed.): Total Parenteral Nutrition, 1st ed., Boston, Little Brown and Company, Inc., 1976, pp. 55–100.

MONITORING DAILY INFUSION OF TOTAL PARENTERAL NUTRITION THERAPY

OBJECTIVES

1. To provide nutrients by vein in order to achieve anabolism and promote weight gain.
2. To deliver TPN in a manner that avoids untoward metabolic complications.

METHOD

ACTION	RATIONALE
1. Begin initial infusion at a slow rate (approximately 60 to 80 ml./hr.).	1. This helps to avoid glucose intolerance.
2. Increase infusion in slow increments (approximately 25 ml./hr./day).	2. This helps to avoid glucose intolerance.
3. Time-tape the TPN bottle and double-clamp the IV tubing; check infusion rate every 30 minutes.	3. This prevents fluid overload and glucose overdose.
4. Administer TPN infusion via infusion apparatus, if possible.	4. This is safer and more accurate.
5. Weigh patient daily, at same time with same clothing.	
6. Keep accurate record of intake and output.	
7. Monitor accurate caloric intake daily.	
8. Measure urinary sugar and acetone levels every 6 hours.	8. This indicates glucose tolerance.
A. If sugar is greater than 2+ report glycosuria.	A. This requires serum glucose measurement and treatment.
B. Use Tes-tape if patient is receiving cephalosporins, large doses of aspirin, or vitamin C.	B. Clinitest tablets may yield a false positive result.
9. Decrease infusion in slow increments—i.e., "wean" the solution.	9. This helps to prevent hypoglycemic shock.

PRECAUTION

Be alert for the signs and symptoms of hypoglycemia, hyperglycemia, hyperosmolar coma, electrolyte imbalance, dehydration, and deficiency states of vitamins, essential fatty acids, and trace elements.

COMPLICATION

Altered fluid administration

REFERENCES

Colley, R., Wilson, J., and Wilhelm, M.P.: Intravenous nutrition—nursing considerations. Issues Compr. Pediatr. Nurs., 2(No. 1):50–83, 1977.

Ryan, J.A., Jr.: Complications of total parenteral nutrition. *In* Fischer, J.E. (ed.): Total Parenteral Nutrition. Boston, Little, Brown and Company, 1976, pp. 55–100.

TOTAL PARENTERAL NUTRITION CATHETER SITE CARE

OVERVIEW

The subclavian catheter dressing should be changed every 48 hours or three times a week on Monday, Wednesday, and Friday. The actual prepping of the skin should be done with gentle but abrasive action to insure removal of all debris and adhesive residue. The entire catheter should also be cleansed. This involves some motion of the catheter so that the underside (including the needle guard and needle, when present) is thoroughly cleansed. Because many TPN patients are malnourished, their skin is particularly sensitive and therefore solutions, bandage materials and tapes should be selected appropriately.

The dressing should always be maintained so that it is aseptic, dry, and air-occlusive. If the dressing becomes loose or wet it should be considered contaminated and changed immediately.

OBJECTIVES

1. To keep the catheter stable, secure, free of debris, and aseptic, thereby minimizing the potential for mechanical and septic complications.
2. To preserve skin integrity at the insertion site.

SPECIAL EQUIPMENT

This consists of the sterile subclavian dressing change kit, containing:
    Three aluminum cups
    One disposable clamp
    Scissors
    Ten sterile gauze pads
    Povidone-iodine ointment
    Two pairs sterile gloves
    One 6″ × 8″ adhesive-backed sterile drape

One bottle acetone
One bottle 1% tincture of iodine
One bottle 70% isopropyl alcohol   } New unopened bottles
One can tincture of benzoin aerosol
One new role 1″ adhesive tape

METHOD

ACTION	RATIONALE
1. Wash hands thoroughly and rinse with surgical scrub solution.	
2. Mask all persons in immediate area. Do not mask patient if this causes respiratory difficulty; instead, have patient turn head away from catheter site.	2. This protects the catheter from nasopharyngeal organisms. The mask also protects the patient from the disturbing odors of some of the prep solutions and the benzoin.
3. Place patient in supine or semi-Fowler's position and remove pillow(s).	
4. Clear off bedside table, cleanse with isopropyl alcohol, and allow it to dry thoroughly.	4. This promotes asepsis.
5. Wash hands again and rinse with surgical scrub solution.	
6. Prepare subclavian dressing change kit (Fig. 137) in a sterile fashion; fill three cups with acetone, iodine, and alcohol.	
7. Squeeze povidone-iodine ointment onto double-thickness gauze pad.	

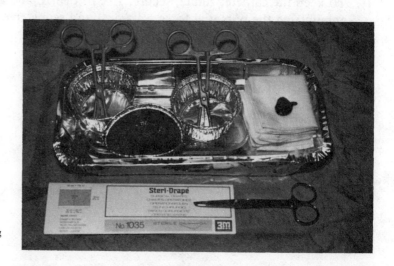

Figure 137. Subclavian dressing change kit.

ACTION	RATIONALE
8. Remove old dressing.	
A. Stabilize catheter to avoid dislodging it.	
B. Pull skin away from tape (rather than tape away from skin).	B. There is less trauma.
C. If gauze sponges over insertion sites do not adhere to dressing (therefore coming off with it) put on sterile gloves, remove sponges, and then change gloves.	
9. Don sterile gloves; trim gauze with ointment to a 2″ × 2″ size, place this outside aluminum cups but well within borders of sterile field.	9. This keeps the ointment and sponges away from solutions and therefore, dry.
10. Observe catheter insertion site for erythema, edema, drainage, or crusting. Culture and report to physician, if appropriate.	
11. Defat catheter insertion site and surrounding skin.	11. Defatting removes debris which could harbor organisms and clears the surface for the iodine.
A. Use an acetone-prepared gauze pad.	
B. Prep in wider to wider concentric circles.	B. This is the "clean to dirty method."
C. Prep only out to border of dressing. The number of gauze sponges necessary varies and is determined by their being clean after prepping.	
12. Prep skin with iodine solution in same manner as above.	12. Iodine is antibacterial and antifungal.
A. Use a 2-minute scrub.	
B. Allow iodine to air-dry.	
C. Concentrate half the time on the insertion site.	
13. Prep skin with isopropyl alcohol solution until all traces of iodine are removed; allow alcohol to evaporate fully.	13. Iodine left on the skin may burn it. Traces of wet alcohol may combine with the povidone-iodine ointment and burn the skin.
14. Apply povidone-iodine ointment on double-thickness gauze to catheter insertion site.	
15. Remove sterile gloves.	

ACTION	RATIONALE
16. Spray surrounding skin with tincture of benzoin; allow benzoin to dry until sticky.	16. Wet benzoin can cause poor adhesion of dressing and/or skin irritation later.
17. Cover catheter with sterile, plastic, adhesive-backed drape.	17. This placement at the catheter hub allows access to it later for IV tubing change.
A. Place drape halfway down catheter hub to create approximately a 1″ border around gauze.	
B. Make sure patient's arm is abducted so that dressing will not bind.	B. If dressing binds it could prevent range of motion.
C. Do not touch adhesive back of drape.	C. This will contaminate it.
18. Apply tape to lateral and upper edge of drape.	
19. Make a ½″ slit in tape to be applied to lower border of drape; place this slit piece of tape up under catheter hub and then seal lower border.	19. This insures occlusion at the catheter hub.
20. Place a piece of tape along lower border, over (and halfway down) catheter hub (Fig. 138).	20. This helps to stabilize the catheter hub.
21. Secure all IV tubing and catheter hub junctions with tape.	21. This prevents accidental tubing separation.
22. Anchor filter (or IV tubing if a filter is not used) to drape on patient's skin.	22. This prevents catheter dislodgment by focusing inadvertent tension here rather than on the insertion site.
23. Label dressing with date and initials. Write on the basic dressing and not on the anchoring tape, which may be removed.	

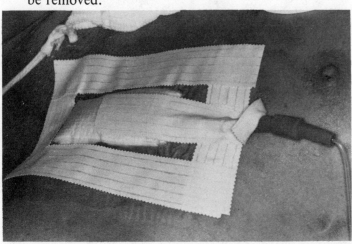

Figure 138. Subclavian dressing.

PRECAUTIONS

1. Substitute alcohol as a defatting agent if the patient is sensitive to acetone.
2. Use povidone-iodine solution if the patient is sensitive to iodine. If povidone-iodone is nonirritating (this is almost always the case) leave it on the skin—i.e., do not remove it with alcohol. Povidone-iodone solution is long-lasting and effective even after drying. Also, its removal by alcohol could create a strong tincture of iodine, which is very irritating to the skin.
3. Substitute one of the adhesive sprays used in ileostomy care (e.g., Hollister adhesive), if tincture of benzoin irritates the skin.
4. Substitute either a sterile, cloth, adhesive-backed tape or try Op-Site if the sterile, plastic, adhesive-backed drape irritates the skin. Op-Site is also waterproof, but it allows moisture vapor beneath it to escape while still affording sterile protection from the environment. If Op-Site is used, omit tincture of benzoin spray and do not surround the upper and lateral edges of the dressing with tape—i.e., only the bottom edge should have tape on it.

RELATED CARE

1. Protect the basic dressing with additional tape if the type of tape used to secure the IV tubing-catheter hub junction and to anchor the filter (or tubing) to the dressing tears the dressing (likely with the plastic drape or Op-Site).
2. Waterproof a cloth dressing (Fig. 139) with a plastic drape in patients:
   A. With tracheostomy or with draining wounds.
   B. In high humidity areas.
   C. With oxygen apparatus that beads moisture.
   D. With nasogastric tubes.

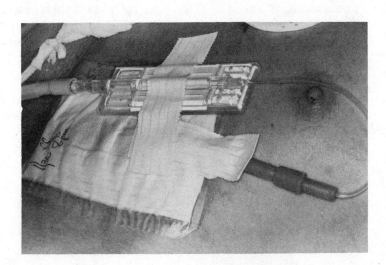

Figure 139. Waterproofed cloth dressing.

COMPLICATION

Sepsis (if dressing not maintained properly)

REFERENCES

Colley, R.: Total parenteral nutrition—nursing approach. *In* Plumer, A.L.: Principles in Practice of I.V. Therapy, 2nd ed., Boston, Little Brown and Company, 1975, pp. 185–213.
Ryan, J.A., Abel, R.M., Abbott, W.M., Hopkins, C.C., Chesney, T.M., Colley, R., Phillips, K., and Fischer, J.E.: Catheter complications in total parenteral nutrition. A prospective study of 200 patients. N. Engl. J. Med., *290*:757–761, 1974.

TOTAL PARENTERAL NUTRITION INTRAVENOUS TUBING AND FILTER CHANGE

OVERVIEW

IV tubing for TPN must be changed every 24 hours. This is a reasonable standard of care, and follows the recommendations of the Center for Disease Control (CDC) in Atlanta. More frequent tubing changes should be unnecessary, and may even increase the risk of bacterial contamination because they involve multiple daily manipulations of the catheter hub-IV tubing junction. It is crucial for the actual procedure to be done aseptically, and that air embolism precautions be taken.

If a filter is used, the choice should be determined by patient and institutional need. There are filters currently available that are fine enough (0.2 micron porosity) to trap both particulate matter and all bacterial and fungal organisms. These filters also have the capacity to eliminate air and to maintain a normal gravity flow rate for 24 hours, even with hypertonic solutions.

This method is written for a gravity infusion; if positive pressure infusion apparatus is used to deliver the infusion, make sure that the pounds per square inch (p.s.i.) pressure tolerance of the filter is not exceeded by the pump.

OBJECTIVES

1. To change the IV tubing and final filter in an aseptic, efficient manner.
2. To minimize the potential risk for microemboli.

SPECIAL EQUIPMENT

TPN infusion bottle
IV tubing—standard adult tubing, unless rate is less than 30 ml./hr.
0.2-micron filter
Aseptic hemostat
Sterile needle
Aseptic adhesive tape
Infusion regulation flow control clamp

METHOD

ACTION	RATIONALE
1. Wash hands thoroughly and degerm with surgical scrub solution.	
2. Make sure TPN solution is as prescribed by physician; check expiration date of solution.	
3. Inspect solution against a strong light for cloudiness, turbidity, or particulate matter; also inspect solution container for cracks (in a bottle) or minute punctures (in a bag).	3. This could indicate solution contamination, in which case its use is contraindicated.
4. Be certain that solution container is waterproof and airtight.	4. This guarantees asepsis.
5. Remove protective covering from IV bottle.	
6. Clamp off IV tubing.	
7. Remove protective covering from IV tubing.	
8. Spike IV bottle.	
9. Invert bottle, fill drip chamber, and prime IV tubing; purge tubing of all air, including air usually trapped in side-arm injection sites.	
10. Insert IV tubing into filter housing and prime filter. Follow manufacturer's specific instructions for priming a filter; all filters differ slightly.	10. Correct filling of the filter is essential to its proper operation.
11. Shut off IV solution and cover end of filter tubing with a sterile needle; label IV tubing drip chamber and filter housing with date.	11. Dating the tubing and filter helps insure that they will be changed on time.

ACTION	RATIONALE
12. Place a tape marked in hourly increments on new TPN bottle. It should be checked every 30 minutes.	12. The time tape allows for easy visualization of flow accuracy.
13. Place a second, extra infusion-regulating clamp on IV tubing. Both IV infusion regulating clamps should be used to adjust the flow rate.	13. If one fails the second one will prevent a "runaway" IV.
14. Place patient in supine position.	14. This helps to prevent air embolism.
15. Remove tape anchoring filter to the dressing and tape securing catheter hub-filter tubing junction; stabilize dressing with one hand.	15. This guards against catheter dislodgment.
16. Turn off patient's TPN infusion and instruct patient to perform Valsalva maneuver before used filter tubing is removed from catheter hub.	
17. Replace used filter tubing with new filter tubing while patient performs Valsalva maneuver.	17. Successful performance of the Valsalva maneuver creates a positive venous pressure that may cause blood backflow through the catheter.
A. Grasp catheter hub with clean hemostat.	
B. Lift hub slightly up off chest wall.	B. Lifting the hub up off the chest avoids contamination.
C. Rotate old filter tubing out gently and twist new tubing in.	C. Most catheter junctions have a Luer slip fit which requires this.
18. Turn TPN infusion on; instruct patient to breathe normally again.	
19. Check all junctions for a secure fit; secure junctions with adhesive tape.	

PRECAUTIONS

1. Integrate air embolism precautions into the method.
2. Integrate aseptic technique into the method.

RELATED CARE

Option: Paint all IV tubing junctions with an antibacterial solution before disconnecting them. Although this has not been required in the above method, it may be a desirable addition in some cases.

COMPLICATIONS

Sepsis
Emboli

REFERENCES

Colley, R., and Wilson, J.: Hyperalimentation: A plus for nitrogen balance. Hamilton, H. (ed.): *In:* Monitoring Fluid and Electrolytes Precisely. Horsham, Pa., Intermed Communications, 1978, pp. 183–188.

Maki, D.G., Goldman, D.A., and Rhame, F.S.: Infection control in intravenous therapy. Ann. Intern. Med., *79*:867–887, 1973.

Rapp, R.R., Bivins, B., and DeLuca, P.P.: In-line filtration of IV fluids and drugs. Am. J. I.V. Ther., *2*:18–23, 1975.

REMOVAL OF SUBCLAVIAN TOTAL PARENTERAL NUTRITION CATHETER

OBJECTIVES

1. To remove the subclavian catheter in a safe, aseptic manner.
2. To assess skin integrity at site, post-TPN catheter removal.

SPECIAL EQUIPMENT

Sterile gauze pads
Povidone-iodine ointment
Isopropyl alcohol
Plastic tape (new clean roll)
Sterile scissors

Sterile forceps
Sterile gloves
Sterile hemostat
Sterile towel
Sterile bowl

METHOD

ACTION	RATIONALE
1. Review patient's record for catheter placement note; check for description of internal venous cutdown or subcutaneous tunnel exit.	1. If either condition exists, the nurse should not remove the catheter.
2. Clamp off intravenous infusion.	
3. Wash hands thoroughly and degerm with surgical scrub solution.	
4. Open sterile towel to create sterile field and place sterile equipment on it.	
5. Fill sterile bowl with alcohol.	
6. Squeeze povidone-iodine ointment onto sterile sponge.	
7. Place patient in a supine position without a pillow.	7. This helps to prevent air embolism.

ACTION	RATIONALE

8. Expose catheter insertion site.
9. Don sterile gloves.
10. Prep catheter insertion site and surrounding skin with alcohol; allow alcohol to dry. Prep in same manner as described in method for "Total Parenteral Nutrition Catheter Site Care."
11. Remove suture at insertion site, using scissors and forceps. If suture is difficult to cut, a pediatric suture set may be easier to use.
12. Remove catheter.
   A. Grasp catheter at distal end with sterile forceps and *withdraw slowly*.
   B. Have patient perform Valsalva maneuver as catheter is withdrawn.
   C. Do not force catheter removal; if it is difficult to remove:
      (1) Stop.
      (2) Tape catheter in place.
      (3) Notify physician immediately.
13. After catheter is removed:

   A. Apply povidone-iodine to insertion site *immediately* while sterile forceps hold catheter.

                    A. Occlusion of this site maintains asepsis and prevents air embolism if tract formation exists.

   B. Observe catheter for correct length and normal tip.

                    B. Expected catheter length varies according to catheter inserted, and should have been noted in the patient's record at the time of catheter insertion.

14. Apply dressing.
   A. Secure dressing with plastic tape.
   B. Layer tape to make a totally occlusive seal.
15. Observe dressing for active bleeding, hematoma formation, or edema. If bleeding occurs:
   A. Apply direct pressure.
   B. Notify physician immediately.

ACTION   **RATIONALE**

16. Label dressing with date and time applied and with notice to leave it on, occlusive, for 72 hours.
17. Activate nursing care plan to re-check insertion site in 72 hours. It should be closed; if not, apply a new occlusive dressing immediately.

PRECAUTION

Integrate air embolism precautions into the method.

RELATED CARE

Culture the catheter if sepsis is suspected. See the method for "Culturing a Total Parenteral Nutrition Subclavian Venous Catheter."

COMPLICATIONS

Catheter embolism
Exudate or fibrin sheath on internal portion of catheter (indicating possibility of infection).

CULTURING A TOTAL PARENTERAL NUTRITION SUBCLAVIAN VENOUS CATHETER _____

OBJECTIVE

To culture the catheter tip in the most effective manner when catheter-related sepsis is suspected.

SPECIAL EQUIPMENT

See equipment list for "Removal of a Subclavian TPN Catheter," plus:
Sterile culture tube
Sterile scissors
Sterile wound culture tube

METHOD

ACTION	RATIONALE

1. Follow method for "Removal of a Subclavian TPN Catheter," steps 1 through 12.
2. After catheter has been withdrawn and is still being kept up and away from skin, proceed with following steps.

NOTE:
*The following steps must be done **swiftly**, as the patient continues to perform the Valsalva maneuver. Failure to maintain this maneuver increases the danger of air embolism. Concern with this persists until the occlusive dressing is covering the catheter exit site.*

3. Milk wound, attempting to express pus, after catheter removal.

   3. Pus could indicate suppurative thrombophlebitis—a very serious complication requiring immediate physician diagnosis and treatment.

4. Culture any pus expressed, using sterile wound culture tube.
5. Note any redness, edema, warmth, or palpable hardness at or near wound.

   5. This could indicate phlebitis, thrombosis, or sepsis.

6. Apply povidone-iodine ointment gauze to insertion site immediately while holding catheter with sterile forceps.

   6. Occlusion of this site maintains asepsis and prevents air embolism if tract formation exists.

7. Observe catheter for correct length and normal tip.

   7. Expected catheter length varies according to catheter inserted, and should have been noted in the patient's record at the time of catheter insertion.

8. Culture catheter tip.
   A. Take second pair of sterile scissors and cut catheter several millimeters inside former skin surface portion.
   B. Drop catheter tip segment into sterile culture tube and recover tube.
9. Apply dressing.
   A. Secure dressing with plastic tape.
   B. Layer tape to make a totally occlusive seal.

ACTION	**RATIONALE**
10. Observe dressing for active bleeding, hematoma formation, or edema. If bleeding occurs: A. Apply direct pressure. B. Notify physician immediately.	
11. Label dressing with date and time applied and with notice to leave it on, occlusive, for 72 hours.	
12. Activate nursing care plan to reassess insertion site in 72 hours. It should be closed; if not, apply a new occlusive dressing immediately.	
13. Hand-carry catheter culture to laboratory immediately after dressing application.	13. This prevents the specimen from drying out.
14. Request that the laboratory perform a semiquantitative culture.	14. This method involves the use of a sheep blood agar plate (see Maki references, below).

PRECAUTION

Integrate air embolism precautions into the method.

RELATED CARE

Complete fever work-up to determine its etiology.

COMPLICATIONS

Catheter embolism

Exudate or fibrin sheath on internal portion of catheter (indicating possibility of infection).

REFERENCES

Maki, D.G., Jarrett, F., and Sarafin, H.W.: A semiquantitative culture method for identification of catheter-related-infection in the burn patient. J. Surg. Res. *22*:513–520, 1977.

Maki, D.G., Weise, C.E., and Sarafin, H.W.: A semiquantitative culture method for identifying intravenous-catheter-related infection. N. Engl. J. Med., *296*(No. 23):1305–1309, 1977.

LIPID THERAPY

Rita Colley, R.N.

ADMINISTRATION OF INTRAVENOUS LIPIDS

OVERVIEW

There are presently two brands of intravenous fat commercially available in the United States—Intralipid 10%, a soybean emulsion and Liposyn 10%, a safflower emulsion. Both are isotonic emulsions (280 m.Osm./liter) and may be administered peripherally. They contain 1.1 calories per ml.

There are two main indications for administering IV fat: (1) to prevent or treat essential fatty acid deficiency; and (2) to enjoy the high caloric yield of fat. Essential fatty acid deficiency is a state that may be more common than formerly believed. Some typical symptoms are thrombocytopenia, thinning hair, dry or scaled skin, and liver function abnormalities. Chemical confirmation of this deficiency state is possible.

Infusion of IV fat requires specific guidelines. Stability of the emulsion needs to be maintained in order to prevent infusion of fat particles that may not be visible to the naked eye.

OBJECTIVE

To administer intravenous fat in a safe, efficient manner, with full awareness of possible complications.

SPECIAL EQUIPMENT

500-ml. bottle Intralipid 10%
"Cutter Saftiset" IV tubing (supplied with Intralipid)

METHOD

ACTION	RATIONALE
1. Before infusing:	
A. Inspect emulsion for frothiness, separation, or oily appearance.	A. These could indicate a cracked emulsion; administration would then be contraindicated.
B. Allow refrigerated emulsion to come to room temperature; this takes only a few minutes.	B. Cold emulsion causes pain and could produce white blanching of the skin.

ACTION	RATIONALE
(Only Intralipid must be refrigerated.	
2. Use specific IV tubing administration set provided with each bottle of IV fat; prime and connect in usual fashion.	2. Special IV tubing does not contain diethylhexyl phthalate (DEHP); fat could leech DEHP from regular IV tubing, although clinical problems have not been reported from this.
3. Infuse IV fat as a separate infusion or as a Y-type infusion connected to catheter hub. Always check compatibility of any Y-tube set-up with the pharmacist.	3. This prevents mixing with other solutions, which could cause emulsion instability.
4. Follow manufacturer's recommendations for rate and dose. Suggested guidelines for adults are as follows. A. Initial rate: 1 ml./min. for first 15 to 30 minutes (Intralipid), and for first 15 minutes (Liposyn). B. First day maximum rate: 500 ml. in 4 hours (Intralipid), and 500 ml. in 4 to 6 hours (Liposyn). C. Usual daily maximum rate: 2.5 grams/kg (Intralipid), and 3 grams/kg. (Liposyn). D. Caloric limitations should not exceed 60% of total caloric intake.	4. This allows time to notice adverse reactions and avoids overdosage.

PRECAUTIONS

1. Do not filter IV fat; it would clog the filter and might crack the emulsion.
2. Never place additives into IV fat; they could crack the emulsion.
3. Keep Intralipid refrigerated until use to maintain the stability of the emulsion; Liposyn does not require refrigeration.
4. Observe the patient carefully during the first 15 to 30 minutes of infusion; note any adverse reactions that might occur and report to physician immediately.
5. Do not interrupt IV fat infusion and/or reuse an opened bottle, since IV fat could become easily contaminated.

RELATED CARE

1. Review the *current* package insert regarding product information before administration of this drug.
2. Assess serum opacity 4 to 6 hours after terminating infusion. Serum will appear cloudy or opaque if the fat has not cleared the blood stream.

COMPLICATIONS

Thermogenic reaction	Altered hemodynamic state
Blood dyscrasias	Flank pain
Dyspnea	Anaphylaxis
Hyperlipemia	Headache
Cyanosis	Sleepiness
Flushing	Nausea
Dizziness	Vomiting
Hyperthermia	Sweating
Transient increases in liver enzymes	Chest pain

SUPPLIERS

Abbott Laboratories, North Chicago, IL, (Liposyn 10%)

Vitrum of Sweden (Intralipid 10% distributed in the U.S.A. by Cutter Laboratories, Inc., Berkeley, CA)

REFERENCES

Abbott Laboratories, North Chicago, IL, The I.V. High Energy Source, Liposyn 10%, 1979.

Cutter Medical: Berkeley, CA, Cutter Laboratories, Inc., Intravenous Nutrition Handbook. 1978.

Fischer, J.E.: Hyperalimentation. *In* Rob, Charles (ed.): Advances in Surgery, Vol. II, Chicago, Year Book Medical Publishers, 1977.

Miles, Richard: Personal Communication. (Cutter Medical, division of Cutter Laboratories, Inc.) 1978.

SAFETY

INFECTION SURVEILLANCE IN THE CRITICAL CARE UNIT

Elaine Larson, R.N., M.A.

OVERVIEW

Infection control measures in the critical care unit may or may not effectively reduce the incidence of nosocomial acquisition of infections. The impact of measures instituted must be evaluated continually in conjunction and cooperation with the total hospital infection surveillance program.

A formal infection control and surveillance program should ideally be developed by an Infection Control Practitioner (ICP). However, in the absence of an ICP, a nurse with expertise and interest in infection control should be designated as a liaison between the unit and other hospital departments, especially between infection control committee members and personnel concerned with surveillance. Responsibilities of the ICP (or nurse designated by the infection control committee) include the steps presented in the method, below.

OBJECTIVES

1. To identify endemic and epidemic organisms which are present in the critical care unit.
2. To be informed of infection rates in the unit.
3. To evaluate the effectiveness of infection control measures instituted and practiced in the unit.

METHOD

ACTION	RATIONALE
1. Review monthly infection reports from hospital infection control officer.	1. A monthly review helps to note trends in infection within the unit and identify the presence of epidemic or endemic strains in the unit rapidly.
2. Establish, review, and maintain unit infection control policies with hospital infection control officer and infection control committee. The hospital infection control committee should review these policies and procedures annually.	2. This ensures the updating and conformance of policies and procedures with accepted standards of practice, and aids in compliance with Joint Commission on Accreditation of Hospitals standards.
3. Review and interpret critical care unit policies and collected data with personnel in unit.	

ACTION	RATIONALE
4. Assist with defining unit infection control needs.	
5. Interpret infection control needs and communicate them to appropriate departments and personnel.	
6. Coordinate efforts to evaluate effectiveness of unit infection control practices.	
7. Use environmental sampling judiciously and sparingly. This includes cultures of such fomites as walls, floors, irrigating fluids, electrodes, sinks, etc. Valid reasons for environmental sampling are to: A. Search for fomites of a specific organism which is causing nosocomial infection problems. B. Document necessity for improved cleaning procedures. C. Increase personnel sensitivity and awareness of potential role of environment in infection control.	7. Results are difficult to interpret and do not necessarily reflect direct risk to patients.
8. Minimize air sampling, as it is of limited use. Use only to: A. Establish quantity of airborne organisms in case of unit crowding. B. Establish quality of airborne organisms in case of an epidemic situation (Fig. 140).	8. Results are difficult to interpret; airborne contamination plays a relatively small part in nosocomial acquisition of most organisms.
9. Establish critical care unit standing policies for routine patient culturing at sites of clinical symptoms of infection, as follows. A. Respiratory: when purulent, bloody, or foul tracheal secretions are present. B. Wound or skin: when purulence, redness, and/or induration are present with or without insertion of catheters, tubes, etc. C. Urinary: when urine is foul-smelling or cloudy.	

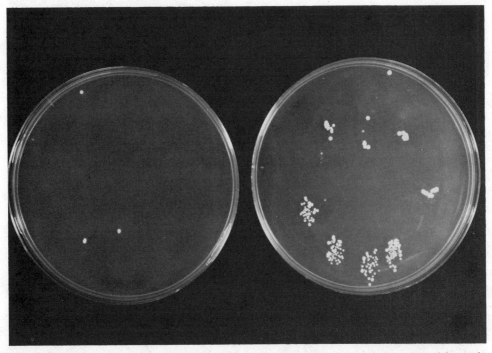

Figure 140.   The transmission of organisms via air and hands. The culture plate on the left shows bacterial growth after an hour's air sampling using the Mattson-Garvin slit air sampler. There are three colonies of skin flora present. The culture plate on the right shows bacterial growth from an ICU employee's fingers. The organisms are too numerous to count. Both samples were taken in a six-bed medical-surgical ICU during the same time period. Plates were incubated at 37° C. for 48 hours.

ACTION	RATIONALE
10. Integrate microbiologic culture reports of patients into nursing assessment and care.	10. This aids personnel in becoming informed of organisms present in the unit.
A. Teach personnel the normal flora of body sites, symptoms of infection, and common opportunistic and more virulent pathogens.	A. This enables personnel to interpret culture results adequately.
B. Note antibiotic sensitivities of organisms reported. Notify physician if patient is receiving an antibiotic to which the organism(s) present is resistant.	B. An antibiotic will be ineffective if organism(s) present are resistant; inadequate or inappropriate antibiotic usage encourages the growth of resistant strains.

PRECAUTIONS

These are an integral part of the method.

RELATED CARE

1. Review and revise policies annually, utilizing appropriate resources.
2. Involve support services in development of protocols regarding environmental and equipment cleaning, and encourage compliance.

COMPLICATIONS

Late detection of infection sources, agents, and infections
Infection

REFERENCES

Brand, L.: A practical approach to infection surveillance in the intensive care unit. Heart Lung, 5:788, 1976.

Hargiss, C.: Personal communication. Seattle, University of Washington Hospital, 1978.

Northey, D., et al.: Microbial surveillance in a surgical intensive care unit. Surg. Gynecol. Ob., 139:321, 1974.

U.S. Department of Health, Education and Welfare: Guidelines for determining presence and classification of Infection. In: Outline for Surveillance and Control of Nosocomial Infections, Appendix II. Atlanta, U.S. Department of Health, Education, and Welfare, 1976.

INFECTION CONTROL IN THE CRITICAL CARE UNIT

Elaine Larson, R.N., M.A.

OVERVIEW

Approximately one in four patients in critical care units acquires nosocomial organisms if the stay is more than 3 days, with the risk increasing as the stay is prolonged. Because personnel are the key to infection control, all control measures implemented must place major emphasis on the role of the multidisciplinary health care personnel.

Methods for three measures for infection control—personnel, equipment, and environment—are presented. The objectives are the same for all three methods.

OBJECTIVES

1. To minimize the risk of infection to the critically ill patient by:
   A. Meticulous hand washing and personal hygiene of personnel.
   B. Appropriate sterilization, cleaning, and monitoring of equipment which contacts the patient.
   C. Instituting, maintaining, and monitoring housekeeping procedures, especially those related to floors, sinks, storage, and utility rooms.
2. To prevent patient-to-patient spread of organisms by means of personnel, fomites, contact, or air.
3. To segregate patients of potential hazard to others by:
   A. Establishing and maintaining isolation policies for the unit.
   B. Practicing satisfactory containment technique.

INFECTION CONTROL MEASURES: PERSONNEL

METHOD

ACTION	RATIONALE
1. Establish hand washing policies and dress code for unit. A. Educate all new employees concerning these policies. B. Provide intermittent (biannual) re-education of personnel. 2. Provide adequate hand washing facilities.	

447

ACTION	RATIONALE
A. If a soap dispenser is not used, use soap rack with adequate drainage and small bars; dispensers and soap racks must be cleaned routinely.	A. Contaminated dispensers have been associated with nosocomial infections. Soap, especially in a pool of liquid, may support the growth of microbes.
B. Check sinks for splashing; if splashing occurs: (1) Lower water pressure; or (2) Erect splash guards; or (3) Insert faucet filters; however, they must be cleaned every month.	B. Splashing will contaminate clothing. (3) Filters can harbor organisms.
3. Provide an acceptable hand washing agent; most soaps or antiseptics are acceptable. A. Choose an agent using following criteria: (1) Effectiveness against organisms most commonly found in unit. (2) Cost effectiveness. (3) Having least undesirable side effects (skin drying, burning).	3. Although some antiseptics are more active against certain organisms, technique and frequency of hand washing are as important as the agent used.
B. Agents include: (1) Hexachlorophene. This may be preferable if staphylococci are a problem.	(1) Hexachlorophene is effective only against gram-positive organisms; its effectiveness is increased with duration of use.
(2) Iodophors. These are preferable if gram-negative organisms (e.g., *Escherichia, coli, Serratia, Klebsiella, Pseudomonas*) are a problem.	(2) Iodophors are effective against gram-negative and gram-positive organisms, fungi, and some viruses.
(3) 70% alcohol. Its use should be limited to those occasions when hand washing facilities are poor or unavailable.	(3) 70% alcohol will adequately disinfect skin in 15 to 20 seconds, but is very drying.
(4) Other agents. (a) Bar soaps adequately remove transient organisms.	

ACTION	RATIONALE
(b) Chlorhexidine (Hibiclens) is effective against both gram-negative and gram-positive organisms; its residual effectiveness lasts up to six hours (in the absence of recontamination).	
(c) Aqueous benzalkonium chloride (Zephiran) is *not* an acceptable skin cleanser.	
4. Employ effective hand washing technique.	4. Hand washing is the most effective infection control measure available.
A. Lather and rub with friction for at least 15 seconds under a stream of warm water.	
B. Rinse and dry with a paper towel.	
C. Turn off faucet with another dry paper towel.	C. Organisms are spread from a contaminated faucet through a wet towel.
D. Wash hands before each patient contact.	
E. Remove all rings other than plain bands.	E. Organisms are difficult to remove from crevices.
F. Remove cracked or chipped nail polish.	
5. Prevent skin drying and dermatitis of hands.	5. Dry, cracked skin harbors more organisms.
A. Alternate agents or use bar soap if a hand washing agent is too drying.	
B. Wear gloves, especially during high risk procedures such as intravenous cannulation and wound care.	
C. Use hand creams with caution.	C. Hand creams are easily contaminated and are a known cause of nosocomial infections.
(1) Use small containers with "squirt" lids (*not* lids that will unscrew).	

ACTION	RATIONALE
(2) Discard when empty, or clean thoroughly and refill routinely.	
(3) Avoid hand cream application immediately after hand washing while in critical care unit; apply while off duty (coffee or lunch breaks, times away from direct patient care).	(3) This decreases the chance of causing infections due to contaminated hand cream and may reduce the residual effect of antiseptics.
6. Protect patients from organisms spread on clothing and hair. A. Wear scrub attire or other washable clothing not worn outside the hospital, and which is changed daily. A clean gown or lab coat must be worn when leaving unit. B. Wear hair pulled back or covered. C. Have visitors don clean gown when entering critical care unit; upon leaving unit, gown is discarded.	6. Clothing and hair are demonstrated fomites of infection.
7. Minimize traffic in unit (especially during sterile or invasive procedures).	7. Increased movement increases bacterial movement in the air.
8. Ensure that entry into unit is through a "clean" area (not through a dirty utility room, for example).	
9. Require participation of all unit personnel in hospital employee health program. A. Keep records of immunization, chest x-rays, or tuberculin tests up to date. B. If renal dialysis or transplant patients are cared for in unit, adopt policies for hepatitis surveilance of personnel and patients.	
10. Exclude personnel and visitors with bacterial infections from the unit;	

ACTION	RATIONALE
these include common cold, influenza, hepatitis, herpes, and staph or strep infections.	
11. Maintain an infection control orientation and education program for all personnel in consultation with and supervised by Infection Control Practitioner (see "Infection Surveillance in the Critical Care Unit").	11. This helps to increase staff awareness regarding their responsibility in infection control.

INFECTION CONTROL MEASURES: ENVIRONMENT _____

METHOD

ACTION	RATIONALE
1. Ensure, as much as possible, that the critical care unit is ventilated adequately.	1. Certain organisms (staphylococci, pneumococci, tubercule bacilli, and others) are known to be airborne.
A. Air should be exchanged at least 12 times each hour.	A. This removes airborne organisms, preventing accumulative build-up.
B. If window fans or air conditioners are used, have filters changed routinely (at least twice a year).	B. Contaminated fans can be sources of nosocomial microbial acquisition.
C. Avoid open windows in critical care unit.	C. Contaminated outside air can increase the risk of infection to patients during invasive procedures.
D. In rooms with regulated air flow ("isolation" rooms), keep door closed, and fans off.	D. Regulated air flow is ineffective when outside air is allowed to enter or inside air is allowed to exit.
E. Avoid shaking of linen, and violent curtain pulling.	E. Organisms become airborne.
2. Collaborate with housekeeping personnel in setting up critical care unit procedures, especially regarding:	2. This decreases the possibility of nosocomial infections acquired through contact with contaminated surfaces.
A. Mopping technique with schedule.	
B. Terminal cleaning after patient leaves unit.	

ACTION	RATIONALE

C. Cleaning of surfaces and pa-
    tient areas. All surfaces should
    be cleaned daily and *immedi-
    ately* after contaminated with
    blood or other body fluids.
D. Cleaning of sinks.
E. Cleaning agents.
F. Methods for evaluating clean-
    ing effectiveness.

3. Segregate clean and dirty areas;
    place linens and other clean supplies
    in least trafficked, most protected
    areas.

4. Prohibit from admission, when pos-
    sible, patients with influenza and
    viral upper respiratory infections,
    especially during epidemic seasons.

    4. These may cause severe pulmonary
        complications in the debilitated pa-
        tient whose defense systems are im-
        paired.

5. For infected patients requiring in-
    tensive care, use hospital standards
    outlined and accepted for isolation
    techniques. Single room isolation
    facilities must be provided, prefer-
    ably with hand washing facilities.

    5. Effective isolation techniques cannot
        be carried out in curtained cubicles.

INFECTION CONTROL MEASURES: EQUIPMENT _____

METHOD

ACTION	RATIONALE

1. Incorporate infection control prin-
    ciples into all patient care activi-
    ties associated with infection risk.
    A. Procedures of particular con-
        cern include:
        (1) Insertion of intravascular
             needles and catheters.

        (2) Use of respiratory therapy
             equipment.
        (3) Insertion and care of
             urinary catheters.

1. Decreases risk to patients, visitors,
    and staff.

        (1) These have been demon-
             strated to be the major
             causes of nosocomial infec-
             tions.

ACTION   RATIONALE

    (4) Use of thermometers.
    (5) Care of intubated patients.
    (6) Wound care.
    (7) Total parenteral nutrition (hyperalimentation).
  B. Carefully assess need for invasive techniques.
  C. Help maintain strict asepsis when such procedures are performed in unit.
  D. Evaluate written procedures of these activities to ensure that they delineate infection control measures.
2. Establish and maintain a cleaning schedule for emergency equipment, including defibrillator, pacemakers, intubation, and resuscitation equipment.

PRECAUTION

Hexacholorophine has been demonstrated to cause neurologic toxicity in infants and in adults after massive exposure of mucous membranes.

REFERENCES

Altemeier, W. et al. (ed.): Manual on Control of Infections in Surgical Patients. Philadelphia, J. B. Lippincott, 1976.

American Hospital Association: Infection Control in the Hospital, 3rd ed. Chicago, American Hospital Association, 1974.

Berk, J., et al.: Handbook of Critical Care. Boston, Little Brown and Company, 1976.

Infection Control. Chicago, Standards Adopted by Board of Commissioners of Joint Commission on Accreditation of Hospitals, 1975.

Kimbrough, R.D.: Review of recent evidence of toxic effects of hexachlorphene. Pediatrics, 51 (Suppl.):391, 1973.

Larson, E.: Hands: The healers and killers. Topics Clin. Nurs., 1:59, 1979.

Levenson, S., and Laufman, H.: Infection hazard of surgical intensive care: Isolation procedures in the surgical intensive care unit. In Kinney, J.M. (ed.): Manual of Surgical Intensive Care. Philadelphia, W.B. Saunders.

Steere, A., and Mallison, G.: Handwashing practices for the prevention of nosocomial infections. Ann. Intern. Med., 83:683, 1975.

U.S. Department of Health Education and Welfare: Isolation Techniques for Use in Hospitals, 2nd ed. Atlanta, U.S. Department of Health, Education, and Welfare, 1975, Superintendent of Documents. Stock No. 017-023-00094-2.

Kit Stahler, R.N., M.S.N. and
Neil Miller, Ph.D.

ELECTRICAL SAFETY FOR PATIENTS AND MEDICAL DEVICE OPERATORS

OVERVIEW

A simple analogy can be made between electricity and the cardiovascular system. Electricity and blood can be envisioned as having distribution and return systems. Current (amps) corresponds with blood flow, and voltage (volts) with blood pressure. The current produces the physiologic effects from an electric shock.

Conductors are materials through which electricity easily flows. Examples are copper wire, blood, and ionic fluids. Insulators resist the flow of current; these include glass, rubber, and intact dry skin. Electrolyte gels are used to decrease skin resistance so that voltages generated internally can be detected externally through the intact skin.

Grounding is the most important principle in electrical safety. A ground is a low resistance electrical pathway to the earth. Its purpose is to limit or carry away undesirable leakage (stray) current from the metal cabinet of electrically operated devices. Remember to ground equipment and not the patient.

Electricity has both positive and negative physiologic effects. Positive or therapeutic effects occur from its controlled use, as in nerve stimulation, electroshock therapy (EST), defibrillation, cardioversion, and cardiac pacing. Negative or hazardous effects occur from contact with devices that have stray currents on their metal chassis. The shock resulting from contact with currents greater than 1 milliamp is termed macroshock. Causes include frayed or damaged power cords and plugs, faulty equipment, and two-wire power cords. Everyone is susceptible. Effects range from a tingling sensation to severe thermal burns.

Microshock involves contact with current less than 1 milliamp. It may be hazardous if a conductive pathway delivers all the current directly into the heart; thus, patients with a central conductive catheter are susceptible. Wire catheters directly into or in close proximity to the heart include temporary pacemaker lead wires, esophageal and tracheal electrodes, and thermistor probes. Leakage current levels of only millionths of an ampere can induce ventricular fibrillation.

The recent explosion of health care technology has vastly increased the knowledge, capability, and sophistication of patient care and has further increased the potential of electrical shock for patients and personnel. Therefore, operators of complex electronic equipment should understand the accompanying electrical hazards and initiate appropriate measures to

454

safeguard patients, themselves, and others. The combination of practical and theoretical knowledge associated with this milieu should be part of the nurse's knowledge base. Overall responsibility of the critical care nurse includes an understanding of the following:

1. Why the device is being used, what it does, and its clinical function.
2. The basic operating principles and mechanics of the device—how it works and how it is applied.
3. The device's unique problems and hazards, appropriate precautions necessary to avoid adverse effects, and how to recognize its failures.
4. Psychologic relationships between the patient, equipment, and operator which may create insecurity, fear, or overdependence.
5. One's own limitations, especially of how and when to request help, training, or service assistance.

OBJECTIVES

1. To provide an electrically safe environment through application of basic electrical principles and associated precautions.
2. To identify nursing responsibilities associated with the safe and effective use of equipment.
3. To utilize clinical engineering in an effective equipment control program to conduct periodic testing, maintenance, calibration, and pre-equipment use inspection, plus consultation during equipment procurement, and staff education.

METHOD

ACTION	RATIONALE
1. Use electrically operated equipment that has been inspected for safety within the last 6 months. The tag on the device should indicate the date of the last inspection.	1. This helps to avoid using hazardous equipment that is malfunctioning or deteriorating. Equipment can still operate with unobservable defective ground connections.
2. Inspect equipment for electric hazards, such as: A. Cracked or frayed line cords and cables. B. Inadequate strain relief. C. Broken or defective connectors, knobs, and switches. D. Damaged or lack of U.L. listed three-prong plugs (identified by a green dot).	2. This is done in order to identify, remove from service, label, and report hazardous equipment.

ACTION	RATIONALE
3. Insure that all equipment is plugged into properly grounded receptacles (wall outlets) that are tested at least annually to insure adequate ground connections.	3. This protects the patient from hazards associated with leakage (stray or faulty) current.

4. Isolate patient from ground.
  A. Use equipment with isolated patient inputs (monitors with isolated front ends).
  B. If the patient is in an electric bed, make sure the bed is either double-insulated or equipped with an isolation transformer.
	4. This prevents the patient from acting as an inadvertent pathway to the ground by effectively separating him/her from the power distribution system.

5. Remove discontinued and unused electrically operated equipment from bedside.	5. This decreases the possibility of accidental damage or failure, resulting in electrical hazards.
6. Prohibit use of ungrounded, patient-owned electrically operated equipment (e.g., razors, radios, hair dryers, fans and *rechargeable* battery-operated units.	6. This eliminates the risk of introducing unsafe equipment into the patient's environment.
7. Turn equipment to "off" position before unplugging.	7. This prevents arcing (sparks) which may cause fires or a secondary startle reaction.
8. Remove plug from wall outlet by grasping plug rather than line cord; pull steadily and straight out.	8. This prevents unobservable and potentially dangerous damage to the line cord and plug.
9. Insure that there are meaningful and ongoing continuing education sessions provided jointly by Staff Development and Clinical Engineering Departments.	9. This promotes a continuing awareness of the safe use of complex electrical equipment in the clinical environment.

PRECAUTIONS

1. Avoid:
    A. Use of equipment that fails inspection.
    B. Use of extension cords.
    C. Use of cheater adapters.
    D. Use of equipment that shocks, sparks, or smokes.
    E. Ungrounded equipment in the patient's environment.
    F. Use of patient-owned appliances in the patient's environment.
    G. Simultaneous contact with the patient and equipment housing.
    H. Storage and spillage of liquids on electrical equipment.
    I. Dangling or kinking patient cables and power cords.

   J.   Draping power cords on pipes or plumbing, or laying them on a wet surface.
2. Do not depend upon equipment failure to warn you of hazardous currents.
3. Identify and remove equipment causing 60 Hertz (cycle) interference on cardiac monitors.
4. Also see "Electrical Safety Precautions for Patients with Direct Conduction Pathways to the Myocardium."

RELATED CARE

Maintain log of records provided by Clinical Engineering Department regarding preventive maintenance, electrical safety checks, and maintenance performed.

COMPLICATIONS

Macroshock: startle reactions, neurologic dysfunction, burns, and ventricular fibrillation
Microshock: ventricular fibrillation

ELECTRICAL TERMS

Alternating current (AC): An electrical current which reverses its direction of flow periodically. In the U.S., AC current cycles or reverses exactly 60 times a second. 60 cycles per second and 60 Hertz (Hz) are synonymous. Related terms are line power, line cord, wall current, interference.

Ampere (amp): A unit of electrical current; the number of electrons passing a given point per second. Fuses and circuit breakers help protect against potentially hazardous current overload.

Chassis: The metal housing, frame, or cabinet of electrical devices.

Circuit: A closed electrical pathway. Electricity does not flow through an open system.

Conductor: A material through which electricity easily flows.

Direct current (DC): An electrical current which flows through a circuit in one direction. It is produced by a battery (chemical reaction). Battery-operated devices include defibrillators, monitors, oxygen analyzers, and pacemakers.

Fuse: A disposable switch that opens and stops the flow of electricity whenever the electrical current is too high. A circuit breaker is similar but is reusable.

Ground: A low resistance electrical pathway to the earth. The ground wire connects the chassis to the earth. One grounds equipment, not the patient. Related terms are three-pronged plug, safety, green, or ground wire, sink or water pipe, and radiator.

Insulator: A material highly resistant to the flow of electricity. There are no perfect insulators.

Leakage current: Current that has strayed from its usual pathway and is seeking ground. Source: AC. Associated terms: chassis fault and damaged or poorly designed equipment.

Voltage: Electrical pressure or potential, the driving force that causes current to flow.

Watt: The electrical measure of power.

REFERENCES

American Association of Critical Care Nurses: Position paper on the roles of professional nursing students and faculty in critical care units. Heart Lung, 5(No. 2):193–194, 1976.

Andreoli, K., et al.: Comprehensive Cardiac Care: A Handbook for Nurses and Other Paramedic Personnel, 2nd ed. St. Louis, C. V. Mosby, 1977 pp.141–143.

Electrical safety. Health Devices 3:ES 3–23, 239–261, 1974.

Jackle, M., Ceronsky, C., and Petersen, J.: Nursing students' experience in critical care: Implications for staff development. Heart Lung, 6(No. 4):685, 1977.

Mylrea, K.C., and O'Neil, B.: Electricity and electrical safety in the hospital. Nurs. '76, 6:59, 1976.

ELECTRICAL SAFETY PRECAUTIONS FOR PATIENTS WITH DIRECT CONDUCTION PATHWAYS TO MYOCARDIUM ⎯⎯⎯

OBJECTIVE

To establish minimum essential precautions that reduce electrical hazards to patients with direct cardiac conductors.

METHOD

ACTION	RATIONALE
1. Wear rubber gloves when working with conductive pathways to myocardium.	1. Temporary pacemaker catheters and saline-filled central venous, pulmonary artery, and left atrial catheters provide low resistance current pathways to the myocardium.
2. Avoid contact with conductive ends of catheters while touching electrical equipment or metal parts of bed.	2. Minute alternating current levels can induce ventricular fibrillation.

ACTION	RATIONALE
3. Use only properly grounded equipment in vicinity of these patients.	3. This reduces the risk of leakage current that may be conducted directly to the myocardium.
4. Ensure that defibrillation equipment is immediately available.	4. There is a potential risk for stimulating the myocardium in the vulnerable period of the cardiac cycle which could produce ventricular fibrillation.
5. Provide continuous dysrhythmia monitoring of patients with direct cardiac conductors.	5. This permits observation and determination of dysrhythmias and their appropriate treatment.
6. Use a 5% dextrose in water infusion for fluid-filled catheters inserted to or in myocardium.	
7. Provide special attention to the following for temporary transvenous pacemaker catheters.	
A. Use battery-powered rather than line-operated devices when being connected to pacemaker terminal.	A. This reduces the possibility of transmitting leakage current.
B. Check for strong electrical fields; these are usually evidenced by erratic deflection of sense/pace indicator needle to left.	B. This may interfere with demand function.
C. Protect pacemaker, catheter, and connections from moisture.	C. Moisture or fluid may cause malfunction of the pacemaker.

PRECAUTIONS

1. Maintain constant alertness for potential risk sources.
2. Minimize electrical equipment in use.
3. Also see precautions for "Electrical Safety for Patients and Medical Device Operators."

RELATED CARE

1. Insure that inspection and preventive maintenance programs are performed.
2. Maintain a log of pacemaker battery usage.
3. Also see related care for "Electrical Safety for Patients and Medical Device Operators."

COMPLICATIONS

Macroshock: startle reactions, neurologic dysfunction, burns, and ventricular fibrillation
Microshock: ventricular fibrillation

REFERENCES

Hoechst Pharmaceutical, Inc.: The Heart and Electrical Hazards: Directions in Cardiovascular Medicine. Somerville, NJ. Hoechst Pharmaceutical.
Hoenig, S.A., and Scott, D.H.: Medical Instrumentation and Electrical Safety: The View from the Nursing Station. New York, John Wiley & Sons, 1977.
Medtronics, Inc.: External Pacemaker. Minneapolis, Medtronics.

ORGAN DONATION

ORGAN DONATION

Peggy J. Reiley, R.N., M.S.

OVERVIEW

Critical care nurses play a vital role in facilitating organ donation by recognizing potential organ donors. This section will deal mainly with kidney donation, since it is the organ transplanted most often. Although the donation of tissues such as eyes, skin, and bone will not be presented in detail, reference will be made when appropriate.

Since 1971 all 50 states have adopted a form of the Uniform Anatomical Gift Act. This act legally provides anyone above the age of 18 with the right to indicate willingness to become an organ donor at the time of death, or authorizes the next of kin to donate useful organs. This intent is made known in the form of a signed document, witnessed by two people. In many

·Renew a life·   UNIFORM DONOR CARD

Please fill out and carry this card with you at all times.

of _____
              (Print or type name of donor)
In the hope that I may help others, I hereby make this anatomical gift, if medically acceptable, to take effect upon my death. The words and marks below indicate my desires.

For the purpose of transplantation, therapy, medical research or education, I give:

(U)____Any Needed Organs or Parts

(KE)___Kidneys and Eyes Only

(K)____Kidneys Only

(E)____Eyes Only

Limitations or special wishes, if any:_____

_____

Signed by the donor and the following two witnesses in the presence of each other:

DATE SIGNED _____ DATE OF BIRTH OF DONOR _____

STREET _____

CITY _____ STATE _____

SIGNATURE OF DONOR _____

WITNESS _____

WITNESS _____

This is a legal document under the Uniform Anatomical Gift Act or similar laws.

Figure 141. Both sides of a Uniform Donor Card.

states, laws have been passed whereby the intent to become an organ donor can be indicated on the driver's license. However, the Uniform Donor Card (Fig. 141) has gained increasing acceptance and provides legal authorization to remove organs.

RECOGNIZING POTENTIAL ORGAN DONORS

OBJECTIVE

To facilitate organ donation by recognizing potential donors and respecting medicolegal parameters.

METHOD

ACTION	RATIONALE
1. Legal evaluation:	
A. Ascertain if written permission has been obtained for donation of organs by potential donor or next of kin.	A. In order to remove tissues or organs, appropriate permission must be obtained.
B. Ascertain if Medical Examiner's permission has been obtained for use of organs, when appropriate.	B. The Medical Examiner's permission for the donation of organs is necessary in such cases as those that involve death within 24 hours of admission to the hospital, a homicide, suicide, or any other unnatural cause.
2. Medical evaluation:	
A. Note age of potential donor.	A. There are age limits that preclude organ donation. In most instances, the maximum age for kidney donation is 60; tissue, such as bone, also has age limits. However, age does not usually interfere with eye donation.
B. Assess health history for any pre-existing disease processes of potential donor, particularly history of: (1) Hypertension. (2) Diabetes mellitus. (3) Malignancy. (4) Hepatitis.	B. The existence of any of these disease processes may interfere with the donation of kidneys (with the exception of a primary brain tumor in the case of malignancies).

ACTION	RATIONALE
C. Assess for presence of infection or infectious process of potential donor; if sepsis is suspected, obtain cultures.	C. Known infection or septicemia interferes with all types of organ donation owing to potential for transmitting the infectious process to the recipients of the graft.
D. Confirm renal status of potential kidney donor by having following laboratory tests performed: (1) BUN. (2) Creatinine. (3) Urinalysis.	
E. Confirm neurologic status of potential kidney donor, ascertaining neurologic death.	E. When pronounced dead on the basis of neurologic evidence, the donor can be taken to the operating room for organ removal.
F. Assist in control for warm ischemia. (1) Maximum amount of time that kidneys can withstand warm ischemia (absence of blood flow in a warm body), and still function successfully when transplanted, is 60 minutes. (2) Neurologic death is not necessary for tissue donations such as eyes, skin, or bone. These tissues can withstand a much longer warm ischemia time.	F. Cardiopulmonary support continues during this time; the kidney organ is not subjected to warm ischemia.

3. Alert organ bank or transplant center in local area when medical and legal evaluation is accomplished and patient is recognized as a potential donor.

PRECAUTIONS

Evaluate the patient's legal status as a "potential organ donor": When a driver's license is coded to indicate that a person is an "organ donor," this is not sufficient data to remove the organs legally; the signature of the donor and of two witnesses is required legally.

RELATED CARE

Contact the transplant center or organ bank in the local area regarding organ, protocols, information, or questions.

COMPLICATIONS

Medical
Legal

REFERENCES

Filo, R.S.: Cadaver Renal Donor Procurement Protocol. Indianapolis, Indiana University Medical Center Renal Transplanation Program, 1977.

Interhospital Organ Bank of New England: Procedures of the Interhospital Organ Bank, Inc., Interhospital Organ Bank, Boston, MA, New York-New Jersey, 1977.

New York-New Jersey Regional Transplant Coordinators Conference: Guidelines and Procedures for Organ Donation and Transplanation, New York, N.Y., Transplant Program, 1976.

Raible, J.A.: System for increasing organ donation. N. Engl. J. Med., *292*:271, 1975.

FACILITATING ORGAN DONATION

OBJECTIVES

1. To support the person/family who is considering organ donation.
2. To ensure that the organ for donation is in optimum physiologic condition to maintain homeostasis and perfusion of the kidneys.
3. To protect the organ against potential infectious processes.

METHOD

ACTION	RATIONALE
1. Share accurate information, appropriate to geographic area, and offer positive support to person/family considering organ donation.	
2. Maintain strict sterile technique: be alert to sources of contamination such as vascular invasive techniques, catheter, tracheotomy, or wounds.	2. Development of an infectious process could, in many instances, eliminate the possibility of the patient being an acceptable organ donor.

ACTION	RATIONALE
3. Maintain an hourly urinary output with a minimum volume of 50 ml.	3. Urinary output of 50 ml. or more is a good indication that the kidneys are being well perfused.
4. Maintain systolic blood pressure at a level that will provide a urinary output of 50 ml. or more. Generally, this will be maintained when the blood pressure is approximately 100 mm. Hg.	4. Prolonged hypotension will result in decreased urinary output and subsequent poor renal perfusion.
5. If, after vigorous hydration, adequate perfusion cannot be maintained, consider use of these vasopressors, in order of preference: A. Dopamine (Intropin). B. Isoproterenol (Isuprel). C. Metaraminol bitartrate (Aramine). D. Levarterenol bitartrate (Levophed).	5. Intropin and Isuprel, although they are vasoconstrictors, do not decrease renal blood flow, whereas Aramine and Levophed have this effect.
6. Consider using mannitol or furosemide (Lasix) if an adequate output of 50 ml./hr. or more cannot be maintained despite sufficient volume replacement and an adequate blood pressure.	6. An adequate urinary output is necessary to provide protection against acute tubular necrosis in the transplanted kidney.

PRECAUTIONS

If adequate renal perfusion cannot be maintained, a rise in the levels of BUN and creatinine may make the patient an unacceptable donor.

RELATED CARE

1. Consult the transplantation center (24-hour availability) for specific protocols.
2. Obtain a physician's written order for initiating select protocol in maintaining homeostasis and kidney perfusion to facilitate organ donation.

COMPLICATIONS

Infection
Altered renal perfusion
Acute tubular necrosis

REFERENCES

Interhospital Organ Bank of New England: Procedures of the Interhospital Organ Bank, Inc. Interhospital Organ Bank, Boston, MA, 1977.

New York-New Jersey Regional Transplant Coordinators Conference: Guidelines and procedures for organ donation and transplantation. New York, N.Y., 1976.

Raible, J.A.: System for increasing organ donation. N. Engl. J. Med., *292*:271, 1975.

Veith, F.J., Fein, J.M., Tendler, M.D., et al.: Brain death. 1. A status report of medical and ethical considerations. J.A.M.A. *238*:1651–1655, 1977.

Veith, F.J., Fein, J.M., Tendler, M.D., et al.: Brain death. 2. A status report of legal considerations. J.A.M.A. *238*:1744–1748, 1977.

ORGAN PREPARATION

OBJECTIVES

1. To continue oxygenation and perfusion of the organ.
2. To provide anticipated medications that may be necessary in organ preparation for subsequent donation.

SPECIAL EQUIPMENT

Portable oxygen tank
Portable ventilator
Ambu bag
Dibenzyline, 100 mg. (if available)

Methylprednisolone (Solu Medrol), 1 gram
Heparin, 10,000 units

METHOD

ACTION	RATIONALE
1. Ascertain that donor has been pronounced dead according to neurologic criteria.	
2. Continue to maintain cadaver by ventilatory and blood pressure support until actual moment of organ removal.	2. Perfused and oxygenated kidneys until the moment of organ removal have a less chance of developing acute tubular necrosis due to ischemia.
3. Prepare following medications for anticipated use:	3. Pretreatment of donors with select medications may have a subsequent

ACTION	RATIONALE
A. Methylprednisolone (Solu-Medrol), 1 gram.	beneficial effect on the transplanted kidney.
B. Heparin, 10,000 units.	
C. Dibenzyline, 100 mg. (if available).	

4. Optional: Once kidneys are removed from a donor, they may be placed on a perfusion machine on which they can be kept viable for up to 72 hours.

PRECAUTIONS

Obtain select protocols, pharmacologic therapy, and/or plan of care for organ preparation from local transplant bank.

RELATED CARE

If a cardiac arrest should occur during the organ preparation phase, begin cardiopulmonary resuscitation immediately, transport donor to operating room, and assist in facilitating an emergency nephrectomy.

COMPLICATIONS

Cardiac arrest
Infection
Tubular necrosis

REFERENCES

Filo, R.S.: Cadaver Renal Donor Procurement Protocol. Indiana University Medical Center Renal Transplantation Program, Indianapolis. Indiana University Medical Center Renal Transplantation Protocol, 1977.

Hamburger, J., et al.: Renal Transplantation Theory and Practice, 1st ed. Baltimore, The Williams and Wilkins Company, 1972.

Interhospital Organ Bank of New England: Procedures of the Interhospital Organ Bank, Inc. Interhospital Organ Bank, Boston, MA, 1977.

New York-New Jersey Regional Transplant Coordinators Conference: Guidelines and Procedures for Organ Donation and Transplantation. New York, N.Y., New York-New Jersey, Regional Transplant Program, 1976.

APPENDIX: SAMPLE FLOW SHEETS AND LOGS

APPENDIX 1—A

INTRA-AORTIC BALLOON PUMP FLOW SHEET

PROBLEM NUMBER _____ PROBLEM NAME _____

PARAMETERS		RESULTS										
TIME												
LOGIC (EP = PE)												
DELAY												
PRIMARY INTERVAL												
FILL TIME												
TRIGGER RATE												
DIASTOLIC AUGMENTATION	4											
DIASTOLIC LOW	3											
END DIASTOLIC LOW	6											
SYSTOLE WITH BALLOON EFFECT	5											
SYSTOLE WITHOUT BALLOON EFFECT	1											
MEAN ARTERIAL PRESSURE												
CUFF B/P												
PULSE												
RHYTHM (EKG)												
CVP												
PAP												
PCWP (MEAN)												
URINE OUTPUT												
VASO - RATE OF:												
VASO - RATE OF:												
CARDIAC OUTPUT												
BALLOON FILLED: AMOUNT OF CO_2												
AMOUNT OF CO_2 REMOVED FROM BALLOON												
L PEDAL PULSE												
R PEDAL PULSE												
L RADIAL PULSE												
R RADIAL PULSE												

LEGEND

LOGIC

EP - EXHAUST PRESSURE
PE - PRESSURE EXHAUST

TRACING

IABP — INTRAAORTIC BALLOON PUMP
CVP — CENTRAL VENOUS PRESSURE
PAP — PULMONARY ARTERY PRESSURE
PCWP — PULMONARY CAPILLARY WEDGE PRESSURE

PULSES

4 + - HYPERDYNAMIC
3 + - STRONG PALPABLE
2 + - WEAK PALPABLE
1 + - INTERMITTENT PALPABLE
D - NON PALPABLE: AUDIBLE WITH DOPPLER
O - INAUDIBLE WITH DOPPLER

SIGNATURES:

FORM 1029X 6/78

INTRA-AORTIC BALLOON PUMP FLOW SHEET

APPENDIX 1—B

TODAY'S DATE	LATEST HAA STATUS & DATE	UNIT	ROOM & BED NO.
HOUR OF INITIATION		DATE OF TREATMENT	DURATION OF TREATMENT
A.M.	P.M.		

☐ STANDARD DIALYSATE COMPOSITION		☐ NON-STANDARD		☐ ADDITIONS IF ANY	
TOTAL SODIUM	135mEq/L		mEq/L	UREA	mg%
SODIUM CHLORIDE	97mEq/L		mEq/L	DEXTROSE	mg%
SODIUM ACETATE	38mEq/L		mEq/L	SODIUM BICARBONATE	mEq/L
CALCIUM CHLORIDE	3.0mEq/L		mEq/L	OTHER	
MAGNESIUM CHLORIDE	1.0mEq/L		mEq/L		
POTASSIUM CHLORIDE	____mEq/L		mEq/L		

TYPE OF DIALYSIZER

TYPE OF ACCESS

☐ CANNULAS	☐ DOUBLE NEEDLE	☐ SINGLE NEEDLE	☐ SELDINGER CATHETER
BLOOD PUMP ☐ YES ☐ NO	☐ SINGLE NEEDLE PUMP	☐ WATER CHARCOAL FILTER	BLOOD FLOW RATE (CC/MIN)

HEPARINIZATION

☐ REGIONAL	☐ CONSTANT	☐ PRIME	☐ LO DOSE	UNITS/HR.
			DESIRED PATIENT CLOTTING TIME	

MACHINE PRIME (N S, PLASMANATE, ALBUMIN, BLOOD)		
	DRY WEIGHT	WEIGHT LOSS DESIRED

NEGATIVE PRESSURE DESIRED

PARAMETERS FOR BP SUPPORT

SPECIAL INSTRUCTIONS (HEMO PERFUSION, SEIZURE PRECAUTIONS, GRADUAL INCREASE OF BLOOD FLOW RATE)

PHYSICIAN'S SIGNATURE

NO. OF MACHINE	FOR LABORATORY USE	LAB TECHNICIAN INITIAL

PATIENT NUMBER

PATIENT NAME

D.O.B.

HEMODIALYSIS ORDERS

DISTRIBUTION:
1 - ORDER BOOK
2 - KIDNEY LAB
3 - PHARMACY
4 - NURSING

UH 0623   JUL 78

1-78-1869

474

APPENDIX 1—C

DRY WEIGHT		DATE ▶							
LENGTH OF RUN /		ON-OFF							
TYPE OF DIALYSER									
ACCESS									
ACCESS CONDITION									
IF FISTULA - SINGLE OR DOUBLE NEEDLE & BRAND									
DIAYSATE CONC – K +									
BLOODFLOW - BUBBLE TIME (SEC) PUMP (C.C.)									
HEPARIN PRIME C.C.									
TOTAL OR REGIONAL HEPARINIZATION									
HEPARIN (C.C./HR.)									
PROTAMINE C.C./HR.									
AVERAGE CLOTTING TIME (MIN.) PATIENT/KIDNEY									
AVERAGE NEG. / HOURS @ THE PRES. / NEG. PRES.									
PATIENT PRIME NS / PLASMA / BLOOD									
WEIGHT		PRE							
		POST							
		CHANGE (+−)							
VITAL SIGNS	PRE	B. P.							
		PULSE							
		TEMP.							
	POST	B. P.							
		PULSE							
		TEMP.							
LAB SENT									
DATE DRAWN/RESULTS OF HAA									
CULTURES									
REMARKS (SEE PROGRESS NOTES) ▶ CHECK BOXES @ RIGHT ▶									
SIGNATURE (INIT.)		ON							
		OFF							

HEMODIALYSIS - COMPOSITE

UH 0538 REV JAN 78

1-78-61

475

APPENDIX 1—D

HEMODIALYSIS LOG

IMPRINT HERE

ON DIALYSIS	DATE		HOUR		OFF DIALYSIS	DATE		HOUR

PREDIALYSIS	POSTDIALYSIS	DIALYSATE FLUID

		BLOOD PRESSURE		DEXTROSE	gm-mg%
		WEIGHT		POTASSIUM CHLORIDE	mEq/L
		BLOOD FLOW		UREA	mg%

HEPARINIZATION:

TOTAL   REGIONAL   PRIMING BLOOD

MONITORING

TIME	BLOOD FLOW	DIAL FLOW	BATH TEMP.	PRESSURES			HEPARIN SYRINGE (cc)	PROTAMINE SYRINGE (cc)	VITAL SIGNS	REMARKS
				NEG.	ARTERIAL	VENOUS				

UH FORM A—302   1-74-2285

476

APPENDIX 1—E

PERITONEAL
DIALYSIS

DIAGNOSIS 1				DIAGNOSIS 2		DIAGNOSIS 3	
					MEDICATION		
TIME	DIALYSIS NO.	VOLUME IN	OUT	FLUID BALANCE	PREVIOUS	PRESENT	REMARKS

PERITONEAL DIALYSIS

APPENDIX 1—F

Jane Smith
1-02-68-374

—IMPRINT HERE—

PERITONEAL DIALYSIS LOG

ON DIALYSIS:			OFF DIALYSIS:		TOTAL HOURS
DATE 3-17-78	TIME 0900		DATE	TIME	

BLOOD PRESSURE	BATH COMPOSITION	
160/100 SUPINE	POTASSIUM CHLORIDE 2.5	mEq/L
165/110 STANDING	DEXTROSE 2.0	gm%
65 Kg. WEIGHT	OTHER ADDITIONS none	

VOLUME OF DIALYSATE SOLUTION

40 liters

MECHANICS OF DIALYSIS:	INFLOW TIME 3 MIN.	DIFFUSION TIME 30 MIN.
	OUTFLOW TIME 15 MIN.	EXCHANGE VOLUME 1.5 LITERS

NOTE: 1. VOLUME MEASUREMENTS MUST BE RECORDED AT THE END OF EVERY (NO.) 2 OUTFLOW CYCLE.

2. WHEN BEHIND IN BALANCE, 1.0 LITER, **REPEAT OUTFLOW CYCLE** AND NOTIFY RENAL FELLOW ON CALL

TIME	INFLOW LEVEL	RESERVOIR	OUTFLOW LEVEL	TOTAL VOLUME	BALANCE	REMARKS
1000	38	3.0	1.0	42	+1	
1045	35	3.0	4.0	42	+1	
1145	32	3.0	5.5	40.5	−.5	Repeat Outflow
1245	29	3.0	10	42	+1	
1345	26	3.0	13.5	42.5	+1.5	

UH FORM A-231 REV. 1/75   1-75-39

APPENDIX 1—G

HYPERALIMENTATION
MONITORING
FLOWSHEET

1. USE A NEW RECORD DAILY.
2. INDICATE UNTOWARD SYMPTOMS USING O FOR
   ABSENCE AND + FOR PRESENCE; DESCRIBE SYMPTOMS
   AND ACTION TAKEN IN PATIENT'S PROGRESS NOTES.
3. FOR CLARIFICATION IN FILLING OUT FORM,
   SEE STANDARD CARE PLAN "MONITORING THE
   PATIENT RECEIVING HYPERALIMENTATION THERAPY."

PROBLEM NO.	PROBLEM																	DATE					

ITEM	FREQ.	TIME																					
		7A	8A	9A	10A	11A	12A	1P	2P	3P	4P	5P	6P	7P	8P	9P	10P	11P	12M	1A	2A	3A	4A	5A	6A
TEMP	Q 4 H																						
PULSE																							
RESP																							
B/P																							
FLOW RATE	Q 1 H																						
SUGAR AND ACETONE	Q 6 H																						
INTAKE	Q 8 H																						
OUTPUT	Q 8 H																						
UNTOWARD SYMPTOMS: CHILLS	Q 1 H																						
AIR EMBOLISM	TUBING CHANGES																						
HYPERGLYCEMIA	Q 2 H																						
HYPOGLYCEMIA	Q 2 H																						
FLUID OVERLOAD																							
CHF																							
EDEMA:																							
PULMONARY																							
CENTRAL	WHEN TURNING PATIENT																						
SACRAL																							
PERIPHERAL																							
OSMOTIC DIURESIS	Q 1 H																						
DEHYDRATION	Q 1 H																						
HYPERALLERGIC RESPONSE																							
INFILTRATION	Q 4 H																						
THROMBO-PHLEBITIS	DRESSING CHANGE																						
THROMBOSIS	DRESSING CHANGE																						
WEIGHT	Q D																						
CALORIC INTAKE																							

RN SIGNATURE	7 - 3:30	3 - 11:30	11 - 7

HYPERALIMENTATION MONITORING FLOWSHEET

INDEX

Page numbers followed by (t) indicate tabular material.

Afterload, 57
Airway management, 191–219
Albumin, 25% normal serum, 358, 360(t)
Allen test for ulnar artery patency, 55
Alternating current, 457
Ampere, 457
Antigravity suit, 123–126
Antihemophilic factor (AHF), 357, 360(t)
Antihemophilic globulin, 357, 360(t)
Aortic pressure, 57
Arterial indwelling catheter site care, 403–413
Arterial pressure, 91–96
Arterial puncture, 43, 49–56
Atrial electrocardiogram with temporary atrial
    pacing electrode, 140–141
Atrial pacing, overdrive, 142–144
Automatic blood pressure monitoring, 60, 105–107
Autotransfusion, 370–372

Balloon for intra-aortic balloon pump, 108–116
Bedside electrocardiogram monitoring, 4
Bennett MA-1, 222(t)
Bennett MA-2, 222(t)
Bleeding, gastrointestinal, 309–327
Blind endotracheal suctioning, 204–208
Blisters, burn, 399–400
Blood and blood component administration,
    355–366
  guide, 359–360(t)
Blood flow of peripheral vascular system, changes
    in, 169–177
Blood pressure, monitoring, 57–107. See also
    Pressure.
Blood pump, for hemodialysis, 273
  use of, 376–377
Blood warming, 373–375
Bourns Bear-1, 223(t)
Burns, 397–402

Cannula, hemodialysis, 260, 273–276
Cardiac output, 60, 100–105
Cardiocentesis, 186–188
Cardioversion, 30–36
Catheter(s), peritoneal dialysis, insertion of,
    278–281
  site care, 282–283
  pulmonary artery, suppliers of, 90
  total parenteral nutrition, culture from, 435–437
    insertion of, 418–423
    removal of, 433–435
    site care, 425–430
  venous and arterial indwelling, site care for,
    403–413
Catheter-over-the-needle set, 43
Catheter-through-the-needle set, 43
Central monitoring station, 5
Central venous pressure (CVP), 57, 58, 75–82
Chassis, 457
Chest drainage unit, disposable, 244–245
Chest physiotherapy, 246–251
Chest tube, 236–245
  disposable, 244–245
  placement, 236–239
  three-bottle closed system, 239–244
Circuit, 457
Circulatory assist devices, 108–126
  counterpressure with G-suit, 123–126
  external counterpulsation, 116–123
  intra-aortic balloon pump, 108–116
Cisternal and lumbar punctures, 296–300
Coil dialyzer, 262–263
Colostomies, 335, 336–342
  irrigation, 344–346
Computerized electrocardiogram monitoring, 6
Conductor, 454, 457
Contaminated wounds, 385–392
Continuous positive airway pressure (CPAP),
    231–235
Counterpressure, external, with G-suit, 123–126

Counterpulsation, external, 116–123
Critical care unit, infection control measures, 451–452
Cryoprecipitate antihemophilic factor (Cryo), 357, 360(t)
Culture(s), from total parenteral nutrition subclavian venous catheter, 435–437
    wound, 389–391

Decubiti, 393–396
Defibrillation, 37–42
Dialysis, peritoneal, 277–288
    catheter site care, 282–283
    flow sheet, 477–478
    insertion of catheter, 278–281
    monitoring, 283–288
Dialyzers, artificial, types of, 261–263
Disposable chest drainage unit, 244–245
Direct current (DC), 457
Drains, wounds with, 385-387

Electrical power for hemodialysis, 264
Electrical safety, 454–460
    with direct conduction pathways to myocardium, 458–460
Electrocardiogram (ECG), 1–29
    atrial, with temporary atrial pacing electrode, 140–141
    bedside monitoring system, 4
    central monitoring station, 4
    computerized monitoring, 6
    lead systems, 16–26
    telemetry, 7, 26–29
    12-lead, 1–3, 8–16
Emerson 3-PV(Post op), 223(t)
Endotracheal intubation, 191, 192–193, 196–200, 215–216
Endotracheal suctioning, 200–204
    blind, 204–208
Epicardial pacing, temporary, 134–137
Equipment, infection control measures, 452–453
Esophageal obturator airway (EOA), 191, 192, 194–196
External counterpressure with G-suit, 123–126
External counterpulsation, 116–123
Extubation, 216–219

Factor VIII (antihemophilic globulin), 357, 360(t)
Fats, intravenous, administration of, 438–440
Femoral vein dialysis, 261
Fick method for monitoring cardiac output, 100, 101–102, 104
Filter change for total parenteral nutrition, 430–433
First-degree burns, 397–398
Fistula, hemodialysis, 260
Fistula/drain site care, 342–344
Fistula/ostomy, 334–352
    containment, 335–342
    odor control, 349–350
    skin care, 346–349
Flow sheet(s), hemodialysis, 474–476
    hyperalimentation monitoring, 479

Flow sheet(s) (Continued)
    intra-aortic balloon pump, 473
    peritoneal dialysis, 477–478
Fluid challenge, 57
Fresh-frozen plasma (FFP), 357, 359(t)
Fresh-frozen red blood cells, 356, 359(t)
Fresh whole blood (FWB), 335, 359(t)
Fuse, 457

G-suit, external counterpressure with, 123–126
Gastric lavage, in hemorrhage, 312–315
    in overdose, 328–330
Gastrointestinal hemorrhage, 309–327
Granulocyte transfusion (WBC), 358, 360(t)
Grounding, 454, 457

Hemodialysis, 259–276
    cannula and site care, 273–276
    equipment, 259–264
    flow sheets, 474–476
    initiating, 264–268
    monitoring, 268–271
    terminating, 271–273
Hemodynamic monitoring, 57–107
    techniques of, 60–61
Hemorrhage, gastrointestinal, 309–327
Heparin infusion pump for hemodialysis, 264
Hollow fiber dialyzer, 261
Hyperalimentation, 417–437
    monitoring flowsheet, 479
Hyperthermia, 301–306
Hypothermia, 301–306

Illeal loop stoma, obtaining urine specimen from, 350–351
Ileostomy, 335, 336–347
Indicator-dilution method for monitoring cardiac output, 60, 101, 102–103, 105
Infection, control measures, 447–453
    surveillance, 443–446
Infection Control Practitioner (ICP), 445
Injury(ies), tracheal, prevention of, 211–214
Insulator, 458
Intermittent mandatory ventilation (IMV), 228
Intra-aortic balloon pump (IABP), 108–116
    flow sheet, 473
Intracranial pressure monitoring, 291–295
Intravenous hyperalimentation (IVH), 417–437
Intravenous lipids, administration of, 438–440
Intravenous tubing charge for total parenteral nutrition, 430–433
Intubation, endotracheal, 191, 291-193, 196–200, 215–216
    nasotracheal, 197
    oral tracheal, 197
Invasive site care (venous and arterial), 403–413
Irrigation, colostomy, 344–346
    wound, 388–389

Kidney donation, 463–469

Laminar airflow (LAF) unit, 417
Leakage current, 458
Left atrial pressure, 59, 96–100
Leukocyte-poor red blood cells, 356, 359(t)
Linton tube, 321–324
Lipids, intravenous, administration of, 438–440
Lumbar and cisternal punctures, 296–300

Macroshock, 454, 457
Magnet, with permanent pacemaker, use of, 165–168
Mechanical ventilation, instituting, 220–226
    weaning from, 226–229
Mechanical ventilators, controls, displays, alarms, and special features of, 222–223(t)
Mesenteric artery line and pitressin infusion, 325–327
Microshock, 454, 457
Myocardium, direct conduction pathways to, electrical safety precautions with, 458–460

Nasogastric tube insertion, 309–312
Nasopharyngeal airway, 191
Nasotracheal intubation, 197
Noninvasive peripheral vascular blood flow measurement, 169–177
Nutrition, total parenteral, 417–437

Odor control, ostomy/fistula, 349–350
Ohio CCV-2, 223(t)
Open burns, 398
Open wounds, contaminated, 387–388
Oral tracheal intubation, 197
Organ donation, 463–469
Oropharyngeal airway, 191, 192
Ostomy/fistula, 334–352
    containment, 335–342
    odor control, 349–350
    skin care, 346–349
Overdose, gastric lavage in, 328–330
Overdrive atrial pacing, 142–144

Pacemaker, permanent, 149–168
    inhibition of, 161–163
    parameters of, assessment of, 149–160
    reprogramming, 163–165
    use of magnet with, 165–168
    temporary, 127–148
        assessment of, 144–148
        atrial electrocardiogram with, 140–141
        conversion from bipolar to unipolar system with, 138–140
        epicardial, 134–137
        overdrive atrial pacing, 142–144
Pacing electrode, 149
Packed red blood cells, 356, 359(t)
Paracentesis, 331–333
Parallel plate dialyzer, 261
Peripheral vascular system, changes in blood flow of, 169–177
Peritoneal dialysis, 277–288

Peritoneal dialysis (Continued)
    catheter site care, 282–283
    flow sheet, 477–478
    insertion of catheter, 278–281
    monitoring, 283–288
Personnel, infection control measures, 447–451
Phlebotomy, 183–185
Physiotherapy, chest, 246–251
Pitressin infusion, 325–327
Plasma, fresh-frozen, 357, 359(t)
Plasma protein fraction, 358, 360(t)
Platelet concentrate, 356–357, 359(t)
Plethysmograph, strain gauge, 169, 175–177
Positive end expiratory pressure (PEEP), 221, 224
    ambuing with, 229–231
Postural drainage, 246–251
Preload, 57
Pressure, arterial, 91–96
    central venous, 58, 75–82
    intracranial, monitoring, 291–295
    left atrial, 59, 96–100
    monitoring, 57–107
        automatic, 60, 105–107
        direct, 60
        transducer systems, 60–61, 68–75
            single, 61–68
    pulmonary artery, 59, 82–91
    pulmonary artery wedge, 58, 87
    right atrial, 84
    right ventricular, 85–86
Pressure-preset ventilators, 220
Pressure transducer systems, 60–61
    multiple, 68–75
    single, 61–68
Pulmonary artery pressure, 59, 82–91
Pulmonary artery wedge pressure (PAWP), 57, 58–59, 87
Pulse generator, 149
Pulse volume recorder (PVR), 169, 172–175
Punctures, cisternal and lumbar, 296–300

Red blood cells (RBC's), 356, 359(t)
Right atrial pressure, 84
Right ventricular pressure, 85–86
Rotating tourniquets, 178–182

Safety, electrical, 454–460
Second-degree burns, intact, 398–399
    nonintact, 399–400
Sengstaken/Blakemore tube, 315–320
Servo, 222(t)
Shock, electrical, 454, 457
Shunts, hemodialysis, 260
Single-needle timed clamping device for hemodialysis, 264
Skin care, ostomy/fistula, 346–349
Stoma, ileal loop, obtaining urine specimen from, 350–352
Stoma/fistula management, 334–352
Stored whole blood (SWB), 355, 359(t)
Strain gauge plethysmograph, 169, 175–177
Subclavian catheter. See Total parenteral nutrition.
Suctioning, endotracheal, 200–204
    blind, 204–208

Tachydysrhythmias, cardioversion for, 30–36
Telemetry, electrocardiogram, 7, 26–29
Thermodilution technique for measuring cardiac
     output, 101, 103–104, 105
Third-degree burns, 400–402
Thoracentesis, 252–255
Three-bottle closed chest drainage system, 239–244
Total parenteral nutrition (TPN), 417–437
  catheter site care, 425–430
  culturing subclavian venous catheter, 435–437
  insertion of catheter, 418–423
  intravenous tubing and filter change, 430–433
  monitoring daily infusion of, 423–425
  monitoring flowsheet, 479
  removal of subclavian catheter, 433–435
Tourniquets, rotating, 178–182
Tracheal injuries, prevention of, 211–214
Tracheostomy, 192, 193, 208–211, 214–215
Tracheotomy, 197
Transducer system, pressure, 60–61
     multiple, 68–75
     single, 61–68
Transfusion(s), blood and blood component
     administration, 355–366
  blood pump, 376–377
  blood warming, 373–375
  reaction, 367–369

Ulcers, decubitus, 393–396
Ultrasound blood flow detector, 169–171

Uniform Anatomical Gift Act, 463
Urine specimen, from ileal loop stoma, 350–351
Urostomies, 335, 336–342

Vascular invasive techniques, 43–56
Venipuncture, 43–49
Venous indwelling catheters, site care for, 403–413
Ventilation, 191–219, 220–235
  intermittent mandatory (IMV), 228
  mechanical, instituting, 220–226
     weaning from, 226–229
Ventilators, 191, 220
  controls, displays, alarms, and special features
     of, 222–223(t)
Ventricular fibrillation, defibrillation for, 37–42
Voltage, 458
Volume present ventilators, 220

Water source for hemodialysis, 264
Watt, 458
Whole blood, 355, 359(t)
Wound(s), burns, 397–402
  clean, 381–384
  contaminated, 385–392
  decubiti, 393–396